Music, Song, Dance, and Theatre

SOCIAL JUSTICE AND YOUTH COMMUNITY PRACTICE SERIES

Series Editor
Melvin Delgado, Professor, Boston University

Series Editorial Advisory Committee
William Bukowski, Professor, Concordia University
Barry Checkoway, Professor, University of Michigan
Constance Flanagan, Professor, Pennsylvania State University
Shawn Ginwright, Associate Professor, San Francisco State University
Ben Kirshner, Associate Professor, University of Colorado
Niobe Way, Professor, New York University
David Moxley, Professor, University of Oklahoma

Urban Friendships and Community Youth Practice
Melvin Delgado

Music, Song, Dance, and Theatre:
Broadway Meets Social Justice Youth Community Practice
Melvin Delgado

Music, Song, Dance, and Theatre

BROADWAY MEETS SOCIAL JUSTICE YOUTH
COMMUNITY PRACTICE

Melvin Delgado

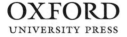
OXFORD
UNIVERSITY PRESS

OXFORD

UNIVERSITY PRESS

Oxford University Press is a department of the University of Oxford. It furthers
the University's objective of excellence in research, scholarship, and education
by publishing worldwide. Oxford is a registered trade mark of Oxford University
Press in the UK and certain other countries.

Published in the United States of America by Oxford University Press
198 Madison Avenue, New York, NY 10016, United States of America.

CIP data is on file at the Library of Congress
ISBN 978-0-19-064216-7

This book is dedicated to Denise, Laura, and Barbara.

CONTENTS

LIST OF FIGURES

Music, Song, Dance, and Theatre

SECTION I

Setting the Context

1

An Overview

Introduction

There is evidence that improving school equity can enhance positive youth development outcomes, and this should not be surprising (Debnam, Johnson, Waasdorp, & Bradshaw, 2014). Schools represent a significant part of youth lives and to ignore them by focusing on out-of-school experiences is difficult and not without its share of perils (Novick, 2015). Schools represent anchors in communities when youth actively seek to be a part of a community's social fabric. Youth spend most of their days outside of school, and afterschool programs have emerged to take advantage of school building availability at the end of the school day (Apsler, 2009).

The performing arts are one arena where youth community practice can be effectively tapped to attract youth both within schools and in out-of-school settings, or what Heath et al. (2001, p. 15) refer to as the "third area between school and family." These settings are highly attractive community-based venues that are nonstigmatizing and serve both youth and their respective communities. The performing arts can supplement or enhance formal education, providing a counternarrative for youth to resist the labels placed on them by serving as a vehicle for reactivity and self-expression (Farrugia, 2016; Sung, 2015).

Youth who may not have strong verbal skills but can engage in movement can gravitate toward dance; youth with good or excellent voices can sing. The performing arts can involve backstage work, and this is particularly attractive to those youth who lack the self-confidence or desire to appear before an audience.

Having youth experience affirming and positive learning experiences can play an instrumental role in their lives and their social peer network (Rhoades, 2016), and the performing arts excel in such a role. Theorell et al. (Theorell, Lennartsson, Madison, Mosing, & Ullén, 2015) studied predictors of continued singing or playing of a musical instrument from childhood/adolescence to adulthood and found that, among several factors, having formal lessons early in life increased the likelihood of lifetime singing and playing.

Early exposure in an affirming and structured environment (activities) can have lifetime benefits, providing a setting and avenue for achieving success and feelings of belonging (Mahoney, Harris, & Eccles, 2006; Mahoney, Larson, Eccles, & Lord, 2005). But not all youth benefit equally through participation (Jiang & Peterson, 2012). Making the community an essential ingredient of a performance helps ensure that the central purpose and message resonates with an audience (Leonard & Kilkelly, 2006a; Stephenson Jr. & Tate, 2015a).

Leonard and Kilkelly (2006b, p. 29) stress how communities are settings and vehicles for performances that tap a common history: "Community is not necessarily a given but it may be made through acknowledgement and/or celebrating a sense of common heritage or place that emerges in the event of live performance. That is where the art of the making comes in. Community is a protean thing that both reflects and creates agency." This narrative takes on significance in the context of youth lives and their communities. This chapter grounds the reader in the appeal and parameters of youth performing arts and the various perspectives that organizations must take into account when tapping this resource in programming.

Broadway Meets Social Justice Youth Community Practice

The "performing arts" is a ubiquitous term, and everyone has his or her own definition and interpretation of what it means. The question of what constitutes a performing art will prove challenging because various perspectives must be taken into account, including the role and influence of a Eurocentric bias. Manchester and Pett (2015, p. 1) address the overlooked perspective of how youth view cultural institutions and how the arts are manifested within these institutions:

> Young people's own accounts of their cultural practices challenge normative definitions of culture and cultural value but also demonstrate how these definitions act to reproduce social inequalities in relation to cultural participation and social and cultural capital . . . cultural policy-makers should listen and take young people's voices seriously in re-imaging the city's cultural offer for *all* young people.

This statement appears all too commonly in discussions pertaining to youth voices. Manchester and Pett argue for including youth voices and explain why it is essential to have social justice appear in the heading.

The performing arts fulfill critical roles in a democracy, and this is often overlooked in any discussion of why supporting the arts with the potential to transform being and enhance in a democratic society. Keeney and Korza (2015, p. 189) address this potential to create a better society:

> Although there is literature on how the arts have been applied to contribute to community betterment, challenges remain in defining the range of

social goods the arts may address. Arts-based change approaches draw upon humans' desire to belong to a group, participate, connect, and contribute to society. These behaviors also strengthen democracies.

This societal transformative perspective is often either ignored or glossed over in discussing the performing arts, regardless of age group. Clay (2006) argues that music can engage marginalized youth in a democratic process, with this engagement being increased through purposeful programming.

Youth practice involving the performing arts can appeal to a cross-section of youth ages, abilities, and social circumstances and must not be limited to a select group with a high probability of success. As noted in Figure 1.1, a number of key factors operate in combination to create a synergistic experience for urban youth engaged in the performing arts when this practice takes into account local circumstances and social justice issues.

Youth community practice is not about "creaming," and it must embrace an inclusive participatory stance. Frazier's (2015) description of the South Bronx's (New York City) DreamYard Project does a wonderful job of showing how

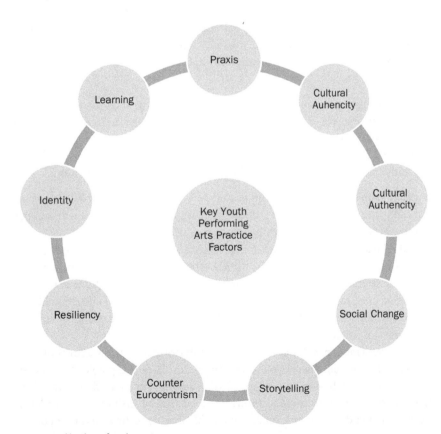

FIGURE 1.1 Youth performing arts

a community organization can offer a range of arts projects and do so while acknowledging how youth community practice can reach youth facing similar difficult social circumstances but with different artistic interests in an affirming and empowering manner. This organization has a big umbrella and incorporates youth with interests in various art forms, not just the performing arts.

A Broadway metaphor captures the promise of music, song, dance, and theatre, and it is appropriate here because of the image that Broadway conjures. The energy, fun, purpose, creative outlet, camaraderie, and determination associated with the performing arts represents a viable and highly attractive outlet for marginalized youth, particularly when their voices are actively sought and they play a prominent role in decision-making that introduces them to social justice values and themes. The arts provide a context and vehicle for lesbian, gay, bisexual, transgender, and questioning (LGBTQ) youth, for instance, to find creative expression and effect social changes (Wernick, Kulick, & Woodford, 2014).

The relationship between performer and audience is an important dimension that must be fostered. Wartemann (2009) emphasizes this interplay in Youth Theater and the simultaneous asymmetry of interaction between actors and audience, raising the question of whether collective creativity is but a theoretical construct or a basic requirement for this form of theatre to achieve its transformative potential. Datoo and Chagani (2011, p. 23) describe the multifaceted ways that communication between a performer and audience can occur when discussing the performing arts:

> Primarily, performance arts and especially mediums such as: dance, theatrical performances employ gestures, expressions, actions (as in acting), speech/voice, and bodily movements etc. These expressions aid to the discourse that individual or a performing group wishes to portray. In this manner, visual and audio aids are economically used to bring effectiveness in expression.

Interactions between audience and performers in all likelihood will be nuanced, and capturing outcomes will be arduous but essential in furthering the use of performing arts to reach youth and their communities.

Moldavanova and Goerdel (2014) expand the construct of sustainability beyond narrow and traditional dimensions to include cultural sustainability and the role that formalized public and nonprofit arts organizations can play in advancing cultural sustainability within communities. Cultural sustainability can be conceptualized by including using arts with youth in situations where their voices are not sought.

Garoian (1999, p. 57) argues that casting performance art as a form of social change pedagogy empowers youth and facilitates them being able "to intervene and reclaim their bodies from oppressive academic practices that assume students' personal memories and cultural histories to be insignificant to identity construction and new mythic representations." Sharing feelings and thoughts can be accomplished in multiple ways that are not threatening, allowing youth to use their preferred method of communication.

"Broadway" captures so much more, making the whole more important than its individual parts. The performing arts provide youth with a chance to channel their creativity and engage regardless of intellectual, physical, and emotional competencies because there are different roles to be filled both in front of and behind the scenes that must come together to achieve a successful performance (Becker & Dusing, 2010; Derby, 2012; Swedeen, Carter &, Molfenter, 2010).

The creation of music, song, dance, and theatre as examples of the performing arts represents but one important dimension of youth practice. These activities can find a receptive audience in youth and their respective communities. Finding appropriate audiences is also of critical importance (Levine, 2008), although this dimension has not received necessary attention in using the performing arts to engage youth. Who should be attending is closely tied to the goals of the performance. One goal cannot be accomplished without serious consideration of the other. The greater the clarity about performance goals, the greater specificity in who should be attending.

Van de Water (2012) provides an excellent critical and historical review of the concept of Theater for Youth Audiences (TYA) in the United States, how it has shaped cultural production for youth, and why it has been so attractive for youth participants and audiences, with lessons for organizations wishing to use theatre to engage and reach youth. Having an "appropriate" audience expands the potential influence of the act or activity to a wider group, thus increasing the reach of youth practice.

Developing an expansive vision of potential audiences is needed. Greene (2015) notes that theatre field trips open up new vistas for youth who do not have the benefit of family traditions of attending theatre. These experiences can be enhanced when trips are to view youth theatre performances. When these performances focus on salient issues in their lives, that experience takes on significance. Adults, too, can be—and often are—beneficiaries of youth performances, although we rarely think of them as a potential audience in youth performances (Bresler, 2010).

Community festivals (Delgado, 2016a) provide an excellent context for reaching out to diverse audiences in venues that are considered safe (psychologically and physically). The case of Queeriosity—a queer youth-led cultural festival held in Brisbane, Australia, is an excellent example of how a festival proved an excellent venue (Taylor, 2012). Youth conferences, too, represent a potential site for performing arts to transpire that can be youth-specific or broader in scope (Agosto & Karanxha, 2012). These youth conferences can reach adults as well, who can either be primary or secondary audiences in these performances. Performances can be tailored to time and space constraints, bringing flexibility and allowing for outreach to community segments without histories of staging performances.

Markusen and Brown (2014) discuss the importance of a proper venue for encouraging attendance at performing arts events. Although they address professional performances and paying audiences, they raise important considerations for where youth performances can transpire, including opening the door to venues associated with professional performances, which can be obtained through in-kind donations. Festivals can be effective for building a collective sense of community by providing an opportunity for wide participation in all aspects of establishing, sponsoring, and attending a performance (Delgado, 2016a; Laing & Mair, 2015).

Introducing a social justice stance broadens the potential appeal of performing arts among youth who are marginalized. Watts and Flanagan (2007) advance a liberation perspective on youth civic engagement and note that this approach is in response to current youth programming that, although having noble intensions, still maintains the status quo. "Fixing" youth is not a sustainable approach in marginalized communities; fixing their situation and addressing the forces that marginalized them *is* viable and sustainable. If the conditions are social, so must the solutions be social (Cote & Allahar, 2006).

Social justice performing arts brings together civic engagement, participation in community civic life, social change, and the capacity enhancement of youth (Harrison, 2010; Karabanow & Naylor, 2015), grounding performing arts within youth community practice, and it does so by emphasizing assets-first, participatory democracy, empowerment, indigenous knowledge, and social justice values.

Youth Performing Arts

The arts, in the broadest sense, have historically played an influential role in shaping human existence and can rightly play an influential role in shaping human services, including the education of social workers and other helping professionals (Moxley & Calligan, 2015; Moxley, Feen-Calligan, & Washington, 2012). Taking this stance opens up this field to innovative social interventions.

The arts can be considered a field in flux for integrating innovative strategies to make a significant contribution to changing communities (Stephenson & Tate, 2015b). Attaching a community prefix to dance, song, and, particularly, theatre and music represents a shift from conventional views of these performing arts to one that is predicated upon local circumstances, history, and expectations, making youth performing arts possible and highly attractive at a local level. The performing arts represent a vehicle for addressing local needs and concerns.

Music and musicians have always been part of communities. Higgins (2012) discusses the role and influence of community music and community musicians; Kuftinec (2003) talks about community theatre; Clift et al. (2015) and Sun, Buys, and Merrick (2012) address community singing; Cheesman (2011) touches upon community dancing. These perspectives differ from conventional forms because of a community's role in shaping how they evolve.

It is impossible to separate the arts from youth (Hickey-Moody, 2013, p. 1): "Young people live through art. Music, film, YouTube, dance, magazines: popular and high forms of art are the language that young people speak." It stands to reason that reinforcing this affinity through youth activities can provide a portal through which youth of all backgrounds can be reached and have their lives enriched in the process. In essence, this portal provides an avenue for marginalized groups to seek social justice (Shaughnessy, 2012).

Sheppard (2013, p. 226), in discussing social justice, quite eloquently captures the potential of the arts to transform a worldview predicated upon a negative or deficit view of youth: "Across multiple contexts, art forms, and social justice efforts, powerful demonstrations paint a picture of a quest for the possible against the prevailing idea that marginalized groups have deficits of knowledge, skills, or worse deficits of culture. Smile, and feel joy, as art replaces this deficit view with demonstrations of agency, creativity, talent, and insight." Youth performing arts can transform youth lives in profound and highly creative ways, and how it does this is only limited by our imagination and commitment to social justice for those youth who are marginalized.

The question of why we should tinker with natural youth interests can rightly be raised. Children and youth have an innate interest in making music. If they are musical without formal training, why should youth community practice formalize and possibly ruin their interests in it? Campbell's (2010, p. 248) answers to this question can also be applied to other performing art forms:

> While children are musical without expert guidance, they become more musical as a result of it. Their lives are enhanced through instruction in and through music as they become all that they can musically be—and more human as a result of knowing music at many levels, in many guises. What children musically do and say is the launch for their further development; I am not campaigning not to "de-school" music but, rather, to bring instruction in line with who the children musically are.

This last sentence is profound and signals to youth practitioners that they must act on the performing arts goals set by youth, emphasizing their importance in decision-making roles. This stance is not new to any social justice–inspired social intervention.

Youth engagement has expanded to include new arenas and approaches over the past 15 years as youth development–inspired programming has found wider acceptance in education, recreation, helping professions, information technology/social media, and sports/movement activity (Agans et al., 2015; Holt, 2007; Sabo & Veliz, 2008; Witt & Caldwell, 2010); the arts (Black, Castro, & Lin, 2015; Fleming, Durham, Lewis, & Leonard, 2015; Hanley, Sheppard, Noblit, & Barone, 2013; Malin, 2015); the sciences (Crowley, Barron, Knutson, & Martin, 2015; Delgado, 2002);

mentoring (Grills et al., 2016; Pryce et al., 2015; Weiler et al., 2015); technology/social media (Bers, 2010; 2012); research (Akom, Cammarota, & Ginwright, 2008); social entrepreneurship (Damon, Bronk, & Porter, 2015; Jennings, 2014; Nicholls, 2006; Osman et al., 2014; Zhang, Lu, Gao, & Chen, 2014); wilderness (Norton & Watt, 2014); and service-learning and civic engagement (Adejumo, 2010; Delgado, 2016a; Kajner, Chovanec, Underwood, & Mian, 2013), to list a few.

Certain activities stand out because of the sheer number of participates, and sports is such an example. It is estimated that 45 million youth aged 8–18 (at least one child in 75% of families) participate in organized sporting activities on an annual basis in this country (Bean, Fortier, Post, & Chima, 2014), making sports the most prominent youth activity in the United States. This level of participation has leveled off and is even decreasing among certain subgroups (Humphreys, Ruseski, & Soebbing, 2014).

Sports have been seen as an attractive way of reaching urban youth of color, particularly when structured around difficult or challenging periods within the day and made accessible to them (Delgado, 2000; Wilson & Hayhurst, 2009). Inner-city schools are increasingly limiting physical education and sports programs due to budget cuts and an increasing emphasis on high-stakes testing (Holt, Sehn, Spence, Newton, & Ball, 2012).

Many different lessons can be taught and learned through sports. Life skills can be taught through sports, and it can be done in a manner that achieves important impact without calling attention to the lessons learned, thus increasing the natural order of learning (Papacharisis, Goudas, Danish, & Theodorakis, 2005). Learning can take place without labeling it as such. Life skills take on even greater value when engaging youth from low-income backgrounds, helping them prepare for economic security as they mature (Lauzon, Christie, Cross, Khan, & Khan, 2015; To, Tam, Ngai, & Sung, 2014).

The performing arts, which incidentally have a very large umbrella, have emerged to fill important voids in the youth practice field but have not benefitted from correspondingly broad conceptualizations, critiques, and publicity, and this book is written to rectify this oversight. The arts help youth and communities respond to disasters and war healing and can be a vehicle for tapping into youth and community resiliency (Kanyako, 2015; Mohr, 2014; Silberg, 2012). There is no area where the arts cannot be applied to marginalized youth because of their ethnicity/race, gender, sexual orientation, and disabilities (both visible and invisible).

Performing arts can also address less "dramatic" needs, too. Jackson, Mullis, and Hughes (2010) report on a program that focused on nutritional education through the use of theatre, dance, and music, bringing a new and refreshing perspective on this important information in the life of youth. This performing arts program ended by having youth participants do a dinner theatre performance where they shared information gained through participation.

Newman and Dantzler (2015, p. 81) summarize a seismic evolutionary shift in thinking about resiliency, with implications for youth, and explain how an emphasis on contextual grounding has changed how we view and respond to this construct:

> For the past two decades, researchers have agreed that resilience refers to the capacity of all individuals to progress, in spite of risks, toward resilient outcomes. Instead of situating risk in youth and their families, current resilience research situates risk within a broader social context, such as racism, war, and poverty. . . . Current resilience research grounds research and practice in optimism for building motivation; positive expectations internalized in youth may motivate them and teach them to overcome risks and adversity.

This paradigm shift bodes well for social justice youth practice because of how it emphasizes environmental factors concerning "risk" or low probabilities of success and how youth respond to these circumstances (James, 2016).

Duckworth's (2016) book *Grit: The Power of Passion and Perseverance* seeks to capture an elusive quality in character that pushes some youth to surmount incredible odds to succeed. Their stories inspire, capturing the spirit of humankind, almost as if they were fulfilling their destiny and no earthly power was going to impede their achievement. Latino youth, for example, too, have grit but this is often overlooked in the academic literature (Guerrero, Dudovitz, Chung, Dosanjh, & Wong, 2016). It is important not to use the concept of "grit" as a way of "blaming the victim" for those who have not persevered because their narratives are just as important as the narratives of those who did succeed. Blaming the victim helps destroy rather than celebrate lives and creates false narratives that perpetuate negative stereotypes.

Ungar and Liebenberg (2011) and Masten (2014) note that there is a tremendous need to assess child and youth resilience across cultures because of how culture influences youth expectations and behavior. Liebenberg and Theron (2015) advocate for the use of innovative qualitative methods to capture the interrelationships among youth, culture, and resilience. It is not a far stretch to see how a cultural grounding shapes avenues for resiliency to unfold. The performing arts may not have the same impact across all youth groups. Community centers using the arts are in an excellent position to incorporate resiliency within assessment and programming (Rhodes & Schechter, 2014).

Masten (2014) argues that a resiliency paradigm is more focused on marginalized youth when compared to positive youth development (PYD), although both share similar historical roots, basic assumptions, key concepts, and goals, which are more associated with grounding positive behavior contextually and developmentally where youth and children spend their time, free and structured. Masten (2014, p. 1044) notes other basic differences:

> What are the notable differences? PYD is by definition more focused on youth whereas developmental resilience science has expanded to life-span perspectives. . . . Relational Developmental Systems Theory [RDST], the conceptual

perspective underlying PYD, nonetheless, is a life-span theory. Similarly, although RDST includes biological levels of organization in integrated developmental systems, PYD has not focused much as yet on measurement at biological levels of analysis. Meanwhile, resilience science is undergoing a rapid transformation, driven by advances in genomics, neuroscience and other biological methods and theory, to forge an integrated multiple levels science of resilience.

Although resiliency and PYD share much in common, the differences should not be blurred or minimized. Each of these perspectives has much to offer youth who have few viable options for engaging in activities of interest and social significance (Clonan-Roy, Jacobs, & Nakkula, 2016).

Performing arts can help young English learners acquire oral language skills in a manner that makes it easier to achieve and does so in a nonstigmatizing way (Greenfader, Brouillette, & Farkas, 2015). Trayes, Harré, and Overall (2012) note that youth performing arts bring benefits, tensions, and frustrations that must be constructively addressed to maximize youth learning and participation. Conroy (2009) specifically addresses the creative tensions between drama, theatre, and disability arts. Learning to navigate tensions and frustrations provides immediate and long-term life lessons (Bower & Carroll, 2015).

Youth performing arts are not the exclusive domain of older children and youth or of performers who are not challenged in a variety of intellectual, emotional, and physical ways. Fletcher-Watson et al. (Fletcher-Watson, Fletcher-Watson, McNaughton, & Birch, 2014, p. 130) note that the arts can be tailored to take into account developmental stages, including even those of babies and toddlers:

> Theatre for early years (TEY) has become increasingly popular around the world in the last 30 years but has struggled with legitimation. Scholars have challenged TEY's validity and have declared performance to children aged younger than 3 years to be frivolous or even impossible. However, new models of aesthetic sensitivity and intersubjectivity have become allied with artistic practice, as artists choose to collaborate with developmental specialists.

Youth performing arts should not be limited or compromised by age or abilities. Even babies and toddlers can engage and benefit from participation (Fletcher-Watson et al., 2014). That may seem radical, but, in actuality, it necessitates a shift in paradigms concerning accessibility and activities.

These activities can also introduce a level of competition, which can be purposeful or unintended. Depending on goals, the performing arts can bring a highly competitive dimension to the work because groups can engage in competition at local, regional, or national levels (Kao & Huang, 2015; Trayes et al., 2012). This viewpoint on competition between groups represents an additional layer beyond competition to be part of a group or program, and some advocates would argue it introduces excitement, travel, and exposure to new surroundings and that the lessons learned through competition prepare youth for a world that is increasingly becoming more competitive.

Barber et al. (Barber, Abbott, & Neira, 2014) stress the importance of youth having at least one organized out-of-school activity that provides purpose in their lives and taps core aspects of their self-beliefs. Mindfulness, too, has an increased presence in the literature regarding its role in shaping and motivating participants to engage and has implications for youth development (Schonert-Reichl, 2014). When life for select youth groups gets very hectic and seems out of control, a space and place that can be an anchor in their days and lives can have profound social meaning (Autry & Anderson, 2007; Futch, 2011). Out-of-school activities can fill this critical role.

The concept of "expertise" has emerged regarding youth learning pathways in and out of school and the importance of these settings in fostering learning (Bell, Bricker, Reeve, & Zimmerman, 2013, p. 119): "We argue that we need to discover and then support the successful learning pathways of youth across social settings over developmental time so that we can promote the development of interests and expertise that may lead to both academic and personal success." There is an acknowledgment that public schools have generally failed certain groups of youth and that much work must be undertaken to make these institutions more responsive to the developmental needs of all students, regardless of their backgrounds and abilities (Eccles & Roeser, 2011; Ginwright, 2015).

The performing arts are a mechanism through which creative expression is encouraged and transpires while concomitantly engaging youth in reflective expression that is transformative at the individual and community levels (Gray, de Boehm, Farnsworth, & Wolf, 2010; Grewe et al., 2015; Lewis, 2014). The performing arts provide the youth community practice field with a social justice-inspired, bold, and highly innovative arena for engaging youth with these interests. It is a brave new world when discussing social justice youth community practice performing arts and what they can contribute to society.

The performing arts can be an effective vehicle for addressing issues that are difficult to talk about, such as HIV/AIDS (Glik, Nowak, Valente, Sapsis, & Martin, 2002) and other sexually transmitted infections (Lightfoot, Taboada, Taggart, Tran, & Burtaine, 2015), as well as the use of alcohol, tobacco, and other drugs (Krieger et al., 2013). Conrad (2008) discusses popular theatre involving risky youth experiences as a participatory form of performing arts that benefits both performers and audiences. Cultural stances can be integrated into highly sensitive issues to make them more relevant.

Daykin et al.'s (2008, p. 26) findings based on a review of the literature came to a similar conclusion: "Our review found evidence of positive outcomes following performing arts interventions and provides insight into some of the impact and process issues associated with arts for health initiatives. The strongest evidence is in relation to the impact of drama on peer interaction and social skills, where we found the largest number of studies." Peer interactions can easily be lost sight of when focusing on how an audience responds to a performance, yet the impact of these peer relationships will last long after an audience leaves.

Youth performing arts are often based on different ontological and epistemological premises, making arriving at a consensus and comprehensive review of the field that much more arduous but essential. Such a review brings with it its share of challenges, such as role of stakeholder influence, processes related to ownership and involvement, and challenges and risks associated with engaging in performing arts interventions (Daykin et al., 2008).

What kind of risks could possibly be associated with performances? Performance anxiety (stage fright) is one of the challenges endemic to the performing arts and probably most widely recognized (Nordin-Bates, 2012); it occurs in performances of music (Brugués, 2011; Kenny, 2011; Osborne & Kenny, 2008), singing (Emmons & Thomas, 2008; Ryan & Andrews, 2009), dance (Walker & Nordin-Bates, 2010), and theatre (Dadsetan, Anari & Sedghpour, 2008; Simmonds & Southcott, 2012). No performing art is immune from creating these types of anxieties, but overcoming stage fright, which is similar to a fear of public speaking, has lifelong implications when successfully addressed. Lessons learned in overcoming these fears can also transfer over to other spheres of youth lives, making the lessons learned that much more significant.

Eurocentrism

There are a multitude of perspectives one can take on the performing arts when thinking of them as potential forms of social interventions, as addressed in the remaining chapters of this book. But the aesthetics of the arts cannot be understood without a philosophical stance, which can either be explicit or implicit, with which to shape conceptualization.

Guarding against the intrusion of Eurocentric epistemologies is critical in the performing arts when dealing with performers who have histories of having been colonialized and marginalized (Carter, 2016). Addressing a Eurocentric stance is significantly relevant when discussing the performing arts because of how it challenges the core and founding principles on which these performances are based (Rakena, 2016).

The power and influence of Eurocentrism is not a recent occurrence, and any individual formally schooled in the social sciences and helping professions will have been exposed to the deleterious causes associated with a centric-bias (Hostettler, 2013). The concept of "Eurocentric intellectual imperialism" captures a stance that is self-evident when discussing the performing arts and other art forms (Leong, 2016). The arts have been looked at as an effective vehicle for decolonizing the academy and have similar potential in shaping discourse within community practice (Mbembe, 2016; Prinsloo, 2016; Rovito & Giles, 2016).

Amin (2009) traces a major shaping force of Eurocentrism to ancient Greece and its predisposition toward rationality. Shohat and Stam (2014) trace its power and influence over many centuries citing the Spanish Inquisition, the expulsion of Jews and Muslims, and the conquest of the Americas as illustrations of why it has such a powerful hold on individuals when thinking about a host of subjects including the arts, both visual and performing.

Eurocentrism views the world from a privileged perspective and sets the stage for a rationale, or ideology, that can lead to colonization, with deleterious consequences for those who have been colonized (Hall, 2013; Shohat & Stam, 2014). Eurocentrism has been used as the rationale for raising the prestige of European culture and civilization at the expense of other cultures and civilizations (Jamsari & Talib, 2015). A zero-sum view captures this particular stance: Europe is the center of the civilized world, if not the universe, and sets the standard from which to measure artistic and nonartistic endeavors (Krossa, 2012).

Pokhrel (2011) argues that Eurocentrism is a systematic distortion of existing realities, and this distortion can be either visible or invisible in how it wields influence. Eurocentrism is a mindset that brings together multiple intellectual propensities that can find many different manifestations, as in the case of the performing arts.

Lal (2012) puts forth an argument pertaining to Eurocentrism's influence on language and the creation of knowledge that raises important considerations for how we shape discourse and how Eurocentrism and colonialization of the mind has deleterious consequences. An overemphasis on the use of English, French, German, and Spanish languages in intellectual work is symptomatic of a Eurocentric hold on what constitutes "legitimate" scholarship. If scholarship uses anything other than these three European languages and, increasingly, English, it cannot achieve "true" worthiness and be considered scholarship.

No knowledge area is exempt from how this worldview shapes perceptions and actions. Eurocentrism can translate into how numerous subjects are thought of and measured: tourism (Cohen & Cohen, 2015), historical conversation (Winter, 2014), archaeology (Tansel, 2015), mathematics (Chahine, 2011), militarism (Morillo, 2014), translation studies (Van Doorslaer, 2012), incarceration (Imani, 2014), trauma theory (Craps, 2013), and personal attributes such as skin color (Hall, 2011) are all manifested. This partial listing illustrates the range of topics influenced by this construct and serves as a testament to its wide appeal and importance.

Vera (2014), in discussing the interrelationship between Eurocentrism and identity regarding Chilean music history, emphasizes the importance of engaging in critique to ground our understanding of context in shaping perceptions:

> In the strict sense, just to speak of the discovery of America implies mythologizing history. The term reminds us of the planetary discoveries; Pluto was effectively discovered in 1930 in that it was not known by humans before that.

Consequently, its use and acceptance supposed forgetting the fact that people previously lived in America. In this way, aboriginal societies were relegated to an undefined space, while Europe was universalized and stood as the representative culture of the West, incarnating the only valid model of civilization by the time.

The emergence of myths and the language used to perpetuate them can be manifested in obvious and not so obvious ways; the effect of a Eurocentric bias on the arts can be very subtle but no less important.

What constitutes "legitimate" song, music, dance, and theatre is deeply rooted in a Eurocentric view of life that provides a baseline or foundation from which to assign value or benefits and to judge other manifestations of performing arts. A critical view toward the influence of a Eurocentric focus toward the performing arts is necessary if these arts are to be attractive to youth of color and fulfill the potential to be transformative in their lives. The term "high art" captures an explicit stand on what is valued and should be emulated, and, just as importantly, all art that falls outside of this realm can be considered "low art."

The following statement from a report commissioned by the Wallace Foundation and produced by Rand Corporation in response to a lack of inclusiveness in audiences highlights how a limited view of the arts reflects an inherent bias and an implicit Eurocentric view (Zakaras & Lowell, 2008, p. xiii):

> Despite decades of effort to make high-quality works of art accessible to all Americans, demand for the arts has not kept pace with supply. Those who participate in the arts remain overwhelmingly white, educated, and affluent. Moreover, audiences for the arts are growing older: Each year, fewer young Americans visit art museums, listen to classical music, or attend jazz concerts or ballet performances.

When performances are irrelevant to a potential audience, they do not wish to partake. Making them relevant necessitates that these audiences play an active role in shaping the performances. This is not a difficult formula to comprehend.

There are current efforts under way to counteract Eurocentrism's influence within the field of education and other systems. These efforts to counter a Eurocentric perspective go by many different terms such as polycentrism, cultural diversity/humility, and multiculturalism, among others. *Afrocentrism* is arguably one of the most popular responses by which African-Americans counter a Eurocentric bias. Afrocentric praxis is in direct response to US society's efforts to minimize or denigrate the history and culture of African-Americans (King & Swartz, 2015).

Performing arts do not have to conform to Eurocentric definitions, thus allowing and encouraging urban youth to introduce their cultural backgrounds into how these activities are operationalized and evaluated (Markusen & Brown, 2014; Rovito, 2012). "Decorum" or the social contract between an audience and performers is not universal, and youth can and should be expected to have a different perspective (Peck, 2015). Art's authenticity is predicated upon encouraging youth to self-express, and this is often tied to life circumstances and the cultural backgrounds of performers and those who sponsor these performers.

Maeso and Araújo's (2015) view Eurocentrism as a paradigm that is useful for interpreting history and current events and a potential future founded on scientific rationality and the role of law. This paradigm is socially constructed and has survived because of its effectiveness in shaping and maintaining a worldview of elite dominance over other groups. A superior–inferior dichotomy simplifies this worldview. This perspective becomes manifested in all spheres of society, and particularly in educational systems that socialize those who are "inferior" or "culturally deprived" and who need to acquire the knowledge, behaviors, and aspirations of those in power.

Eurocentrism shapes how cultural values and beliefs get viewed and manifested. Again, the culture of people of color fares poorly when compared to White European culture. The devaluing of youth, too, is part of this worldview, effectively undermining a significant demographic sector of this community. Nordkvelle (2015, p. 53) draws an interesting parallel between Eurocentrism and adultism:

> The European conquest and domination of the World-System was based on underlying assumptions about its right to dominate, in the same way as adults dominate children. Inventing a European superior identity and an "other" of a lower estate legitimised the conquest of the Americas. In this sense the shaping of a European self was the result of an interactive but uneven relationship.

It is interesting to see how the argument of Eurocentrism can be viewed from an adultism point of view. Youth performing arts eschewing a Eurocentric worldview serves to empower a group of people, but it also empowers youth in the process. The synergistic impact of youth performing arts that are culturally affirming and significant from a social justice viewpoint cannot be underestimated.

Armin (2008, p. 219) issues a charge related to Eurocentrism for youth community practitioners engaged in the performing arts: "The process of systematically locating the Eurocentric deformations in dominant ideologies and social theories, retracing their genesis and bringing out their weaknesses is not sufficient. An outmoded paradigm disappears only on the condition that another paradigm, freed from the errors of the first, is positively expressed." Heavy emphasis on culture shaping youth performing arts is an attempt to respond to this challenge in a relevant and affirming manner.

It is appropriate to end this section on Eurocentrism with a discussion of the European origin of the concept of stigma. Interestingly, Goffman (1963, p. 1) traces the origins of the term *stigma* to the ancient Greeks, and highlights its relevance to urban youth of color: "The Greeks, who were apparently strong on visual aids, originated the term *stigma* to refer to bodily signs designed to expose something unusual and bad about the moral status of the signifier." Urban youth of color are stigmatized because of their appearance and where they live, and the performing arts provide an attractive vehicle for addressing this stigma and the source of it.

Storytelling (Voices from Below)

Gallagher (2014) posits that urban youth and theatre has adults, who wield influence over these youths, must be prepared to question our beliefs, values, and understandings to make sense of why and the various ways they are marginalized in society. Being open to intently listening to their stories is one effective way of challenging ourselves to embrace new interpretations and insights into their lives and struggles.

These stories can find expression in different forms (Lesko & Soundarajan, 2015, p. 99): "Stories are not just what we read from books to children or tell for entertainment around the table; they help us define our lives and ground is in place and describe and define our relationships with other people and humanity more broadly." Mosavel and Thomas (2010) were attracted to Playback Theatre (Project REECH) because of its reliance on storytelling, enactment, and dialogue in low-income neighborhood research focused on identifying major health issues.

Smith (2015) describes the Neighborhood Stories theatre program as creating a bridge between different segments of an urban community through performing stories that validated lived experienced. Strand (2009), although referring to musicians, observes that storytellers view narratives as a way to reflect on events and reality as they are remembered, creating meaning in the process for both performers and audiences.

Performing arts can tell a story without words. Sometimes the story is whimsical in nature; at other times, it is quite profound, with deep social meaning. And stories can be entertaining without embracing a social message. Regardless, there is always a moral to any performance. When stories involve issues of injustices that performers and audiences alike can relate to, they take on greater significance for both (Gallagher, 2014).

Palidofsky (2010) reports on the success of Storycatchers Theater and the role youth played in writing, producing, and performing musicals, including the Fabulous Females, a theatre program for incarcerated girls based at the Illinois Youth Center. Fabulous Females encourages girls to share their traumatic experiences and, through theatre, draw critical connections between these events and the choices they made that led to incarceration. These stories enlighten and empower them to heal, equipping them with tools to help them upon their released back into the community.

Trauma, which is not foreign to urban youth, shapes human perceptions of life, and finding expression for traumatic events is often very difficult (Fisher 2009, p. 108):

> For the survivors of trauma, however, the human desire to provide an account of oneself can become a profoundly troubling process. The traumatic eludes comprehension and communicability. It shatters our self-perception and disables our capacity to process, understand and express what has been encountered.

Expressive methods to facilitate the sharing of trauma-related stories help the individuals sharing these narratives as well as their audiences. Individuals who have traumatic stories that they felt were restricted to them can come to realize that others in the community have also suffered through these painful instances.

Giving testimony is empowering when it involves a group in this sharing act (Solinger, Fox, & Irani, 2010). The concept of "giving testimony" captures a process and narrative that is particularly painful and transformative (Fisher, 2009, p.114):

> In the performance of testimony, the language of the other performs that which exceeds experience and is unknowable. To hear this testimony is, to some degree, to enter into the traumatic in a way that is immediate and unsettling. For testimony, as we have seen, is not an ordered, it is incomplete, fragmentary; revealing an encounter that lies beyond explanation and comprehension. For that reason, the performance of testimony should always remain unsettling and never reassuring.

Fisher's conclusions on the unsettling nature of testimony, including its power, warrant close attention because the transformative goal of social justice youth community practice performing arts is never smooth, and participants, including practitioners and audiences, must be warned about the emotionality of this journey.

There are numerous ways to tap narratives. One method is the use of story circles, and I have found this to be very effective when working with youth from collectivistic value backgrounds. Cocke (2015, p. 148) described the multifaceted benefits of story circles: "Story circles engender appreciation for the unique intellectual, emotional, and spiritual qualities of each participant and develop oral expressions and listening skills. Each individual's story is a present to those in the circle, with the quality of the listening also a gift in return to the storyteller." Facilitators help identify themes with emotional content that can find its way into a performance (Boyes-Watson, 2008).

Sharing a social justice purpose has appeal among marginalized youth and their communities. Sonn and colleagues' (Sonn, Quayle, Mackenzie, & Law, 2014) oral history theatre project (Chronicles) taps into family oral histories and storytelling as key concepts in helping Aboriginal youth develop insights into their identities, thus countering dominant narratives that are demeaning, stereotypical, and non-belonging. Schneider (2008) provides examples of racial and ethnic groups (Alaskan Native, East Indian, Palestinian, Mexican, and African American) and how oral historians, folklorists, and anthropologists research traditional and historical oral narratives, creating insights into cultural and historical knowledge.

Youth contesting or resistance stories offer alternative definitions and explanations that shape how artistic expressions are manifested and perceived (Bell, Desai, & Irani, 2013; Milton, 2011). Youth resistance, assets, and strengths are rarely associated with each other yet they enjoy a close association (Dupree, Spencer, & Spencer, 2015). Understanding youth lives through their own voices is a hallmark of social justice participatory research, teaching, and practice (Dover, 2013). Storytelling is one method for achieving this goal.

Maynes, Pierce, and Laslett (2008, p. 1) ground storytelling as a distinctive method within a historical context and allow us to appreciate how its origin was in response to important social forces occurring during that time period:

> The relationship between the individual and the social has been a problem of perennial concern to social scientists and humanists alike. In the second half of the twentieth century, theorists from various disciplines and often competing tendencies . . . converged around theories that undermined classical understandings of the individual as a purpose social actor. The critiques went to the core of much modern Western social, political, and historical analysis; more deeply, they raised new questions about selfhood as it is understood, articulated, and practiced by individuals.

Storytelling (personal narrative) is an art form and method emphasizing first-person accounts to provide a way for individuals to share their own stories and agencies. The arts represent an attractive vehicle for constructing stories and sharing them with a broad audience.

Maynes, Pierce, and Laslett (2012) argue that storytelling, as manifested through oral histories of the major social movements of the past several decades, has played a critical role in advancing storytelling within the social sciences, particularly in the case of listening to stories by people who historically have been voiceless, thus bringing forth a compelling social justice view of their histories and experiences. These experiences generally go unrecorded, leaving a substantial gap in our knowledge base. Alrutz (2015, p. 112) addresses how youth stories introduce new ways of creating meaning in their lives:

> In many ways, this deceivingly simple practice of sharing and analyzing personal stories constitutes a significant political act. As youth participants begin to recognize personal stories, individual differences, and lived experiences as valuable forms of knowledge, they disrupt traditional social expectations and hierarchical ways of making meaning.

Storytelling can create new insights and social transformation. This method can be manifested through a variety of means, as in the case of the performing arts, and grounded within a cultural context.

Narratives are not bound by a narrow interpretation of how they are conceptualized and delivered, which can have strong Eurocentric biases; this fact opens up this field to a wealth of new methods that can be combined to enhance central messages. Music is a form of narrative without words (mood) that captures a central message when grounded within a cultural tradition (Campbell, 2010, p. 256):

> We need not look very far to recognize the extent to which music is linked with stories, plots, plays, and shows. Children are regular viewers of and listeners to these productions, yet they may not often perceive the role that music plays to enhance the drama and the development of characters. Music communicates sentiment and ambience, as it also supplies motivic material to signal "the good guys" and "the bad guys," the terrifying and the timid.

Although these observations pertain to music, similar conclusions can also be applied to other forms of performing arts. Casting a wider net on what constitutes a narrative facilitates youth community practice and its embrace of a social justice or critical stance and helps integrate various manifestations of culture.

The performing arts entertain and tell a story in the process. Cohen-Cruz (2006, p. 17) discusses grassroots theatre as storytelling: "The signature grassroots approach is personal story-based, which offers people a subjective way to respond to social circumstances." Storytelling captures narrative and plays a critical role in this book as we examine the performing arts as a vehicle for engaging youth, particularly those from ethnic and racial backgrounds that have made them vulnerable to the point where they are feared and treated as second-class citizens.

The arts provide youth with a chance to come together to construct a social justice narrative that encourages creativity and is affirming. This narrative can unfold through music, song, dance, and theatre, although it can also be done through poetry, film, murals, and publications. These methods can be combined with each other and with countless others (Lim, Chang, & Song, 2013).

Lambert (2011, p. 17) discusses the relationships among storytelling, cultures with oral history traditions, and epistemology and the potential for capturing and validating new forms of knowledge that, incidentally, find a receptive audience among youth of color and others who are marginalized:

> In oral culture, we learn completely through story. At the core of literary text and screen/electronic culture, stories are fundament tools of retaining knowledge as well. But what separates the literature culture in text and screen from the oral-centric cultures of story-exchange, is the unit of remembrance is held intact as a story to be expected to not only interpret but retain. To know the songs of your community, to have the ability to explain how the harvest must be tended, how to birth babies, and care for the elders, how to negotiate

with outsiders, is built into stories. The collection of stories becomes your epistemology.

The power of stories and the varied ways they can be shared can be captured through a variety of means, including the performing arts. There simply is no one way that these stories can be transformative, and there is no age group that cannot benefit from engaging in sharing stories—and never more so then when these stories address social injustices (Heggestad & Slettebø, 2015).

Difficult situations present youth of color with opportunities to respond in ways that tap their resilience, character, and coping strategies (Wexler et al., 2014). In essence, "what does not kill you makes you stronger." Using storytelling provides youth with a means through which to articulate and understand their experiences and resilience. It allows them to use their own words, including profanity because it is raw and unfiltered, and metaphors that hold symbolic meaning and facilitate storytelling. Youth tell stories differently from adults.

Storytelling can occur in a variety of highly attractive ways for urban of youth of color, including digitally (Haddix & Sealey-Ruiz, 2012). Alrutz's (2014) book *Digital Storytelling, Applied Theatre, & Youth: Performing Possibility* challenges us to expand their vision of how to deliver youth-focused performing, and, in this case, the use of digital storytelling is a method that holds appeal, particularly for youth interested and versed in the use of technology. Digital storytelling provides a platform for exploring a variety of performative goals (Lea, Belliveau, Wager, & Beck, 2011), and it is a method that has gathered increased popularity over the past decade (Lambert, 2011). Alrutz (2013) and Wales (2012) see tremendous potential in using digital storytelling as an applied theatre praxis with marginalized youth.

Youth can develop core experiences and ideas for shaping how the central messages of their stories will be told. Creating a script with accompanying music and images helps bring their stories to life digitally and involves multiple forms of performing arts (Halverson, 2009; Hull & Katz, 2006; Nelson, Hull, & Roche-Smith, 2008). These stories can cover a range of time periods and can accommodate brief vignettes or more elaborate stories, thus taking advantage the flexibility of digital storytelling (Lal, Donnelly, & Shin, 2015). These narratives can inform and support policy solutions.

The sharing of narratives can be facilitated through the use of technology. The program Youth Fostering Active Community Engagement for Integration and Transformation (FACE IT) does a wonderful job of illustrating the use of photovoice and digital storytelling as a means of using these techniques to engage in dialogue and develop and share youth narratives about their communities (Cushing, Love, & van Villet, 2012, p. 180): "Although dialogue is beneficial and an important part of the participatory process, using Photovoice and digital storytelling took the discussions to a deeper level and enabled the youth to focus on the physical environment of their community." Technology cannot substitute for dialogue, but it can enhance it.

Youth being able to understand their narrative (process of discovery) translates into being able to share it with others (process of transformation). This statement may seem simplistic, but it is quite profound when examined more closely. Techniques such as photovoice and digital storytelling help clarify and deepen stories in a way that conventional methods do not, tapping into youth interests and agency.

Alrutz (2014, p. 13) provides a description of how digital storytelling and applied theatre interconnect to enhance a performance, spotlighting the role and influence of power and social justice in a manner that lends itself to narrative sharing and encourages an audience to be receptive to hearing the story:

> Specifically, digital storytelling as an applied theatre practice relies on the intentional integration of live performance-making with digital representations. The process and products include real-time, embodied theatre and interactive performance elements, as well as digitally mediated representations such as photography, stop animation, recorded voice-overs, and video. The approach is critically engaged, in that it brings attention to issues of power, identity, and inequity.

A critical perspective that is sensitive to power dynamics helps ensure that a social justice basis for a performance guides how digital storytelling and applied theatre unfolds.

Matsuba et al. (Matsuba, Elder, Petrucci, & Reimer, 2010) provide a case study of how youth who are marginalized ("at-risk") can have positive stories to share if provided with an opportunity and encouraged to do so. Storytelling among youth can take a negative slant but can also elicit positive outcomes if the storyteller is encouraged to share examples of strengths, nobility, good deeds, and character. Marginalized youth must be provided with sufficient time and space to allow these stories to emerge because they can be much more proficient at highlighting their mistakes and flaws rather than the shining examples in their lives.

Storytelling is an art form, one practiced by every human being, and often deeply grounded within a cultural context, although it be called many different names. It is not restricted to any one group regardless of their demographics or cultural transitions (Maynes et al., 2012). The telling of a story regarding social injustices, if done with profound feelings, encourages the sharing of emotions in a manner that is easier to express for the storyteller (Banks, 2012; Phillips, 2012). The performing arts represent an attractive vehicle for directing these emotions that encourage a collective response, and the power of the group takes hold.

Stories can capture moments of joy and pain and be told in many different forms through narratives, paintings, songs, dances, and plays. Community practice must capture these stories to inform practice. In youth practice, it requires that practitioners and academics be able to enter the world of youth and do so in a manner that respects them and does justice to their meanings (Wales, 2012).

This book makes a conscious choice to capture these stories through the performing arts, more specifically by featuring stories that focus on social injustices, highlighting youth strengths and assets and not just their plights (Picower, 2012). Stories create shared meanings and purpose when involving a group, allowing members to select aspects that have particular meaning for them. The arts are a storytelling vehicle that must be deeply rooted in local customs and symbols to be successful in maximizing youth potential for social change (Garlock, 2012; Kenny & Fraser, 2012; Morris, 2012).

Capturing community stories to craft a dance performance is an example of how to ground a performance within the historical context and values of a community (Ferro & Watts, 2011). A community focus also provides an opportunity for stories to facilitate collaboration with other religious and human service organizations and thereby increasing the likelihood of achieving lasting social change (Castrillo, 2012).

Practitioners can play an influential role in helping marginalized youth make sense of their place in society by creating a space for them to engage in praxis and providing them with the requisite tools to aid them in socially navigating their environment (Baldridge, 2012; Forrest-Bank, Nicotera, Anthony, & Jenson, 2015; Morris, 2012). Praxis and storytelling come together in a manner that can be quite natural, facilitating exploration, sharing, and a search for answers and eventual social action (Batsleer, 2012; Chávez, 2012; Nembhard, 2012).

Youth are not often encouraged to use storytelling as an art form, even though they are often exposed to stories within their families and cultures and may not think of this as an "art form" (Yoon, 2012). Youth of color, in particular, often come from cultural traditions of storytelling, so this method will not seem alien to them. It is one that they can use in dealing with family and friends, giving expression to feelings that may be arduous to share in conversations or exchanges and facilitating intergenerational relationships.

Cultural Authenticity and the Performing Arts

Social justice youth community practice through the performing arts is based on a foundation that incorporates culture as a central feature. Discussions of authenticity, culture, and the performing arts must go beyond an erudite focus, bringing to the fore serious social and political dimensions. Any discussion of culture raises issues related to authenticity and who has the "right" to validate certain beliefs and practices (Dávila, 2012; Disegna, Brida, & Osti, 2011; Huang & Hsu, 2011).

Casteran and Roederer (2013, p. 153) define authenticity as "a concept that encapsulates what is genuine, real, and/or true." It is not unusual to see the term "organic" associated with authenticity and the process that gives rise to ownership and decision-making (Alonso & O'Shea, 2012). The value placed on ownership and decision-making is closely tied to participatory democracy, and this carries over into defining authenticity.

Authenticity has been conceptualized as being deeply embedded within memory, place, identity, and cultural significance (Waterton & Smith, 2009), and it is associated with an event's significance when tied to attendee expectations and the sponsors of an (Chhabra, 2010). Delgado (2016b) has conceptualized authenticity as the "glue" that brings a community together in pursuit of a common vision or goal.

To take into account the dynamic nature of this concept, authenticity can be viewed as a continuum rather than as a binary "yes" and "no" point-of-view (Gundlach & Neville, 2012). Pine and Gilmore (2007) propose a classification of authenticity as falling into one of five categories: (1) original, (2) natural, (3) exceptional, (4) referential, and (5) influential. This categorization is subject to interpretation and contextual considerations, thus highlighting the challenges faced in making determinations, with implications for how performing arts embrace and use culture in shaping productions.

Cultural authenticity must be solidly based on a consensus of the cultural values that are held by a community or group (Brown & James, 2004; Lytra, 2011; Trinidad, 2012). Oldenburg (1999) addresses the importance of festivals being authentic and not measuring their success or value by economic gain and other factors associated with attendance. This is also applicable to the performing arts. Dávila (2012, p. 189), issues a cautionary note on the quick and uncritical embrace of culture:

> In sum, this book is offered as a rejoinder to the general assumption that culture is always restorative of social identities and as a reminder of how powerfully distorting mainstream representations of culture can be when issues of equity and creative economies are concerned. In my view, these assumptions reproduce an empty and symbolic politics of multicultural representations that do not account for the racial politics involved in creative economies, while ignoring processes of commodification, appropriation, and mainstreaming that are at work.

Culture can be subverted and used to oppress communities, or it can be a key element in the performing arts (Forsyth, 2012; Spracklen, Richter, & Spracklen, 2013).

Cultural authenticity is not restricted to the performing arts and has applicability to community celebrations (Delgado, 2016b). This book has purposefully embraced culture, broadly defined, as a key element of social justice youth practice and the performing arts.

Book Goals

One of this book's primary goals is to expand the parameters of what constitutes youth community practice by proposing a new arena for social justice practice that embraces youth performing arts as praxis (Harlop & Aristizabal, 2013). This will be done through five interrelated goals:

1. Provide an urban-focused youth social justice practice conceptual foundation based on an explicit set of values and ethical challenges that shape a youth community practice program
2. Illustrate through a series of case studies how music, song, dance, and theatre can be integral to a social justice youth community
3. Outline various ways that social justice goals become manifested in youth community practice performing arts
4. Identify future directions for the field of youth community practice involving the performing arts
5. Identify the rewards and challenges of evaluating the effectiveness of music, song, dance, and theatre

These goals are presented as separate entities, but there is a tremendous amount of overlap among them, as there is with all performing arts.

Conclusion

This chapter introduced the potential of performing arts to reach, engage, and positively transform youth lives, including the challenges that youth community practice will encounter in reaching out to marginalized youth through the use of music, song, dance, and theatre to achieve personal and community transformation. These performing arts are tools, and tools are only as good as the person using them. Programs staffed by competent practitioners ensure that youth have the highest chances of succeeding.

Performing arts social justice youth practice has unlimited promise to make important contributions if it is conceptualized, participatory, and implemented to take into account local circumstances and priorities. Yet all forms of social justice youth practice bring challenges, and the performing arts are no exception. This practice is not a panacea, and that can be said about any youth practice.

2

Youth Community Practice

Introduction

Helping prepare youth cognitively, emotionally, politically, and socially to eventually assume "competent" adult roles benefits themselves, their families, communities, and society. These benefits take on greater significance in the case of youth who are destined to be tracked to this nation's underclass. A nation's ability to redirect these youth increases their human, social, economic, and political capital.

The forces shaping youth marginalization can also set the stage for their salvation when the conditions are established that allow youth to appreciate their strengths and potential for achieving social change. They have a vital interest in the outcome. Planning *with* rather than planning *for* has consequences. Social justice's influence on youth community practice makes it particularly conducive for using the performing arts.

Although the actual concept of transitions has been subject to critique, there are varied ways that adults can tap youth strengths, assist them in critical transition periods, and foster their achievement (Cuervo & Wyn, 2014). Some may argue that this is the role of schools and that these institutions should suffice in meeting this goal. Others will argue that schools have failed and that other institutions must fill the void because no generation should be expected to make it without assistance and a supportive environment (Smyth & Robinson, 2015).

An appreciation of youth dreams and nightmares requires a multifaceted and socioculturally nuanced understanding of their situations as well their communities. Understanding their dreams necessitates understanding their nightmares, too. This chapter provides insights into a group that defies simplification and enumeration, but one for whom there is general acknowledgment that their state of being is severely compromised. Youth are a group that a nation must pay close attention to, and I do not mean through surveillance. Arguing for investing in youth does not require debate, although how to allocate funding can be debated. The field of youth community practice and its various manifestations represent an attempt to identify, capture, and harness youth dreams for a better future.

A primary goal of this chapter is to capture the dynamic nature of a field that is ever changing and, in the process of evolving, bringing forth new rewards and challenges (Dimitriadis, 2008). Every one of the five words in "social justice youth community practice" is laden with deep historical meaning, contested definitions, and potentially inherent contradictions. When the words "performing arts" are added, it only magnifies the rewards and challenges.

Youth Community Practice

It is wise to pause and focus attention on the youth community practice field and ground its parameters, international reach, rewards, and challenges both in general and specifically as it relates to the performing arts as outlined in this book. The field of youth community practice encompasses a range of methods and philosophies (Purcell & Beck, 2010). In English-speaking Europe and Commonwealth nations, the field is known as "youth work" (Buchroth & Parkin, 2010; Gormally, 2015; Gormally & Coburn, 2014; Hlagala & Delport, 2014; Jeffs & Smith, 2010a; Sibthorp, Bialeschki, Stuart, & Phelan, 2012) and there, too, it encompasses a variety of approaches, all with their share of rewards and challenges for practice.

Social pedagogy, which is situated between the fields of social work and education, has found favor in non–English-speaking countries with strong national and regional differences (Bryderup & Frorup, 2011; Hämäläinen, 2003; Kornbeck & Jensen, 2009). Social pedagogy, in similar fashion to youth work and youth community practice, also has had to contend with definitional and boundary differences or confusion, thus hampering collaboration across continents (Kornbeck, 2009).

Developing, understanding, and appreciating youth community practice necessitates using frameworks that allow us to break this field down into perspectives or categories. Banks (2010) reviewed the field of youth work and arrived at a framework for assessing this form of practice with direct applicability to youth community practice. Banks's view has youth work falling into one of three distinct perspectives: (1) as an activity, (2) as an occupation, and (3) as a discipline. Youth community practice, too, can fall into these perspectives. When introducing a social justice prefix, it politicizes how this work unfolds with youth.

When youth work is viewed as an activity, it casts this practice as part of a greater constellation of activities that single out youth for engagement. When viewed as an occupation, is signifies a specialty and an identity for a practitioner who wants to be employed in this area. When viewed as a discipline, it encompasses theory that can be taught and learned as a field, laying out the foundations for individuals either wishing to learn certain types of activities or actively seeking work in this field. This perspective opens the field for interdisciplinary contributions.

Beck and Purcell (2010, p. ix) trace the historical origins of youth and community work to ground it within the current-day context and, in the process, highlight many outlets for this form of practice:

> Youth work and community work has a long, rich and diverse history that spans three centuries. The development of youth work extends from the late nineteenth and early twentieth century with the emergence of voluntary groups and the serried ranks of the UK's many uniformed youth organisation, through to modern youth club work, youth project work and informal education. Youth work remains in the early twenty-first century a mixture of voluntary effort and paid and state sponsored activity.

The evolution of youth and community over a lengthy period of time bodes well for its continued evolution into the immediate future, with expansion into new arenas such as the performing arts. Expansion into new arenas will cause tensions as this field challenges conventional wisdom about what constitutes youth practice.

All forms of community practice are exciting but also equally fraught with incredible demands, ethical challenges, and the constant facing of the multifaceted consequences of a socially unjust society (Richardson & Reynolds, 2012). Youth practice stands out because of the magnitude of the challenges of addressing a population group that is too young to vote and that does not have elected officials representing their best interests. This status is compounded when, because their backgrounds make them "different," youth are targeted for surveillance and control.

An overarching framework or umbrella under which to categorize various forms of youth development programs is very much needed. Mapping the universe of practice is an essential step in the direction of understanding the scope of this field, and embracing a common vocabulary and set of constructs facilitates comprehension and communication across academic disciplines, thus advancing the knowledge base. Understanding the key values underpinning these constructs also is essential to fully grasp this field. Youth community practice has the potential to fill this niche and provide the field with a "home" for a variety of social interventions.

Youth practice can be defined as the undertaking of a set of structured activities premised upon an explicit set of values that emphasize the worth of youth and their capacities to create positive change in their lives and their communities. When youth practice embraces social justice, it opens up a rich area of study and practice, one with a long history that entails a deliberative process that focuses on social inequalities (Burkemper, Hutchison, Wilson, & Stretch, 2013; Delgado & Staples, 2008; Ginwright, 2015).

This definition is purposefully both simple and broad to cast a wide net on a multitude of goals, programs, and activities; it raises important implications and challenges for undertaking evaluation and comparing different programs to grasp the significance of this social intervention across different youth groups and geographical settings.

Kemp (2011) argues that when youth development programs seek and achieve transformative results, it simply turns "conventional youth programming wisdom on its head." These programs aim beyond keeping youth out of trouble, seeing it as a waste of valuable resources to embrace a narrow focus. An expanding universe, to continue with this metaphor, is difficult to grasp, and it isn't a stretch to view youth community practice in this fashion. This book chooses to focus on one section of this universe, with an understanding that are other sections that co-exist and can be equally significant. Much can be learned from this section that can also be applied to other sections of the universe.

The Quest for Innovative Youth Practice

The quest for innovation is a staple of community practice and bodes well for this field reaching youth who are often labeled "difficult to engage" (Delgado, 2016a; Jackson, 2014; Stanton, 2015; Teater & Baldwin, 2012). There are groups of youth who have not benefitted from having their abilities and needs understood by policy-makers and funders (Greenberg & Lippold, 2013). This quest becomes essential as the nation's demographics change and communities are dramatically transformed through new incoming groups.

Funding sources have a fondness for innovative programs, and community practice, if it is to expand, must deliver on exiting new ways of reaching and serving communities (Abramson & Moore, 2014; Blanchet-Cohen & Cook, 2014; Puttick, Baeck, & Colligan, 2014). Putting the stamp of "innovative" on a proposal increases the likelihood that it will get attention in an increasingly competitive world of funding.

The community practice field also values innovation when it has potential for reaching underserved populations within a community context (Goldbard, 2006; Keller, 2014; Weil, Reisch, & Ohmer, 2012). The youth practice field is engaged in a never-ending search for ways of engaging youth who stand to benefit most from programming (Bose, Horrigan, Doble, & Shipp, 2014; Fischer, Craven, & Heilbron, 2011; Fredricks & Simpkins, 2012; Peterson, Newman, Leatherman, & Miske, 2014). These "new ways" must survive the quest for evidence-based results that can be documented.

We can argue that, with rare exceptions, all youth fall into the "endangered" category (Luthar & Barkin, 2012), but a conceptual and empirical argument can be made that low-income youth of color residing in this nation's inner cities would qualify as more worthy recipients of attention (Kirshner, 2009, 2015; Matloff-Nieves, Fusco, Connolly, & Maulik, 2015; Woodland, Martin, Hill, & Worrell, 2009). These youth assume added priority when intersectionality is introduced (Collins & Bilge, 2016; Ling & Monteith, 2014), as evidenced in the major racial upheavals occurring across the nation in 2015 and 2016.

Even within this category of youth, there are those who because of their emotional, physical, intellectual, and sexual identities face even greater challenges in socially navigating their daily lives (Balcazar et al., 2012; Mallett, 2012). The social exclusion and targeting of males (Rondón, Campbell, Galway, & Leavey, 2014) has started to get attention in discussions about social interventions that attempt to reach this demographic group. Gender, and we can add varying physical, intellectual, emotional abilities, and sexual orientation, does necessitate specific attention if youth programs are to be inclusive and representative of their communities (Bruening, Clark, & Mudrick, 2015).

Woodson's (2015) *Theatre for Youth Third Space: Performance, Democracy, and Community Cultural Development* introduces a capacity development paradigm, casting theatre into a prominent place in what is called a "third space" (public arena) by emphasizing youth as having agency rather than focusing on their educational, artistic, or social limitations. This assets perspective counteracts a destructive labeling process that emphasizes either deficit or charity views. Obtaining funds to study use of the performing arts with urban youth is arduous, but it is not too arduous to get funding to study criminal activities (Lansford, 2006).

Wylie (2015) argues that youth work in Britain has never experienced a golden age. I like to think that the golden age of youth community practice is near and worldwide. Community practice's reach in the twenty-first century is expanding and is only limited by our imagination (Gutierrez, Gant, & Richards-Schuster, 2014). Fostering the use of the performing arts in social justice youth practice is but one example of how this field can expand in a progressive and engaging manner.

Beck and Purcell (2010) discuss popular education practice in youth and community development because of its potential to achieve important personal transformations in the lives of participants. Photovoice has introduced an exciting method for engaging communities (Ohmer & Owens, 2013). Using photovoice in youth performing arts opens up this method for transformative practice experiences and evaluation (Greene, Burke, & McKenna, 2013). Transformative practice has gained increased currency because of its emphasis on learning and growing using a holistic, as opposed to a fragmented, approach (Beck & Purcell, 2010).

There is strong agreement in youth community practice (which incidentally encompasses a number of notable paradigms and approaches, most notably Positive Youth Development [PYD] and Youth-Led [YL] development) that innovative approaches to engaging urban youth are desperately needed, particularly ones that are social justice–based, consider youth as assets, and actively engage them in decision-making positions within initiatives (Delgado, 2016*b*; Ferrera, 2015; Flanagan & Christens, 2011; Grills et al., 2016; Harris, Wyn, & Younes, 2010; Ho, Clarke, & Dougherty, 2015; Knight, 2015; Sprague-Martinez et al., in press). A narrative youth shift is needed, one that views youth not as problems for a nation but as assets and valuable members of society.

Out-of-school settings allow youth programs to transpire outside of the time period when youth are in a structured school program. These settings can occupy the same physical place as schools but involve different expectations, personnel, and activities, thus differentiating this space from school. The settings also can involve community-based places where youth programming transpires either exclusively focused on youth or as part of overall programming for all age groups.

Out-of-schools settings are best conceptualized as vehicles for achieving ambitious goals (Boyes-Watson, 2008). Community outreach is never a program unto itself, but is an activity that seeks to engage potential participants in a change effort. Out-of-school settings take on significant prominence in youth practice because of their accessibility and potential to create innovative programming that is attractive to both youth and funders.

These settings can potentially create affirming and intrinsically rewarding growth experiences, which are key markers of successful youth programs (Intrator & Siegel, 2014). Yet not every out-of-school setting meets youth needs in a manner that can be transformative in their lives and respective communities. Some settings simply seek to keep youth safe by keeping them off dangerous streets. Although this is not a goal to be minimized, it is insufficient to prepare youth to socially navigate their surroundings and ultimately achieve roles as contributing adults in their communities and society.

Promise and Challenge of Positive Youth Development

It would be foolhardy to discuss youth practice without paying due attention to PYD because of its prominence in this field (Clary & Rhodes, 2006; Silbereisen & Lerner, 2007). PYD has managed to bring together governmental and nongovernmental entities throughout the world in an unprecedented manner (Bozlak & Kelley, 2015). This has served to bring much needed resources and attention to a significant shift in youth practice paradigms, a shift that only increases in importance over time.

PYD has not suffered from a lack of scholarly attention (Arbeit et al., 2014; Benson, Scales, Hamilton, & Sesma, 2006; Bowers et al., 2015; Jenson, 2012; Nakkula, Foster, Mannes, & Bolstrom, 2010; Shinn & Yoshikawa, 2008; Silbereisen & Lerner, 2007; Vasudevan, 2015; Zaff, Jones, Donlan, & Anderson, 2015). PYD's success is not restricted to out-of-school settings and can be found within schools, too, further increasing its reach beyond the conventional focus on out-of-school settings (Lewis et al., 2016; Smith, West, & Bozeman, 2015). There are no realms that PYD cannot effectively address nationally and internationally (Ferrer-Wreder, Adamson, Kumpfer, & Eichas, 2012; Hamby, Pierce, Daniloski, & Brinberg, 2011), and there is recognition that it will "take a village" to achieve the goals associated with PYD and other forms of practice.

Youth of color, particularly African-American/Black and Latino, face challenges related to health inequities, and participation in PYD activities can aid them in increasing their human capital, which translates into other forms of capital (Atkiss, Moyer, Desai, & Roland, 2011; Maley, 2012; Norton & Watt, 2014).

The argument can be made that there is insufficient research on PYD when looking at the field from a more nuanced perspective (Masten, 2011), and there is a call for methodological and theoretical advances to further our understanding of the interplay of youth activities and their ecology, how youth thrive, and how PYD empowers them to achieve successes (Kurtines et al., 2008; Lam & McHale, 2015; Tolan, 2014).

All youth activities are not created equal regarding commitment and potential outcomes. Although sports and arts programs are particularly appealing to youth, research indicates that sports are associated with high stress. Larson et al. (Larson, Hansen, & Moneta, 2006) found service-learning activities attractive for acquisition of teamwork competencies and the development of positive interrelationships and social capital. Activity selection must be closely associated with programmatic goals, with keen attention paid to the expectations and competencies that youth wish either to enhance or acquire. The increasing number of newcomer youth in the United States is generally unreported in this expanding PYD literature.

There is no indication that PYD has peaked in popularity, and this stands as a testament to its importance among youth practice professions and the social sciences. There are many causes that can incorporate PYD. Schusler (2013) illustrates the potentially broad reach of PYD by using environmental action, which can be considered congruent with PYD goals and principles, to aid educators and practitioners in addressing social justice by tapping youth interest in this topic. Environmental action, to be viable, must address how youth conceptualize it and must focus on issues that are most salient in their lives and those of their families, friends, and communities (Delgado, 2016*a*).

Halverson (2009) brings together PYD and artistic production through the use of interrelated strategies that rely on a dramaturgical process that entails engagement in telling, adapting, and performing stories with personal meaning and helping to shape identity. This transformative process helps youth with stigmatized identities to develop more positive views of themselves (demystification) and can support individualistic and collectivistic self-conceptions, critical values that shape worldviews (Goffman, 1963; Green, 2013).

Personal transformation is a key theme in social justice community practice performing arts. There are multiple challenges that confront practitioners and evaluators alike in tapping how this transformation has evolved and its significance (Preston, 2009*b*, pp. 305–306):

> Firstly, there is a need to be alert to the useful and sustainable features of a project for participants and organizations involved. This might well not be predetermined or expected but emerge within a project. Secondly, practitioners need to develop effective strategies for evaluating that which is not easily measurable; the development of people's consciousness and agency long after a project has completed. . . . Finally, there is a need for practitioners to have a clear distinction between "ideals" of transformation and the "reality" in a

given setting and to develop critical analyses of applied theatre intervention and their impact.

Although Preston is referring to theatre, his comments have relevance to performing arts in general. Capturing lightning in a bottle is difficult, yet there is no denying the existence of lighting. Capturing and measuring it will prove formidable, but it is a worthy goal.

PYD is enhanced when strengths are purposefully identified, fostered, and aligned with community assets, particularly in the case of marginalized youth (Coulter, 2015 Lerner, Buckingham et al., 2015). Youth character is another key construct associated with PYD, with implications for how programming unfolds (Ruch, Weber, & Park, 2015). PYD has brought with it a tremendous breadth of view in understanding youth and increasing their embrace of pro-social behavior and competencies across a number of social arenas and the "5 C's" (see next paragraph), thus increasing their chances at achieving success (Law, Siu, & Shek, 2012).

Fostering self-regulation is a significant part of PYD and can be either an explicit or implicit programming goal (Morgan, Sibthorp, & Wells, 2014). Fostering emotional regulation, too, is associated with PYD, and many in the field consider it critical in achieving any significant measure of success with youth in compromised situations (Buckley & Saarni, 2009).

The 5 C's provide a well-rounded perspective on development—Competency (musical, academic, and social), Confidence, Connection, Character, and Caring (Geldhof et al., 2015)—and each of these constructs brings with it both a wealth of theoretical and empirical knowledge for expanding the richness of the field and also corresponding research challenges in understanding their significance. Critical and creative thinking are considered core elements of PYD, and cognitive competence wields significant influence within and outside of educational settings, having applicability across the entire life span (Sun & Hui, 2012).

The performing arts are an attractive outlet for this competence, along with other PYD activities. Youths' embrace of the value of responsibilities also plays an influential role in their development. Salusky et al. (2014) identified the process of assuming responsibility as consisting of four stages: (1) voluntarily taking on roles and obligations, (2) a willingness to experience challenges and the strains associated with them, (3) a willingness to carry out obligations, and (4) the internalization of a self-concept that translates into responsible behavior in other contexts. Each stage has cognitive and concrete actions that can be examined and reinforced through carefully planned programming.

PYD scholarship has enriched our understanding of how youth thrive and how best to structure in- and out-of-school programs to maximize their engagement and existing resources to help them and their communities (Geldhof et al., 2014). It has shifted focus from youth as sources of problems, a fundamental point, to youth as having potential and capacities and being worthy of society investing in them because they have tremendous talent (Gavin et al., 2010; Spencer & Swanson, 2013).

This shift is no small conceptual or political matter because society has a proclivity for viewing youth, as a group, as being needy. PYD can incorporate youth cultural backgrounds, as in the case of American Indian/Alaska Native youth, by tapping culture as a strength (Jones & Skogrand, 2014, 2015; Kenyon & Hanson, 2012). Bi-culturalism, as is the case of Latino youth, is an asset rather than a limitation or deficit, and, once conceptualized as such, it provides community practitioners with endless possibilities for programming (Acevedo-Polakovich et al., 2014). Bi-culturalism prepares youth to be global citizens in a world that is increasingly in need of citizens who can thrive in a complex society.

All youth possess strengths. Can youth practice address challenges while not losing its focus on strengths and assets (something that is never simple)? How do we ensure that we do not lose the forest for the trees? Jones and Skogrand (2015, p. 43) answer these questions in the affirmative: "Recognizing challenges and deficiencies while focusing on positive aspects will serve to bring communities together with a vision for the future." And, using theatre to uncover strengths is attractive from a social justice and gendered perspective (Lind et al., 2010).

Reconceptualization of who qualifies as "youth" has also resulted in youth-serving organizations changing, too, to become more responsive. Intrator and Siegal (2014, p. 27) note how creating a spark in youth is essential in successful organizations:

> Youth development begins by sparking interest and then engaging young people cognitively, behaviorally, and emotionally so that they put forth the concentrated and purposeful effort necessary for achievement.

Organizations must take a holistic or comprehensive view of youth if they hope to keep them meaningfully engaged and able to maximize potential benefits from participation (Crnic, 2012). This view must also involve youth dealings with local police forces, as evidenced by the number of police shootings and killings involving youth of color. This stance will prove controversial, but it is essential if programs are to remain relevant in their lives (Moore et al., 2016; Sekhon, 2016; Tolliver, Hadden, Snowden, & Brown-Manning, 2016).

Zeldin and Camino's (1998) statement, as quoted by Zeldin, Camino, and Calvert (2012), that "there is nothing as theoretical as good practice" captures the sentiment that practice-informed theory and research in the field of youth community practice reinforces how practice dictates scholarly attention. PYD's popularity has not gone without serious theoretical, philosophical, and methodological critiques, which are essential for any field to progress.

Questions have been raised about the universality of PYD when addressing intersectionality and contextual grounding, which necessitate an active social change agenda to be an integral part of any form of programming due to the presence of social forces of oppression (Cho, Crenshaw, & McCall, 2013). It is insufficient to address youth needs without corresponding attention to and action on the social forces that are undermining their progress.

Collins and Bilge (2016, p. 2) provide a definition of intersectionality that captures the complexity of this construct and its importance in discussing marginalized youth:

> Intersectionality is a way of understanding and studying the complexity in the world, in people, and in human experiences. The events and conditions of social and political life and the self can seldom be understood as shaped by one factor. They are generally shaped by many factors in diverse and mutually influencing ways. When it comes to inequality, people's lives and the organization of power in a given society are better understood as being shaped not by a single axis of social division, be it race or gender or class, but by many axes that work together and influence each other. Intersectionality as an analytic tool gives people better access to the complexity of the world and of themselves.

Undervalued youth in this society are complex and misunderstood; an intersectionality perspective provides a frame through which to understand and respond to them.

Taylor (2012) offers a stinging critique of PYD and its efforts at social engineering in addressing undervalued youth and society's efforts at engaging in acting-out behaviors without addressing the environmental forces operating to marginalize and stigmatize these youth. Where is PYD and the Black Lives Matter movement? The impact of violence in the lives of urban youth of color cannot be ignored in urban-focused youth community practice of any kind.

Culture-specific processes, which have tremendous relevance to youth of color and can result in positive youth outcomes, have not received the attention they deserve in PYD research and scholarship, and this limits PYD's potential impact on youth community practice (Evans et al., 2012). Intersectionality and contextual grouping requires that youth culture and operative realities inform assessments and interventions (Lesko, 2001). Borden et al.'s (2006) literature review on Latino youth development, although dated, concluded that the literature on PYD has generally overlooked this important group. Although progress has been made, more must be accomplished for Latino youth, particularly for those who are undocumented.

Any efforts at youth programming, particularly those focused on urban youth of color, must take into account culture (and subculture) in shaping the conceptualization of interventions, and the concept of culture must be broadly defined and inclusive of multiple views since it is not monolithic.

Debies-Carl (2013) critiques youth study paradigms as falling into three major categories: (1) youth phenomena clustered under what can be considered a monolithic conceptual umbrella; (2) a propensity to focus almost exclusively on style and consumption of goods; and (3) a belief that there is a lack of reasoned and rational behavior, with a corresponding ineffectiveness in achievement of concrete or real social change. Youth subgroups are often underestimated and trivialized, thus undermining any effort at a comprehensive appreciation of the subject.

Praxis and reflexivity introduces a politically charged analysis in discussing the relevance of PYD for those who are highly marginalized. Praxis is not possible without critical and creative thinking (Tsai, 2012). Providing the requisite space (time, activities, place, and support) for this to transpire is essential and can possibly result in a shift in epistemological thinking that facilitates embracing social justice values and principles (Rieger & Schultz, 2014).

PYD research has rarely taken into consideration racial identity, a prominent asset, and this limits its understanding of what constitutes a normative process among African-American youth for positive youth development (Evans et al., 2012). A similar statement can be made concerning other youth of color. Racial socialization (preparation for confronting bias, cultural socialization, and egalitarianism) is another dimension that has generally escaped focus and has particular saliency for youth of color in undervalued communities (Hughes et al., 2006).

Spirituality can be an integral part of community practice (Hill & Donaldson, 2012; Zhang & Wu, 2012) and is found within PYD (Lerner, Roeser, & Phelps, 2008). Benson and Roehlkepartain (2008) argue that spiritual development is a missing priority in youth development. Even though spirituality can be a significant factor and an important dimension in the lives of youth, it can be simply overlooked in programming (Cheon & Canda, 2010; Scales et al., 2014). Spirituality must be grounded in a local context to be successful, and youth of color have not benefitted from PYD spirituality research (Nicolas & DeSilva, 2008). Spirituality can take on various manifestations and should not be confused with religious beliefs (King, 2008).

How spirituality is expressed in youth practice and the performing arts is open to creative interpretation, and this brings exciting and important dimensions to these art forms. The performing arts of music and dance can bring social meaning within the context of spirituality, language, and culture, as evidenced among Native Americans (Jones & Skogrand, 2015). Belly dancing is another example of how innovative thinking involving youth programming and an openness to engage spirituality is possible (Kraus, 2012, p. 59):

> Belly dance is spiritual for some people who participate in this artistic dance form. . . . Results show dancers who situate spirituality within the music, physical movement or connections with other dancers experience spirituality soon after they get involved in belly dance. However, spirituality within the dance takes time to develop for those dancers who find spiritual significance in their connections with audience members during performances. These findings suggest that when a practitioner begins defining belly dance as spiritually meaningful is partly related to the particular aspects of belly dance a dancer associates with spirituality.

Belly dancing introduces a form of dancing with capabilities for expanding our horizon of understanding of spirituality and brings a dimension to dance that is rarely discussed within youth community practice.

Spirituality is not limited to particular settings, time periods, population groups, or manifestation (as in the case of belly dancing) that can be marshaled in service to youth. Woodley (2013) notes that belly dancing provides an opportunity to learn about another culture and to share of oneself and the struggles that seem to be part of our everyday life, including those that are oppressive. This flexibility is a curse and a blessing for practitioners. It can be integrated in highly effective ways, but it can be quite challenging to evaluate its presence and effectiveness.

The most serious criticism of PYD programming is reserved for its lack of a social justice focus because not all youth who engage in programming face similar challenges (Delgado, 2016a; Spencer & Spencer, 2014). Travis and Leech (2014, p. 93) advocate for empowerment-based PYD as a means of counteracting a depoliticized (apolitical) approach toward youth engagement and advance a model that emphasizes an enhanced role of community within this field as a means of ensuring that youth activities have meaning in their lives and positively impact their community:

> A shift occurred in research about adolescents in the general population. Research is moving away from deficits toward a resilience paradigm and understanding trajectories of positive youth development. This shift has been less consistent in research and practice with African American youth. A gap also exists in understanding whether individual youth development dimensions generate potential in other dimensions. This study presents an empowerment-based positive youth development model. It builds upon existing research to present a new vision of healthy development for African American youth that is strengths-based, developmental, culture-bound, and action-oriented.

There is a close relationship between youth feeling disempowered and engagement in behavior that is dysfunctional and compromising to their well-being (Pearrow, 2008). Disempowerment can also lead to behavior that resists (oppositional resistance) control by adults.

Some youth social justice scholars would cast these behaviors as desistance or resistance and social activism (Aidi, 2014; Dimitriadis, 2014; Tuck & Yang, 2014). The famous English author Oscar Wilde (Wilde & Dowling, 2001), although not labeling it as desistance, stated this concept quite well in the following quote: "The best among the poor are never grateful. They are ungrateful, discontented, disobedient, and rebellious. They are right to be so."

Resistance does not have to involve overt acts (Dimitriadis, 2008, p. 79): "Resistance refers to the everyday practices and symbols marginalized groups use to 'claim space' for themselves in and against oppressive circumstances.

Resistant practices are often not seen by participants as explicitly political. Their incipient political importance is often located by scholars and researchers." Understanding these acts, including their motivation and manifestation, needs local grounding and youth voices to interpret them.

Empowerment is a strategy for self-governance to act on self-interest (Kwon, 2013). It must also seek to change the social circumstances that led to disempowerment and find a response to oppression (Epstein, 2013). Viewing communities as a context, a goal for achieving change, and as a method helps bring together youth assets and social ecology and reinforces social justice action in the performing arts.

Social justice youth development (praxis, social change, community development, youth leadership development) is a direct response of a branch of this field to be more attuned to the needs of marginalized youth (Christens & Dolan, 2011; Conner, 2012; Iwasaki, 2015; Geiser & Quinn, 2012; Quijada Cerecer, Cahill, & Bradley, 2013). The same objective can be introduced by using "critical," with all of its social-political history (Johnston-Goodstar & Sethi, 2013).

Youth are very astute about their sociopolitical position in a society dominated by adults. In the case of marginalized youth, they confront the abuses of power and indifference by adults in authority on a daily basis and do not have to be convinced of their marginality (Hankey, 2014; Powell, 2014; Spencer & Doull, 2015). These challenges are also faced by youth organizers in their efforts to achieve legitimacy within the social activism field because this arena is dominated by adults (Conner, 2016; Delgado & Staples, 2008).

The integration of youth with disabilities within PYD programs must assume a prominent goal if PYD hopes to be a field that is inclusive and not one limited to only those without physical and mental challenges (Becker & Dusing, 2010; Olsen & Dieser, 2012). Youth with disabilities have not found a prominent place within PYD programmatically or in the scholarship, thus representing a group that has very few options for engaging in after-school activities because of the challenges they face in obtaining transportation and, depending upon disability, aides who can assist them in participating in activities. Youth work, too, has not escaped this criticism (Taylor, 2012).

Wylie (2015, p. 53) issues challenges pertaining to funding and youth work in Britain, but this conclusion is equally applicable to the funding scene in United States:

> Despite the best efforts of families, schools or voluntary groups, little is likely to change for the better in many young people's lives, or in what youth work can do to support them, until central and local government re-discover their own enabling and leadership roles. But young people and their needs will still endure. It is especially incumbent on those in leadership roles in youth work to develop more coherent, consistent and compelling arguments to campaign on their behalf. And, bound together by common values, to demonstrate a greater sense of solidarity with others in the sector as well as with the young.

Innovation is possible without requisite funding, but there is no denying that it can play a role in shaping momentum.

Youth with disabilities face incredible obstacles in reaching their potential (Carter, Brock, & Trainor, 2014; Gorter et al., 2014). These obstacles have much to do with our prejudices about their interests and capabilities. These youth are resilient, and resiliency as a social construct, despite its popularity among scholars, must be expanded to include people with disabilities and tap their definitions of what it constitutes (Runswick-Cole & Goodley, 2013). Youth of color who are deaf are rarely discussed in the professional literature, often being treated as if they simply do not exist (Moore & Mertens, 2015). This insidious invisibility poses serious consequences for them and their respective communities and is applicable to other visible and invisible disabilities.

Wooster (2009) addresses the importance of defining what is meant by "inclusion" in the performance arts and presents the case study of the Odyssey Theatre, a group of learning disabled and non–learning disabled performers. He emphasizes the value of thinking of performance as an art form with both artistic and social worth and of paying special attention to its role in empowerment and leadership.

Band et al. (Band, Lindsay, Neelands, & Freakley, 2011) raise the important point of not setting up youth with disabilities to fail at the performing arts; although the authors were addressing professional companies, their conclusions concerning the need for necessary supports and the possibility of introducing a new model based on aesthetics has applicability at all levels of production, including at the school or amateur level. For some youth with disabilities, being exposed to the performing arts may represent a potential source of full- or part-time (summer) employment (Carter et al., 2010).

Some performing arts lend themselves to integrating youth with disabilities better than others (e.g., music vs. classical ballet). I remember watching a dance troupe that integrated a performer in a wheelchair in a manner that was quite natural and amazing at the same time, making the performance memorable.

The emergence of the concept of "critical disability" brings into discussion issues of oppression based on abilities and how this interacts with other forms of oppression in the lives of youth with disabilities (Slater, 2013). Intersectionality takes on even greater prominence when dealing with urban youth of color, LGBTQ youth, those with disabilities, and the undocumented (Banales, 2012; Daley, Solomon, Newman, & Mishna, 2008; Grady, Marquez, & McLaren, 2012; Irazábal & Huerta, 2016; Revilla, 2012; Sládková, Mangado, & Quinteros, 2012). Intersectionality is a concept that helps bring together academics and practitioners in service to youth who are marginalized.

The introduction of the prefix "critical" to youth practice puts practitioners and academics on notice about an injustice that has occurred and the need for actions that seek to undo this injustice (Giroux, 2011). This prefix radically transforms an intervention and has sociopolitical influences throughout all stages of the research informing this intervention and the practice. Youth practitioners must ask how PYD can be used with all forms of youth activities. Questions have been raised about how the 5 C's can be manifested in sports (Martinek, 2005), and how sports can address social justice.

There is no subject that cannot be addressed from a social justice perspective, including physical education (Randall & Robinson, 2016). The role of the 2015 University of Missouri football team in bringing down a university's administration because of racial injustice is rare in the annals of United States sports, but shows sports potential to address social justice. The example of New York City's New Renaissance Basketball Association and gun violence illustrates how a sporting activity, in this case basketball, can serve a social justice issue by bringing further attention and a message—in this case a positive one—to a major social issue in the lives of youth (Korman, 2015). The Rens, as they are called, have attached a bright orange patch to their jerseys to bring attention to gun violence.

Jones et al. (2011) addresses why "It is plausible that sport does not provide a homogenous experience for all young people. Rather, the different rules, structures, coaching styles, motivational climates, and organizational nuances observed across sports may provide young people with diverse developmental experiences and PYD outcomes." A comprehensive discussion of sports and PYD must not be restricted to boys. Rauscher and Cooky (2016) address girls' participation in sports from a feminist or critical perspective to understand the potential and pitfalls when PYD is applied to girls and sports. Sport still favors males; this can be seen across all sports and is evident in how the women's national soccer program, although as successful as the men's team, still is less heavily funded. Discussion related to issues of sexism must be integral to any form of sports programming.

Sports that are team-oriented help youth acquire valuable teamwork or group skills and learn important lessons that can be used later in life (Camiré, Trudel, & Forneris, 2014; Forneris, Bean, & Halsall, 2016; Newman & Alvarez, 2015). Sports participation has been found to influence other aspects of youth engagement as well (Zarrett et al., 2009). How well the lessons learned and PYD competencies transfer to other social-political spheres in youth lives needs considerably more research and attention (Turnnidge, Côté, & Hancock, 2014; White, Wyn, & Albanese, 2008).

Sports and injuries are closely related (Sabato & Caine, 2016). Bean, Fortier, Post, and Chima (2014) reviewed the literature on organized sports and their impact on youth and their families and found that there are negative consequences to youth engaging in athletics (injuries, mental health issues, poor well-being, alcohol and other drug abuse, attrition/burnout) and to their parents/families (financial burdens, time investment, emotional well-being, stress, and familial relationships strains). Emergency room visits resulting from sports injuries cannot be ignored, just as intentional school-related injuries cannot be ignored (Amanullah, Heneghan, Steele, Mello, & Linakis, 2014). When injured, low-income athletes must seek medical attention, and their chances of receiving quality health care are not the same as their middle and upper middle class counterparts, making recovery more arduous to achieve, with increasing lifelong consequences.

A willingness to accept these risks must be openly acknowledged by youth and their parents/legal guardians. The waivers that are presented for signature generally focus on the potential of physical injuries and totally overlook the psychological and financial implications of sports on participants and their families. These multifaceted costs take on greater prominence when discussing low-income families that can ill-afford additional stressors in their lives.

Coakley (2011, p. 306) raises a caution concerning sports as a development strategy that can also apply to other activities, including the performing arts:

> There is a widespread belief that sport participation inevitably contributes to youth development because sport's assumed essential goodness and purity is passed on to those who partake in it. Promoted and perpetuated by sport evangelists and kindred spirits, this belief inspires the strategy of using sports to create among young people the attributes needed to achieve personal success.

Coakley's concerns strike at the basic premise that any activity is better than no activity, but a poorly conceived activity can be worse than no activity because of how it may repel youth from participating in other activities in the future.

Grills et al. (2016) stress how Afrocentric values and culture can shape PYD to make it of increased relevance to these youth of color:

> Positive youth development is critical for African American youth as they negotiate a social, political, and historical landscape grounded in systemic inequities and racism. One possible, yet understudied, approach to promote positive youth development is to increase African American youth consciousness and connection to their Afrocentric values and culture.

Using Afrocentric values and culture lends itself to the performing arts because of how youth can be valued in shaping participation and performances.

Culture and context are closely intertwined and work together to shape youth identity, participation expectations, actions, and implications for efforts to reach out and engage them (Harris & Lemon, 2012; Rivas-Drake et al., 2014; Xing, Chico, Lambouths, Brittian, & Schwartz, 2015). Vila's (2014) *Music and Youth Culture in Latin America: Identity Construction Processes from New York to Buenos Aires* examines the interplay between music and culture and how music helps youth reflect on who they are, with implications for other forms of art.

Marginalized Youth

There are countless ways of speaking about youth who are at difficult stages in their lives or who have made choices that have compromised their chances at success.

How adults label these youth says a great deal about our values and worldview. These views may be conscious or unconscious, yet there is no denying their impact in shaping social policies and programs. I prefer the term "marginalization" for many different personal and professional reasons.

Marginalization is a concept that most social scientists and human service providers will be familiar with. It applies to youth as a group and it takes on even more significance when introducing intersectionality (Balcazar et al., 2012; Ling & Monteith, 2014). McCready (2004, p. 142) discusses the process of marginalization of gay and gender nonconforming Black male youth and the importance of successfully addressing the intersectionality of homophobia, racism, and heterosexism for these youth in helping them navigate educational systems. He notes that it is essential to identify the influence of these forces before actions can be taken to alter attitudes and behavior:

> If more queer youth of color are willing to risk harassment and abuse by openly identifying as gay, lesbian, bisexual, or transgender, then we as urban educators [and youth community practitioners] should be willing to risk stepping out of our comfort zones to unravel the complexities of their lives.

Intersectionality provides a lens for grounding youth experiences in a manner that incorporates daily lived experiences, thus making it necessary to take into account oppressive forces in any analysis and intervention plan.

The "lived experience" of transgender youth of color highlights the reality of multiple oppressions in their lives in a very stark manner. Viewing this oppression without taking into account the role of resilience does a disservice to these youth (Singh, 2013; Singh, Meng, & Hansen, 2014). Sharing their stories allows them to raise issues of oppression; resilience becomes an important mechanism by which they can inform others of their lives, and it facilitates them obtaining both validation individually and a sense of collectivity or belonging, an important dimension in all youth lives.

The performing arts are an excellent collective mechanism to help youth achieve these goals. There is power in numbers; this is never more true than when you believe you are the only one at the margins of society and then discover that others join you in these feelings.

A great deal depends on how "at-risk" is defined and then operationalized (Kronick, 2013). It is safe to say that, regardless of how it is defined, the emphasis remains on the individual and not on society. Riele (2006) argues that by labeling youth as being "at-risk" we further marginalize them by blaming the victim rather than asking why they are marginalized in the first place and shifting the onus away from youth and onto society.

Youth with spoiled identities are conscious of how society distrusts and fears them and how they have been labeled and socially isolated (Bateman, 2011; Cauce, Cruz, Corona, & Conger, 2011; Cherng, 2015; Kuper, 2015). Spoiled identities translate into youth becoming isolated and limited in how, when, and where they can seek help when they find themselves in difficult situations. The performing arts must eschew using an "at-risk" label because such a label is demeaning and only further marginalizes youth (Conrad, 2005).

There's a relationship between perceived racial discrimination, well-being, and achievement among African-American youth (and other youth of color), and this should not be surprising (Seaton, Neblett, Upton, Hammond, & Sellers, 2011; Syed, Azmitia, & Cooper, 2011). Adult-imposed identities on youth are not necessarily incorporated by them, but that does not take away from the social consequences of these acts. Youth may engage in resistance acts to counteract these efforts (Ball, 2012; Creasap, 2012; Delgado, 2016a), and music and song also can be manifestations of this resistance (Tremblay, 2016).

The definition of marginalization is not simple, and that should not be surprising. A simple definition, although attractive, would do a disservice to a complex and highly charged construct that is deeply rooted in this society. Certain groups of youth have been singled out by society to be feared, monitored, and punished as a result of an infraction, and youth of color who reside in the nation's inner cities are a prime example (Akom, Cammarota, & Ginwright, 2008, p. 1):

> Social science research on Black and Latina/o youth has been dominated by studies that focus on "problem" adolescent behavior. These studies are largely related to public policy concerns about crime and safety in poor urban communities. Typically, they explain youth crime, delinquency, and violence as individual pathological behavior, or from cultural adaptations that stem from social disorganization in poor urban communities. The social disorganization thesis explains how gross disinvestments in urban communities ultimately lead to the erosion of community and family values and to behaviors that create and sustain poverty. Scholars argue that urban youth learn "ghetto related" behaviors, including disrespect for authority, indifference toward educational achievement, and lack of work ethic from other urban residents who have given up on legitimate means for economic security.

This focus has social-economic-political consequences for youth of color and their communities. Resilience is rarely associated with these youth, yet it is present if we understand the social forces they confront on a daily basis (Aisenberg & Herrenkohl, 2008; Dill & Ozer, 2016).

Dimitriadis (2008, p. 11) addresses an implicit bias that equates "urban" with violence, youth, and a disregard of laws: "Indeed, 'urban' is itself a highly contested term. Although it has come to symbolize a kind of racial code word for pathology, it is also the terrain upon which the most significant and important youth culture movement of the late-twentieth century was born—hip-hop." Hip-hop is a message and vehicle for transforming the lives of urban youth.

A youth definition from an adult perspective may not coincide with that of youth, and that is why the cultural-social context that youth find themselves embedded within shapes their view of themselves and why they feel embattled (Blatterer, 2010). The definition of "youth" as a unitary category has been dominated by a biological domain that deprecates social, psychological, economic, and cultural domains (Griffin, 2013).

A gender binary view has faced considerable pushback, but the same cannot be said about the definition of youth. Contextual grounding does not apply when a biological domain dominates thinking on the subject, giving the impression of precise and clearly delineated boundaries. Intrator and Siegel (2014) discuss the shifting definition of adolescence and the challenges of arriving at a consensus definition: "It is becoming widely accepted that the length of adolescence is extending to the mid-to late twenties—a period sometimes called emerging adulthood—and the pathways to becoming independent adults have become more ambiguous and numerous." "Emerging adulthood" has a strong socioeconomic status connotation. Marginalized youth do not have the "luxury" of an extended period of youth, but instead one that is severely shortened.

White, Wyn, and Albanese (2008) note that marginalization is a systematic process taken by those in authority and a chance occurrence: "The systematic marginalization of young people (and their communities) is marked by the disintegration of connections with mainstream social institutions (such as school and work), and a tenuous search for meaning in an uncaring and unforgiving world." Youth marginalization is heightened when it is grounded spatially (segregated), and there are few social places where this marginalization is more obvious than in a nation's cities (Ferrare & Apple, 2012).

Cities often have a well-deserved history as being places with higher levels of tolerance for people with obvious differences (small-town America is often romanticized). If you are "different," it is not a view that readily emerges because of how pronounced the marginalization can be. Cities, because of their high concentration of youth and their attractiveness for youth who are "different," provide ample opportunities for engaging these youth and for developing a collective sense of community beyond just geographical similarities. Population density and segmentation facilitate the use of limited resources.

Changing demographics has resulted in a nation that is increasingly grayer and browner: the browning of the nation has thrust African-American/Black, Asian, and Latino youth into a demographic majority for those 18 years of age and younger (Delgado, 2016a). With changing demographics comes a ripple consequence, which brings to mind a South African proverb: "When the music changes, so does the dance" (Heppner & Jung, 2012). This proverb signifies the importance of activities responding to changes in demographic composition and doing so in an affirming and culturally syntonic manner. For this book's purposes, youth will cover latency to 20 years of age, with extra attention being paid to those 13 to 19 years of age.

Critical Youth Practice and Social Justice

There is also an awareness that "one-size programming" does not fit all youth, calling attention to the importance of contextualization and the matching of youth experiences, demographic profiles, expectations, abilities, cultures, and awareness of social justice issues with the most appropriate youth practice vehicle for engaging and maximizing their outcomes (Stanton, 2012; Staples, 2012; Weis & Dimitriadis, 2008). Conrad (2015) argues that there is a moral imperative to undertake socially innovative interventions when social justice is a guiding principle and that anything less does a disservice to communities. Opportunities to make significant differences in the lives of marginalized youth are few and far between, and practitioners and academics must not let these moments or opportunities pass.

Critical praxis within education and the social sciences, particularly anthropology, geography, psychology, and sociology, has its historical roots with Karl Marx and the legacy of the subsequent Frankfurt School (Anderson, 2011; Azmanova, 2012; Collins, 2012; Honneth & Reitz, 2013; Kehily, 2014; Kress, Degennaro, & Paugh, 2013). These historical roots have evolved since then. The Frankfurt School responded with the development of critical theory to counteract positivistic and technocratic schools of thought, with critical theory coming to play a prominent role in shaping current-day discourse on social justice and youth as one example (Wishart & D'Elia, 2013).

Its present day evolution has seen a number of prominent educators and social scientists influence its modern adaptation, most notably the work of Paolo Freire (Brazilian) and Antonio Gramsci (Italian), although not as well-known as Freire in the U. S., in two different continents, bringing together of reflection, theory, and action, and referred to as praxis or critical praxis (Beck & Purcell, 2010). Critical youth studies brings together various disciplines and views within this age and socio-political-philosophical stance (Agger, 2014).

The emergence of critical youth studies brings together those with interest in hearing the voices of youth who have been relegated to the fringes of society and providing a home, forum, and vocabulary for working with and for youth in their efforts to achieve social justice (Ibrahim & Steinberg, 2014; Kelley & Kamp, 2014). Praxis and agency are key ingredients in critical youth studies, which embraces intersectionality in analysis and the crafting of actions (Grady et al., 2012). Coffey and Farrugia (2014) argue that a youth agency construct remains ambiguous due to ontological and epistemological confusion, although this ambiguity has not hindered its popularity among social scientists.

A critical perspective has manifested its influence in a variety of ways, sometimes without the prefix of "critical" to signal this philosophical stance. The introduction of human rights into discussions of social justice is not unusual in scholarly publications. Rubin (2012) argues that this nation's embrace of No Child Left Behind (NCLB) legislation and the increased emphasis on high-stakes standardized testing, with its accompanying emphasis on uniformity of thought and the eschewing of creativity, has resulted in a decrease in youth critical thinking skills and a corresponding de-emphasis on social justice. Excelling in school often means not engaging in critical thinking (Landy & Montgomery, 2012).

Richards-Schuster and Pritzker (2015) advocate for applying the United Nations Convention on the Rights of the Child (CRC) as a means of strengthening youth participation in civic engagement and other realms. Human rights must be integrated into any and all forms of education because no segment of society is immune from having its rights violated (Becker, 2012; Spero, 2012). A similar stance can be applied to social interventions.

Any discussion of a social justice/critical paradigm and youth community practice must not exclude academics. Academics must challenge institutional bias and acts of oppression toward marginalized youth and other groups, and there is a concerted call to action to accomplish this goal (Goodall Jr., 2012; Hastings, 2012; Kindall-Smith, 2012; Nembhard, 2012). Academics in collaboration with youth and communities is viable and has considerable potential for future undertakings (Parchment, Jones, Del-Villar, Small, & McKay, 2016), although it is always challenging to accomplish.

Lavie-Ajayi and Krumer-Nevo (2013) advance the need to offer a critical counter-narrative to conventional youth practices, and critical or social justice youth work with marginalized youth must embrace two distinct yet interrelated goals: (1) individual development, including the enhancement of abilities, and (2) collective critical consciousness and the promotion of social justice. It can be argued that individual development cannot occur without a concomitant grounding within a social justice frame of reference and subsequent social action.

Lavie-Ajayi and Krumer-Nevo (2013) offer a three-part model stressing ecology (streets as a physical and political spaces), use of counter-narrative, and the role of the youth worker as social capital agent. This interrelationship is essential to maximize the potential of critical youth work to achieve social change for a generation that faces incredible odds against achieving success.

Sharing narratives is often the first step in a deliberative process that shows the commonalities of how social injustices have changed youth lives and those of significant family and friends. The arts give voice to the stories of social issues, drawing attention to and creating catharsis after a major community event, and doing so in a way that serves to engage and unite people in a nonthreatening manner (Chappell & Faltis, 2013; Orleans, 2012). The intensity of a social justice message is often accompanied by feelings of hope, unity, and determination (Christens & Speer, 2015; Spero, 2012). Using the performing arts to convey this message presents a viable method to increase its significance.

The performing arts are about much more than a performance within a community context or a work of art. In addition to the importance of the artistic or aesthetic contribution, a performing arts production also is community- and participatory-centered. Rogers (2012) advocates using the performing arts and cultural geography in illuminating how people make sense of their lived experiences and the space where they transpire. In cases of marginalized youth, how this experience gets manifested in the performing arts illustrates how social injustices shape the geography (place) of where they can or cannot go, with their life being narrowly geographically defined.

Contextualizing programs is essential because youth practice models are often developed without regard to adaptation considerations for a variety of geographical settings; programs require many different approaches, rather than the typical "one-size fits all" approach, and the saying that to "plan is human; to implement is divine" comes to mind, reflecting the importance of context in shaping outcomes.

Gentrifying urban neighborhoods present different challenges from neighborhoods that are losing populations due to disinvestments, as in Detroit, or neighborhoods that are shifting in demographic composition, as in the case of Watts, Los Angeles, which has have gone from predominantly African-American/Blacks to Latinos, with high percentages of undocumented immigrants (Chimurenga, 2015).

PYD as a paradigm encourages youth to engage in school and make contributions to their communities, and these contributions generally cover a wide range of types (Chase, Warren, & Lerner, 2015; Hershberg, Johnson, DeSouza, Hunter, & Zaff, 2015). These contributions and services generally tend to have a nonconfrontational quality to them and do not embrace a social justice/social change stance that challenges the status quo.

Social protest is a legitimate form of community service, and it must have a prominent place among the constellation of other forms of youth community service or civic engagement (Clay, 2012; DeJaeghere & McCleary, 2010; Kirshner, 2015; Rogers, Mediratta, & Shah, 2012; Shange, 2012). A 2010 inventory of youth social action organizing in the United States identified 160 active campaigns, up from 120 in 2004 (Torres-Fleming, Valdes, & Pillai, 2010), illustrating the appeal of this method for youth.

It becomes critical that the performing arts not reinforce stereotypes or further marginalize youth and the communities they are intended to reach (Amoabeng, 2012; McLean, 2014). There are a number of excellent examples that challenge stereotypes while advocating for the use of the performing arts as a vehicle for achieving social change, thus highlighting the potential for achieving positive changes.

Shepard's (2012) *Play, Creativity, and Social Movements: If I Can't Dance, It's Not My Revolution* does a wonderful job of illustrating (visually and narratively) how social activism, social justice, and the arts can serve as vehicles for drawing attention to and participation in urban social justice causes and for integrating marginalized groups, including youth, in social protest. Rivera-Servera's book (2012) *Movements of Hope. Performing Queer Latinidad: Dance, Sexuality, Politics* also does a superb job of illustrating the interrelationships of identity, intersectionality, social justice, cultural traditions, and the importance of various performing arts in bringing these different elements together in a cogent and coherent form.

Social justice service and actions take on tremendous importance in the case of marginalized youth and have a prominent place within the constellation of youth community practice approaches (Delgado, 2016*b*; Matloff-Nieves et al., 2016). Social injustices in their lives and in those of their families and friends become important motivators for engendering civic responses that can be classified as social protests. Relationships developed while engaging in protest, including friendships, and lessons learned take on significance and serve to create camaraderie.

Social Media

Social media expands the reach of the performing arts. Goldbard (2006, p. 65) addresses the limited physical and virtual access that marginalized communities face in engaging in cultural expressions, thus setting the stage for the importance of social media:

> Members of marginalized communities lack public space for their cultural expressions. Speaking concretely, they seldom have institutions, facilities or amenities equal to those available to more prosperous neighborhoods or communities. In terms of virtual space, they are likely to lack equal access to mass communications media and therefore any meaningful opportunity to balance the sensationally negative pictures of themselves pervading commercial media.

Creating spaces for cultural expression may represent one of the most significant contributions community practitioners can make to a community. This goes hand in hand with creating hope and eventual social change. Social media is an equalizing and democratizing force that can be marshaled in service to youth performing arts.

Barron et al.'s (Barron, Gomez, Pinkard, & Martin, 2014) book *The Digital Youth Network: Cultivating Digital Media Citizenship in Urban Communities* illustrates how digital media has permeated virtually all aspects of institutional and noninstitutionalized society and groups, with no group more affected than youth who have embraced this form of communication. Its appeal and potential can permeate other aspects of their lives.

Adults usually think of social media as a way of facilitating communication (Jones & Mitchell, 2016). As noted by McGough and Salomon (2014), when viewed from a youth perspective, there are numerous benefits that they can achieve through its use: an increase in critical thinking skills, content knowledge, connectedness, and interpersonal and leadership skills. Social media takes on significance among youth and connects them across geographic boundaries.

Social media provides youth with an opportunity to expand the impact of their work beyond a narrow audience. Youth media, particularly when guided by a critical media literacy perspective, bridges audiences across a large geographical terrain and provides a vehicle for youth practice (Johnston-Goodstar,

Richards-Schuster, & Sethi, 2014). YouTube, for example, is a participatory media platform that provides youth with a place to "create, connect, collaborate, and circulate," increasing potential reach across communities (Chau, 2010). It is a platform that youth are very familiar with.

Conclusion

Viewing youth as capital is contrasted with the conventional view of them as a liability. Successfully addressing youth translates into preparing a generation to address challenges now and in the future. The rewards of achieving this goal are considerable. This goal brings challenges, too, and particularly so when discussing marginalized youth because it entails challenging the status quo and putting youth in a position of being challengers and threatening. The potential rewards far outweigh the limitations and challenges.

Youth community practice in its various manifestations has been presented as a viable approach for reaching youth, and the performing arts have been singled out as having proved their success with marginalized youth. Although these arts may not be the preferred mechanism for engaging youth when other approaches are available, within the performing arts there is a range of viable and attractive approaches that will appeal to different youth interests.

3

Youth

Introduction

Helping prepare youth cognitively, emotionally, politically, and socially to eventually assume "competent" adult roles benefits themselves, their families, their communities, and society as a whole. These benefits take on even greater significance in the case of youth who are often destined to be tracked to this nation's underclass. A nations' ability to redirect these youth increases their human capital and that of their families, neighborhoods, and society as a whole.

Youth are a distinctive group regardless of how we define them from an academic perspective, although defining who belongs to this group is subject to intense debate and has social consequences once agreement is reached. Urban youth are keenly aware of how they are viewed, and their resistance to these perceptions are often thought of as hostile actions (Emdin, 2010). They are feared as if they were adults, yet they have none of the power of adults.

This chapter sets a foundation for viewing youth from various significant social-cultural-demographic perspectives, including how they are defined for the purposes of this book, with an emphasis on those who are marginalization (stigmatized), their demographic profile, and their relationships with adults in authority. Each perspective will reappear throughout this book in various forms to do justice to its importance in shaping social justice youth practice and the performing arts.

Labels and Youth

It can be argued that many a career has been made by focusing on youth, particularly when addressing them as a threat with poor impulse control (hedonistic/risk takers) and in desperate need of close adult supervision, if not surveillance; this is especially true for particular subgroups that are perceived as threatening and are facing challenges related to intersectionality (Cammarota & Romero, 2011; Fine & Torre, 2004; Ruck, Harris, Fine, & Freudenberg, 2008; Weiss, 2011).

This nation has a love–hate relationship with its youth. At one level, we consider youth the "future of a nation" and we extol their importance in positioning the country to compete globally; at the same time, we say that the nation is in trouble because our youth are not prepared to assume the mantel of leadership in the future. If youth are the future of a nation—and the world, for that matter—why not invest the time, energy, and resources that are needed to ensure that they have an increased likelihood of a positive future?

The label "at-risk" is very popular in the youth and human services scholarly literature, and it increases the appeal of these books, making youth that much more worthy of attention by drawing attention to their plight. There is a certain degree of ease in using this label when youth are low-income, of color, and reside in segregated urban communities.

The same argument can be made by attaching the label of "epidemic" to a social problem to raise it to a level worthy of political attention and corresponding funding. The "at-risk" label is often selectively applied to reinforce certain narratives or stereotypes. Has it ever been used with stockbrokers who are "at-risk" for committing major fraud or university administers who may be "at-risk" for malfeasance? Of course not. It is a label reserved for a very select and important population group, one that is relatively easy to label.

Some critics of the at-risk label have proposed using "marginalized" instead as a way of shifting the attention back to society and away from youth without losing focus on them and introducing the question of why are they on the margins of society (Riele, 2006). The onus in this situation is placed on explaining the social forces at work rather than on youth vulnerabilities and deficits, a view that implies that there is something about them or what they have done that makes them at-risk and worth fixing. Moral panic and the term "blaming the victim" comes to mind because it illustrates scapegoating by a society intent on punishing a group for engaging in resistance acts (Krinsky, 2008).

The prevailing sentiment among helping professionals is to express concern for youth with "problems." Hammond (2010, p. 1) comments that the underlying assumptions pertaining to this stance must be examined: "'having a problem' suggests that problems belong to or are inherent in people and, in some way, express an important fact about who they are. The existence of the problem provides the rationale for the existence of professional helpers and a developed language by professionals to describe the problematic areas of concern. The power to label youth as "having a problem" is substantial, representing one of the greatest challenges in shifting discourse from a focus on them as problems to society as the problem maker.

A book on youth and the performing arts is predicated upon embracing a positive and affirming view of youth and supporting the idea that youth are worthy of investment and willing to engage in activities. It seems as if thousands of books have been written or will be written on youth from a deficit perspective, and this is a narrative that society feels comfortable with and understands, although it may have deleterious consequences for youth (Giroux, 2011, 2012, 2014). This is a sad commentary on the power of negativity in shaping adult views of youth, with a focus on those who are most stigmatized. It also serves as a warning about the barriers that must be surmounted if a counter-narrative is to prevail.

Youth are not a monolithic group even when focusing on specific demographic factors. Race and ethnicity, which are arguably the most popular ways of categorizing people regardless of age, represent broad constructs that can accommodate various dimensions and make comparisons across groups arduous. Efforts to understand youth more comprehensively require a clear and definitive definition. Youth is a socially constructed category and subject to all of the vicissitudes and limitations of any social construct.

Youth are complex beyond demographics and difficult to categorize into simple groupings that are not based on their operative reality and self-identities. The idea of the United States being a nation of immigrants is taken to new heights as outgroup relationships result in new identities when measured against conventional definitions. The nation's demographic composition is rapidly changing, making simplistic categories dangerous when setting policies and guiding youth program development.

Youth are best understood within their lived context while taking into account their geographical setting. Most youth live in cities, and so do the vast majority of youth of color. They are relegated to certain sections of cities (contested spaces) that we have developed a range of labels to describe, with "inner-city," "blight," "slum," and "ghetto" being arguably the most popular. Youth have been marginalized socially and geographically, and segregation has its social, economic, and political price.

Although I am a big advocate for acknowledging the enhanced value of cities in the lives of youth, these geographical settings (and the state of mind they engender) can also increase the challenges they face and must not be romanticized (Tienda & Wilson, 2002, p. 3): "Urban living can alleviate many of the hardships associated with rural poverty and underdevelopment, but in the context of rapid social transformation, it can also increase the challenges of normative youth development." The "rural myth" is just that: a myth that has been perpetuated over time. Rural life has never been easy or safe, nor is it today (Brass, 2014; Hofstadter, 1955; Kelsey, 1994). There is good reason rural residents uproot and move to cities in search of better opportunities.

Urban living brings with it a host of challenges and benefits, and the latter is missing in any serious discourse on the subject that impacts the social identity of those who reside within urban boundaries. Social identity is impacted by numerous factors, including where an individual lives (White, Wyn, & Albanese, 2008). Place can be a repellent, but it can be a draw when there are positive associations.

"Place attachment" refers to the significance and emotional connectedness that we ascribe to a physical place. This attachment is reinforced when ethnicity/

race are synonymous. When communities become contested places and spaces, residents with place attachment can feel threatened along a variety of dimensions. Gieseking and Mangold (2014, p. 73) make an important observation regarding place, identity, and the construction of autobiographies:

> Why do we feel that we belong in some places and not in others? Place and identity are inextricably bound to one another. The two are co-produced as people come to identify with where they live, shape it, however modestly, and are in turn shaped by their environments, creating distinctive *environmental autobiographies*, the narratives we hold from the memories of those spaces and places that shaped us.

It is not a stretch to see the power of place in shaping youth identity and why urban youth of color incorporate their neighborhood as part of their identity. Contesting place and the youth who occupy that space highlights their marginalization and their place of residence. Labels shape perceptions and even identities.

Definition of Youth

Much thought has been given to defining youth in this book, and this should be the case in any work advocating social interventions that involve youth in a prominent manner. One approach is to keep it simple and provide a straightforward and short definition, but this does a disservice to youth community practice because of the complexities involved in defining youth; another approach is to be very erudite and give an entire chapter to a subject that can easily have multiple volumes devoted to it.

I have elected to take a more ambitious approach, but not one as erudite and ambitious as a comprehensive definition—a middle-of-the-road approach to inform but not overwhelm. A reader-friendly definition will be provided, but not before a social context is presented that draws upon a variety of academic traditions and stances on the subject and how local sociocultural circumstances shape this definition.

A number of academic disciplines have long tackled the problem of providing a definition of what constitutes "youth" so there is a long tradition in this realm (Jones, 2009). Studying youth and adolescence as a critical period also has a long anthropological tradition (Bucholtz, 2002).

Why is a multidimensional definition of such importance in the social sciences, humanities, and helping professions? At a fundamental level, it facilitates communication and investigation because everyone is on the same page, paragraph, sentence, and word. We all agree on what is being discussed and measured, although this level of clarity is rare and never more so than when discussing what constitutes an age group.

At a more advanced level, clear definition facilitates much needed collaboration across academic disciplines and professions, evaluation, and research, which is essential to maximize existing resources and mobilize political will. This level of interaction leads to much-needed sophisticated theory development that can inform practice. The following brief sample illustrates the variety of interdisciplinary-based approaches.

The French sociologist Pierre Bourdieu (1978), as quoted in Jones (2008), said "Youth is just a word." This provocative statement forces us to pause and discuss the consequences it has for this age group and the nation. If we substitute "women" for youth, it would result in heated debate and conversation, but this is not the case for youth. Having a second-class status relegates youth to an invisible state of being, and efforts to change this bring forth social and political backlash.

Savage's (2007) book *Teenage: The Prehistory of Youth Culture 1875–1945* illustrates the social forces at work in shaping adult views of youth, and how youth culture transcends time, identifying an interconnectedness that youth practitioners and academics must first acknowledge and then take into account in present-day views of this age category.

Savage traces the emergence of the concept of "teenager" as a discreet age group to the mid-1940s and the post World War II period, with the rise and influence of consumerism and mass marketing to this group. Dimitriadis (2008, p. 13) challenges what constitutes a "youth": "Youth is a highly contested term— historically evolving, often assumed to be stable, and deployed in a range of ways with concrete effects for the most vulnerable populations."

Jones (2008) identifies seven key themes emerging over the past several hundred years as academics debated the concept of youth and illustrates why it is not a straightforward process to arrive at a consensus definition: (1) *science versus nature* (myth versus enlightenment education); (2) *biology versus culture/nature versus nurture* (biology as deterministic versus social/cultural contexts); (3) *age generation or social class* (structural versus individualistic influences); (4) *conflict versus consensus* (generational conformity versus conflict); (5) *structure versus agency* (free to choose or constrained); (6) *structure versus process* (considered from an age generation or transition to adulthood); and (7) contributors or dependent (assets versus deficits).

These perspectives, with the possible exception of the first, are all alive and well. The later perspective stands out and will in all likelihood continue to cause considerable debate into the foreseeable future. Each perspective brings its own approaches to social interventions so that these views have implications for how "best" to think of youth and how the performing arts can be tapped in this cause.

White and Wyn (2008, p. 5) address the debate on youth as a universal versus social construct and explain why it is important to settle this issue because of its implications for social policies and youth programming:

> This shift has led to a considerable debate within youth studies about the extent to which youth is a universal stage of life or whether it is a social construct and, like adulthood, gains its parameters and meaning from social conditions.

The debate about social change is closely connected to this because, according to some interpretations, both youth and adulthood are changing.

There are strong arguments to be made for a social construct point of view, particularly in light of current debates about when youth can be considered financially independent, now that a high percentage of young adults live at home because of financial constraints. Recent methodological advances have strengthened adolescent theoretical models (Crosnoe & Johnson, 2011).

Youth community practitioners must challenge basic assumptions and understandings of how we define children and youth and be open to new conceptions that are more grounded in their operative reality (Woodson 2015, p. 24):

> The words *children* and *youth* do not just describe or mark physical bodies, time passed, or experienced gained, these terms exist as complex theoretical concepts created and recreated ideologically and contextually . . .. Understanding *children* and *youth* as key words does not require subscribing to hard and fast rules, rather, youth workers of all stripes need to recognize that both our own and our communities' conceptual models limit our understandings of what and who young people are and/should be.

It is simpler to use age-related terms, such as "children" and "youth," and expect everyone to be in agreement about what these terms mean both practically and symbolically. But reliance on such broad terms does a disservice to any field focused on these population groups.

Leccardi and Ruspini (2012) in their book *A New Youth?: Young People, Generations and Family Life* acknowledge a range of influential social forces that have prolonged the status of youth and influenced their relationships with the intimate and distant world around them and describe how these relationships allow them to forge new freedoms but also entail consequences. Furstenberg (2000) viewed the 1990s as a particularly significant historical period during which research and scholarship explored the causes and ramifications of extending the period in which adulthood is achieved.

This generation is unlike any previous ones, and that can be said for all generations. Yet accepting this premise means that we should be prepared to make necessary modifications to existing programs and activities to make them of increased relevance to this generation.

Cote and Allahar (2006) propose viewing youth from one of three historical perspectives: (1) conceptions of youth through a lens of historical changes, (2) a historical view of youth within a country's history, and (3) youth within a current-day political and economic context. All three are interconnected, yet each brings a unique view of the forces and circumstances at work in shaping adult perceptions of youth. Youth perceptions of fellow youth are often missing in the first two perspectives and must be sought if we are to provide a window into how to shape messages to reach youth and provide a grounding of this topic.

The World Health Organization (WHO; 2013, p. 1) defines "youth" in an international context while acknowledging the existence of differences:

> YOUTH is best understood as a period of transition from the dependence of childhood to adulthood's independence. That's why, as a category, youth is more fluid than other fixed age-groups. Yet, age is the easiest way to define this group, particularly in relation to education and employment, because "youth" is often referred to a person between the ages of leaving compulsory education, and finding their first job.

The 15 to 24 chronological years used by the WHO covers a developmental period that goes beyond that used in the United States, thus pointing out how this age range varies significantly across countries and continents, making cross-national comparisons difficult.

Society's emphasis on viewing youth as "adults in waiting," which can be traced back to the Middle Ages, is reflected in how social policies are developed to the detriment of youth, their communities, and society (White & Wyn, 2008, p. 105):

> Across all areas of formal and informal policy formation and practice, there is a range of practices affect how young people live their lives. These practices are commonly based on the view that young people are not as important as youth, but as future adults. These policies often draw on the language of youth development to assert that young people are important because they represent the future and social capital of our society. . . . As many commentators have pointed out, policies that locate young people's value in their future as adults also tend to emphasize "governmentality" . . . that is, they provide a rationale for monitoring and controlling young people's lives in the interest of protecting the future of young people and of the society.

A shift in thinking of youth not as a nation's future but as a nation's present does not negate their future contribution but instead serves to emphasize their potential for present-day contributions: contributions can be both current and future, and these are not mutually exclusive. Life is rarely an either/or proposition and requires a nuanced understanding.

Kirshner (2015, p. 5), a leading proponent of youth activism, reinforces the importance of the here-and-now view of youth and how values shape adult views of how youth engagement is perceived: "The argument for engaging young people as partners in public work, rather than objects of policy, is rooted in a set of normative values. Youth should be treated as 'citizens of the future'; they are citizens now who experience, interpret, and sometimes resist the policies that organize their everyday lives." These policies are rarely affirming and empowering of marginalized youth.

Youth and their self-identities are subjects that are synonymous and worthy of attention in any form of social intervention. Expressing and refining identity becomes an essential developmental dimension of youthhood, including exploring other social identities and expanding their knowledge base about other groups, and also serves to reinforce their basic cultural belief systems (Barber, Abbott, & Neira, 2014). One can be hard pressed to find alternatives to the performing arts that can be as effective and attractive in shaping positive identities and, in the process, engaging wide audiences (Sonn, Quayle, Belanji, & Baker, 2015).

Positive identity is a construct with tremendous relevance to positive youth development and can be enhanced through participation in out-of-school programs (Noble-Carr, Barker, McArthur, & Woodman, 2014; Rahm, Lachaîne, & Mathura, 2014; Tsang, Hui, & Law, 2012). Identities can go far beyond a narrow focus on ethnicity and race (Holloway & Valentine, 2014; Nortier & Svendsen, 2015; Reynolds, 2015). Assisting youth in achieving this identity clarity naturally provides practitioners with ethical challenges. To understand youth means understanding how they define themselves, particularly in situations where their identity does not conform to conventional definitions.

An age-based definition is arguably the most common and easiest way of defining youth, and it is predicated upon a belief that all youth share the same age-based developmental tasks and challenges (Moje, 2015). There is a leap of faith in accepting this premise because taking an age-based definition also presupposes that social-cultural circumstances remain constant.

We should introduce another youth dimension, which is place- and urban-bound. For the purposes of this book, the term "urban youth" seeks to capture a population group; a geographical setting; a cluster of capacities, assets, and strengths; and a social state of being that systematically marginalizes a group of youth because of their social-economic class, ethnicity/race, sexual orientation, and abilities. This covers a great deal of territory and captures a state of mind and exposure to forces in shaping this definition.

The power of Madison Avenue is such that the concept of "urban youth" has emerged to capture a lifestyle that can be marketed, particularly in selling clothing and music that are fashionable and represent an urban way of life that is attractive and to be copied (if at all possible) regardless of where one resides (Dimitriadis, 2008). Jordan and Weedon (2015) argue that White males are the biggest consumers of Black culture as represented through various cultural symbols, most notably music. The appropriation of Black culture is dramatically different from using this culture as a window through which to develop a better understanding and appreciation of another group.

Marginalized Youth as a Focus

Language and labels play an influential role in shaping attitudes and society's responses to the social circumstances that individuals may be confronting.

Whether we label certain youth groups as "at-risk," "vulnerable," "anti-social," "angry," "in need," "under-privileged," "throwaway," "disconnected," "dissatisfied," "damaged," "multi-problem," "disadvantaged," "pre-delinquent," or "marginalized" is predicated upon assumptions (biases) and values shaping youth policies and programming (James, 2012; O'Connor, Hill, & Robinson, 2009).

Pica-Smith and Veloria (2012) note that "at-risk" is a label most frequently used with youth, is socially constructed, and its popularity in the scholarly and popular literature is undeniable. They reported that 6,811 articles used the term "at-risk" in their titles in the ERIC database, with the Psycho Info database listing 10,099 such titles. A Google Scholar search found 1,380,000 documents. A Google Images search uncovered 13,500,000 entries. The magnitude of these publications is indicative of the power of this label across audiences and shows why it influences social policies so strongly.

Foster and Spencer (2011) argue that a label of "at-risk"—or "resilient," for that matter—does a disservice to youth because it is an inappropriate way to capture youths' past, current, and future prospects. The prefix attached to youth goes beyond semantics and reveals important assumptions and values concerning the causes of the "problem," setting the foundation for social policies and interventions that incorporate this prefix and actions predicated on this assumption.

A historical understanding of this construct's evolution is needed to appreciate its current meaning. Pica-Smith and Veloria (2012, p. 34) provide an evolutionary insight into the underlying premises shaping its present popularity:

> While the term has not been operationalized, it would appear to represent a tangible construct instead of a socially constructed one that has been critiqued for reifying a new social identity of risk that pathologizes youth of color and poor youth. . . . When the term "at risk" became popularized . . . it was simply a new manifestation of a cultural deficit model . . . the construct has placed the locus of dysfunction in individuals of color, single-parent families (especially mothers who are not married), low income communities, and people with disabilities. The discourse of risk ignores institutionalized structures of inequality and a systemic analysis of what places youth at risk. Therefore, we argue that the construct of risk and "at risk" must be deconstructed, interrogated, and problematized in order for students to develop a critical consciousness that extends beyond the individual level of analysis.

Practitioners and scholars must worry about the power of labels and the importance of deconstructing their meaning (Besley, 2009). Labels may focus attention, but is this the kind of attention that the marginalized need?

A shift from a deficit view to a strength/asset/resiliency focus requires a different set of values and vocabulary, and it manifests itself in very concrete and highly visible social political actions (Delgado, 2016a). Its manifestation goes beyond merely a different worldview to encompass concrete results that are open to evaluation and reporting of findings in a manner that can impact practice and social policies (Hammond, 2010, p. 6):

- Feel special and appreciated—strong sense of hope and optimism
- View life as a dynamic journey that involves them writing the next chapters by how they perceive themselves and who they invite on the trip
- Have learned to set realistic goals and expectations for themselves
- Rely on productive coping strategies that are growth fostering rather than self-defeating
- View obstacles as challenges to confront—not avoid

"Label Jars not People" is much more than a throw-away slogan, striking as it does at the insidious outcomes of stigmatizing labels when applied to human beings because it places the onus of social circumstances on the individual facing challenges, or blaming the victim.

The concept of marginalization has been salient for the past 10 years nationally and internationally and in a variety of ways, and it promises to continue to do so in the immediate future (Nicholas et al., 2016; Park & 朴宰亨; 2015; Poteet & Simmons, 2016; Sandhu, 2015; Shelton, 2015). Its appeal has to do with capturing a realization that many different youth groups may share commonalities in how society views them as "surplus" and as being pushed to the margins of society.

Bringing together disparate groups facilitates focusing on common social forces that are compromising their futures (and one might also add those of their families) and undermining the social fabric of the communities where they reside. A focus on poverty and protective factors helps achieve this goal (Madsen, Hicks, & Thompson, 2011).

There has been a criminalization of childhood in this country, with youth of color having a long tradition of being singled out for suspicion (Kwon, 2013; Tilton, 2010). The school-to-prison pipeline concept is definitely focused on urban African-American and Latino youth (Dunn, 2013; Malone & Malone, 2015; Meiners, 2010; Wald & Losen, 2003). It highlights how certain youth groups are targeted from very early on and how social forces shape institutional responses. Many different societal institutions play a role in making this pipeline, with schools playing a particularly influential early role in tracking youth toward dead-end jobs at best and prisons at worst (Adams-Taylor, 2014; Erevelles, 2014; Ginwright, 2011; Kirshner, 2015; Pane & Rocco, 2014; Winn, 2011).

Youth self-identities suffer because of marginalization, and this has lifetime implications if ignored (Ferrer-Wreder et al., 2002). The concept of "throwaway youth" captures how certain youth groups are simply viewed as surplus and expendable by society (Pyscher & Lozenski, 2014). If youth of color believe they have a future worth living for, this translates into embracing positive choices in attitudes and behaviors and effectively places them in an advantageous position in navigating their social environment (Caprara et al., 2014; Johnson, Jones & Cheng, 2015; Walsh, 2008).

These youth can draw upon rationales for alternative behaviors from their "tool boxes." If the only tool they have is a hammer, it stands to reason that everything starts to look like a nail in their world. Having additional tools allows them to assess the most appropriate tool for the situation on hand. The more tools youth have, the better, because this provides them with options to use the right tools at the appropriate time and in the appropriate circumstances.

This does not mean that youth or adults may not have a favorite tool. If violence is the only way a person knows to respond to stressful situations, we must ask why this is the preferred method for handling stress. If other ways of handling stress are learned, this provides the individual with options that will not compromise his or her status in society. This may seem simplistic, but violence triggers can be deconstructed and substitutes provided.

This way of thinking results in further integrating youth into the social fabric of their community, which can influence the behaviors of their social peers and friendship network if viewed from a social ecological perspective. The opposite is also true. Youth performing arts must not be conceptualized as a vehicle for rescuing or fixing youth who are marginalized (Cahill, 2008; Ersing, 2009). Rather, the arts should be viewed as an alternative to conventional ways of thinking about youth engagement (Lauver & Little, 2005).

Technological advances have opened the door to using the performing arts to create excitement for audiences and serve as an attractive recruitment mechanism for youth, including their introduction to dance (Anderson, Cameron, & Sutton, 2012). Jensen (2011) sees tremendous potential for how theatre can encourage youth and provide opportunities for tapping into the spaces and technology in their daily lives, creating new aesthetic possibilities and a vehicle to attract them to this performing art form.

It is as artificial to separate out youth from adults as it is to view them as existing outside of their communities. It is not uncommon for youth to have many influential adults in their lives who share similar marginalization, thus challenging youth practitioners to broaden the scope of their interventions and take into account this situation to help ensure the success of interventions (Ramphele, 2002, p. 29):

> Successful interventions to enhance youth development need to incorporate strategies that enhance self-esteem in young people. Children on the street, abused young people, and marginalized groups in all cultures suffer from poor self-esteem. It becomes doubly difficult for them if their own parents, teachers, and other caregivers face the same problem.

This calls for a social justice orientation that helps these youth understand (praxis) the forces leading to their marginalization, but also points to strategies that can assist them and their families in changing these conditions and altering the forces that create them. Praxis outcomes maximize social justice youth community practice.

Marginalization is not restricted to any age group, but youth and older adults share a higher probability of being targeted. There is a higher chance of intersectionality involving these groups, thereby increasing the physical, social, psychological, political, and economic consequences of being marginalized, including death. Marginalization can never be considered a "lifestyle choice."

As already noted, the category of youth covers a distinctive age range from 10 to 18 years, although one can lengthen or shorten this time period. There will be instances in this book when material addressing a different age range will be covered because of the particular relevancy of the scholarship and findings to the central thrust of this book.

Tienda and Wilson (2002, p. 11) emphasized the importance of youth being welcomed and made to feel as if they belong and are openly affirmed by society: "As young people grow up, their integration into society is a prerequisite for their normative development and well-being. Integrating a sense of acceptance and belonging is crucial to accomplish integration." The social exclusion that youth experience profoundly shapes their feelings of worth, undermining their identity and social agency and their eventual success as they enter adulthood.

Brief Portrait

This section touches upon demographics and provides a narrative about what these numbers mean for youth practice. The introduction of the topic of demographics very often creates uneasiness and probably for good reasons. Numbers are followed by more numbers and then supplemented by graphs of various kinds. Numbers are sterile: they do not have faces or stories to tell. But there is power in numbers, because they provide a different story, one that facilitates interpretation.

This section limits itself to several demographic statistics in the hopes of establishing a foundation for why urban youth of color are worthy of specific attention. It is necessary to point out that relying on demographics to paint a portrait of youth is unidimensional and provides an incomplete picture, yet it is a dimension that must be a part of any conversation on youth.

According to the Pew Hispanic Center, based on 2012 statistics from the US Census Bureau, there were 17 states where Latino children constituted at least 20% (or 1 out of every 5) of the kindergarten population. This is more than double the number of states (8) listed in 2000 (Krogstad, 2014). It does not take a demographer to understand the meaning of this statistic as we trace this cohort over the next 15 years until they enter the post high school period, with each developmental stage bringing its own demands and challenges.

The increasing numbers of multi- or bi-racial youth means that all the key concepts integral to social justice community practice must take their presence into account, and this will bring challenges in applying concepts that historically have focused on single ethnic and racial groups, such as ethnic identity (Fisher, Reynolds, Hsu, Barnes, & Tyler, 2014). And this in turn will have implications for positive youth development (PYD) and other forms of youth community practice, such as the performing arts. Tapping into cultural strengths necessitates new paradigms that are multiracial, such as Afro-Mexican culture and dance, and has implications for programming and the development of youth social agency (González, 2004; Vaughn, 2005; Vinson, 2005).

Exercising agency is very popular, and it has found a receptive home in youth practice with a social justice focus (Delgado, 2016*a*). Kirshner (2015, p. 6) points out powerful inherent contradictions in this society and how they effectively and systematically hamper youth of color from succeeding and exercising agency both currently and as they age into adults:

> Youth activism is fueled by a series of contradictions that implicate American society as a whole. The first is a structural contradiction: low-income youth of color are exhorted to work hard and fulfill their responsibilities to go to college, but for many this is a remote possibility . . .. This structural contradiction is accompanied by a developmental contradiction: most youth are developmentally ready to participate under conditions of support, but lack opportunities to do so. Think of this as a lack of fit between paternalistic societal institutions and young people's rapidly growing cognitive capacities and desire for personal agency. Both structural and developmental contradictions are shaped and twisted by the persistence of racial caste in an allegedly color-blind world.

The personal agency of low-income youth of color is at best a mirage when these structural contradictions are overlooked or ignored. Social justice youth community practice can increase agency by providing the space for praxis.

It is appropriate to end this section with a striking message by Cote and Allahar (2006, p. 137) about the challenges adults must successfully surmount if future generations are to be effectively positioned to exert a positive influence on their communities and the nation:

> It may be trite to say that the best hope for the future lies with new generations, but unless the liabilities plaguing the current generation of young people are rectified, that hope is not accompanied by moral and political will. What is called for is renewed energy and vision among adults, for it will take energy and vision to turn the tide against the forces oppressing young people, and by implication oppressing future humans as they come of age.

A belief in a better future is essential for all human beings. If we are to argue that there is one group where this belief or dream is essential, it would be among a nation's youth (Howard et al., 2011; Kabir & Rickards, 2006).

Undocumented and Newcomer Youth

Immigrant and refugee youth face many of the same challenges that native youth of color face but with additional challenges due to their citizenship status and the current political climate in this country. Their status within the urban communities they finally settle in is socially compromised, making adjusting to their new home and developing social relationships—which is difficult to begin with—even more arduous (Fine & Jaffe-Walter, 2007). Out-of-school participation by Latino newcomer youth is low when compared to those who are native-born, and a potential valuable resource goes under-used by them (Yu, Newport-Berra & Liu, 2015).

Newcomer youth, particularly the undocumented, cannot be separated out from the environment they live in, and cities are a significant factor here (Boyes-Watson, 2008). Glick, Schiller, and Schmidt (2016) challenge current urban narratives and call for a counter-narrative to prevalent dominant epistemological frameworks on the "sociability' " of residents who are often referred to as "different" or "foreign," with detrimental impact on them. They propose four interrelated parameters that shift the thinking and the conversation:

1. A view of urban space from differential and multiscalar power trajectories
2. An analysis of narratives and silences concerning the subjects of diversity and cultural differences to take into account different positions and the exercise of power
3. An understanding that different "temporalities make visible or invisible the presence, agency, and interconnection of various actors engaged in 'city-making' "
4. An embrace of the importance of "the social" to help ensure that concepts of diversity, variation, mobility, and conflict are understood as part of urban life and not considered exclusively an attribute of "the other."

Newcomers can become an integral part of the social fabric of urban centers, and the more accepted they perceive themselves to be, the faster this process unfolds, thus opening up opportunities for them to make important contributions. This can be facilitated when schools are willing to openly address transnational experiences (Sánchez, 2007). Newcomers' experiences can be both exclusionary and inclusionary in their new land, and the arts can provide a medium through which to find creative expressions of their hopes and challenges (Davis, Yuval-Davis, Kaptani, & Kaptani, n.d.).

The concept of "heritage language" is increasingly appearing in the literature to capture the importance of language in the lives of newcomer youth and its role in shaping and strengthening cultural identity as a buffer against the negative stereotypes that these youth will encounter as they transition to their new country and home (Chappell & Cahnmann-Taylor, 2013). Language does not just communicate; it can also be symbolic, capturing sentiments by using words or terms that simply cannot be translated into another tongue and still keep the original meaning and emotional sentiments.

Storytelling and the arts represent an attractive mechanism for integrating heritage language and the symbols associated with it as part of a personal narrative that can be shared with peers and an audience of non-peers in performances (Chappell & Faltis, 2013). Kirova and Emme (2008) provide a culture-specific example in the use of *fotonovela* (a novel using photographs and brief narratives) with immigrant children, describing it as a method that can enhance multigenerational relationships.

Conclusion

An appreciation of youth dreams and nightmares requires a multifaceted and socioculturally nuanced understanding of their situations as well their communities. Understanding their dreams necessitates understanding their nightmares, too. This chapter provided insights into a group that defies simplification and enumeration, but there is general acknowledgment that their state of being is severely compromised. The forces shaping youth marginalization can also set the stage for their salvation when the conditions are established that allow youth to appreciate their strengths and potential for achieving social change. They have a vital interest in the outcome. Planning *with* rather than planning *for* has consequences, and the next chapter introduces social justice youth community practice values and ethical conflicts and their influence on the use of the performing arts.

4

Key Values, Ethical Challenges, and Social Justice Youth Community Practice

Introduction

Social interventions are vehicles that bring values to life. A discussion about values and corresponding ethical dilemmas and conflicts is never done without serious deliberation, and this should not be limited to academics either. All parties must engage in deliberative discourse, and, in the case of youth practice, youth take center stage in this dialogue, which is a rare experience for them. Reflection and deliberation serve youth well as they age into adulthood.

A post-performance dialogue phase is rare in conventional performing arts but critical in bringing audiences and performers together to engage in discourse (Capila & Bhalla, 2010). Adding a collective dimension brings added significance for youth who have limited options for engaging in dialogue with adults in a safe environment.

Youth practice is highly contextualized and predicated on explicit or implicit values guiding all dimensions from conceptualization to evaluation. How these values are debated and operationalized generates ethical tensions and conflicts; it is impossible to discuss one without discussing the other and bound to elicit a range of emotions.

Values and concepts/constructs take on a life of their own and can evolve in varied ways from their original meanings. This can be an oversimplification, but it is important to understand how values get shaped by the environment and the times we live in. Epstein (2013, p.72) argues that empowerment as a value and form of practice was not originally intended to increase abilities in daily life, but rather to meet the more ambitious goals of targeting oppression and collective mobilization:

> The concept of empowerment has been vulgarized, coming to refer to usual improvements in individual functioning, thus encouraging social work as well as nursing, rehabilitation medicine, and many other fields to claim that

they pursue political and social change by simply going about their daily chores without actually measuring empowerment outcomes. Improvements in the activities of daily living, socialization, psychological coping, and physical rehabilitation are not what Freire, Fanon, King, Friedan, and their contemporaries had in mind when they pressed for the empowerment of people.

This is not to say that empowerment cannot manifest itself in self-efficacy. The concept was developed to address significant social change and, more specifically, as part of a group coming together in pursuit of a common goal. The introduction of the collective adds an important dimension.

Empowerment is integral to virtually all forms of youth practice, including the performing arts, and this stance often goes unchallenged by practitioners and academics. Empowering youth to have greater decision-making power increases the likelihood that this will result in ethical challenges when discussing newcomer youth from cultures that place a high priority on parents wielding decision-making influence (Delgado, Jones, & Rohani, 2005). Empowering youth without simultaneously threatening parents or legal guardians is an ethical balancing act with a value that enjoys almost universal acceptance but in reality must be modified to take into account cultural backgrounds and levels of acculturation.

Common values are subject to debate concerning composition, degree of power, prioritization, and even existence and level of commonality. Engaging in this debate is time and effort well invested; when clarity is achieved on the "essential" or "core" values, an important aspect of youth practice and the performing arts is established and a foundation is laid for examining and debating other factors, such as activities emanating from the agreed upon values.

Quality youth programs do not just happen, and no day goes by when staff do not encounter difficult value challenges that, when handled successfully, add quality to the programming and positively shape outcomes (Edwards, 2014). Leadership is essential in these circumstances. Larson and Walker (2010) address how leaders in effective youth programs address challenges (racial, ethical, and other types) in creating high-quality programs.

Role and Purpose of Values

Values are generally relegated to a conversation often undertaken by adults about what youth consider to be important in their lives. This looks very good in grant applications because it signifies clarity about the basic premises that a program is based upon. Conventional views cast youth into learner and/or audience groupings and not into teacher or performer roles. Include them as artists, citizens, and assets represents a radical expansion of roles based on an embrace of values (Woodson, 2015).

Values are critical to all aspects of life and social interventions, and youth practice is no exception. Values are not restricted to interventions focused on the performing arts either. How values are operationalized differs according to local circumstances, settings, and activities, which makes identifying them challenging and navigating conflicting values difficult. Organizational culture is greatly influenced by the values of those in leadership (Chen, Lune, & Queen, 2013).

Larson and Walker (2010, p. 347), based on research on challenges faced by youth program staff, note that possessing an ability to "balance—to weigh and address diverse considerations while keeping youth at the center—are vital practitioner skills for creating and sustaining program quality in the ongoing life of a program." This balance is not easy and can be facilitated when staff embrace an explicit value stance that can be easily articulated and acted upon.

An explicit understanding of the values guiding social interventions, including having them prominently displayed and being prepared to discuss or even debate them, helps practitioners in the decision-making process and in navigating the turbulent waters associated with community interventions. Youth values, too, must be made explicit and incorporated into the program.

Values do not exist in a vacuum; they play a significant role in shaping a social intervention from its conception to its implementation and eventual evaluation. This is the case in discussions of social justice or critical youth practice and the performing arts, and even more so when we introduce intersectionality and social justice into program activities. Bazo (2010) provides an excellent case example of intersectionality in describing how Boston's True Colors: Out Youth Theater at the Theater Offensive used theatre to engage youth who are gay, lesbian, bisexual, and transgendered (GLBT). This model integrates goals related to personal, social, and artistic expression; empowerment; and social activism.

The youth practice field has developed an extensive following and a consensus "that joint work, common values, shared power, and a focus on collective issues contribute significantly to positive outcomes" (Zeldin, Christens, & Powers, 2013, p. 385). From an international viewpoint, Daniel et al.'s (Daniel, Dys, Buchmann, & Malti, 2016) study of Swiss adolescents and social justice values identified the significance of sympathy and friendship quality in shaping how these values are perceived and acted upon in programming.

A collectivistic value can be incorporated into positive youth development (PYD) video games when these games emphasize cooperative competition and teamwork to make them attractive to youth from collectivist cultural backgrounds (Adachi & Willoughby, 2013). Teams engaged in video competitions introduce communication and cooperation elements while stressing competition in the process. The participation of youth of color in extracurricular activities, as in the case of low-income Mexican youth, is influenced by cultural values that must be taken into account in programming (Dawes, Modecki, Gonzales, Dumka, & Millsap, 2015).

A discussion of youth programs must also address how values permeate all aspects of program activities, including sports, which we often narrowly think of as simply physical exercise and competition (Whitehead, Telfer, & Lambert, 2013). Values cannot exist without ethical dilemmas and corresponding conflicts; this chapter sets a context for social justice youth practice and the performing arts. Although values, ethical dilemmas, and conflicts will be treated separately, in reality they are highly integrated, making addressing them that much more difficult for the field.

Making the implicit explicit increases the likelihood that youth are not undermined and further marginalized in the process of being engaged. This process may appear simplistic, but in reality it is quite arduous and unsettling for both adult staff and youth. Implicit values may be buried deep in our unconscious; because of this, we respond automatically, without having a clear understanding of why we do what we do. Making implicit values explicit is difficult enough for one individual to undertake; it becomes extremely complicated when done collectively because this is a subject that is rarely discussed in an open and participatory manner.

This group process helps participants understand various ways of thinking about values without engendering feelings of being right or wrong. Discussions will carry over into other spheres, and this is positive for all participants and staff, serving as an indicator of a program that is dynamic and searching for the best approach to social justice.

Key Values

Efforts to distill key practice values to a select few are bound to prove troubling and controversial, and rightly so, because of the instrumental role that values play in shaping all aspects of a social intervention. The process of distilling them to a select group ("highly desirable") is a worthy exercise requiring serious thinking, research, and debate, and what social intervention cannot benefit from such scrutiny?

Arriving at these cores values is a journey worth undertaking, but it will also bring forth ethical dilemmas and challenges because choices must be made on how to conceptualize a social intervention. Social justice youth performing arts benefit from closer scrutiny and debate, including what constitutes evidence of success—an increasingly important factor in securing of external funds. For this book, six values were selected (see Figure 4.1), although there is no consensus in the youth practice field on the composition of this list. These values were selected based on my experiences in practice and the academy, a review of the literature, and discussions with youth and colleagues in this field.

CULTURAL COMPETENCE AND HUMILITY

The performing arts embrace culture as the foundation upon which to undertake a performance. It can be argued that cultural competence/humility is so important

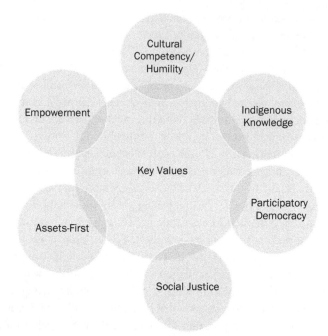

FIGURE 4.1 Key values

that it should permeate all values. In the case of this book, it is of sufficient importance to permeate all the values that social interventions are based on while also
holding a prominent position itself. It is an appropriate starting point for this difficult and most likely contentious discussion on values. No social intervention is
value-free, and this must be acknowledged.

The concept of cultural competence/humility has universal qualities, and few
in the social sciences and helping professions are unfamiliar with its various definitions and why it is so important. The goal of cultural competence/humility is
not disputed since social interventions must not make youth feel bad about their
identity.

Whether we can ever really achieve cultural competence is debated, and this
accounts for the emergence of cultural humility as a preferred concept in many
circles (Chavez, 2014; Gallardo, 2014; Isaacson, 2014). In striving for cultural competence, the journey is embraced and celebrated, but the ultimate destination will
always be out of reach. Culture is dynamic (with no consensus on its constitution)
and evolves to take into account social circumstances, and this is exciting and
daunting.

Youth are immersed in various forms of culture, including ethnic and racial,
which is the most common ways we think of culture. And youth have their own
culture as well because of their age and shared experiences, a culture that brings
with it language, symbols, clothing styles, and choice of music and dance, and this,

too, evolves and changes. Geographical settings, such as cities, also shape culture. Culture is dynamic and changes according to social circumstances. Viewing cultural competency/humility in youth practice requires a broader understanding of its significance and how it shapes youth performing arts.

Culture plays a prominent role in the performing arts, although it may not be open to scrutiny. The earlier discussion on Eurocentrism in Chapter 1 highlights how a European stance shapes what is considered worthy of admiration and duplication, and we can add social-economic class to this implicit bias. The explicit introduction of cultural values in social justice youth practice and the performing arts provides "material" for shaping how a performance's central message resonates with youth and the audiences they wish to attract and inform.

SOCIAL JUSTICE

Although social justice was addressed in Chapter 2 and will be addressed throughout this book, here we discuss it with a specific focus on the performing arts. One of the central arguments in this book is that social justice can and must be a critical element in any form of performing art focused on youth at the margins of society. This stance is not unique to any form of art. Social justice must also be a part of youth-focused service-learning and civic engagement, as well as other practice foci (Delgado, 2016*a*).

The aspirational ideas embedded in social justice goals can be powerful motivators that serve as the basis for youth performing arts and other activities seeking social change (Hytten & Bettez, 2011; Staples, 2012). Bell and Desai (2014) put forth a persuasive argument that the arts, in all of their manifestations, must be a critical element in social justice practice, providing a highly engaging mechanism for giving voice and direction to social justice messages.

Elam (2001, p. 1) succinctly lays out the potential relationship between social justice and theatre: "Repeatedly, in the modern and postmodern United States, oppressed people and new political movements have turned to the theater as a means to articulate social causes, to galvanize support, and to direct sympathizers toward campaigns of political resistance." Academics and practitioners need not go to great lengths to substantiate introducing social justice values into theatre or any other performing art.

Shepard (2012, p. 263), in discussing play, creativity, and social justice, listed the influential interplay of factors that highlight that social change can be applied to the performing arts, social justice, and other forms of youth practice:

- It helps activism feel invigorating
- It animates culture
- It helps keep things light—even dark times
- It fosters creativity, which can help achieve movement aims
- It recognizes pleasure

- It creates and supports stories
- It expands the public commons and makes democracy more colorful
- It helps garner media attention to new narratives of action, helping actors propel their culture tales into the larger public discourse
- It reduces alienation
- It cultivates humor
- It creates hope
- It gets people to think
- It supports individual and community strengths
- It fosters nonhierarchical leadership networks
- As a low-threshold activity, it brings people into organizing
- It helps combat mechanisms that control the body and inhibit political activity
- It makes social change work feel compelling and inviting.

Shepard's list can be applied to any performing art that has a social justice purpose. Butler (2014) provides an excellent example of how youth art-as-activism is able to integrate social justice issues into an artist residency program.

There are various ways of thinking about social justice. Thinking of social justice as a journey rather than as a goal or destination works best for me, and I have found it works well when discussing this value with youth who, if they are lucky enough to reach old age, have a long period ahead of them to see its potential manifestation. Breaking down social justice goals into smaller goals, as in any social change effort, makes it easier for youth to see how they will get to an end destination.

Having social justice goals be "immediate," "specific," and "winnable" can offer other life lessons regarding social change and youth-led activism (Ho, Clarke, & Dougherty, 2015). Valuing social justice necessitates that youth development skill sets or competencies break down social change strategies rather than focusing on developing enthusiasm and indignation as a rallying cry for engagement (Eliasoph, 2014). The lessons learned, including the framework guiding the action, have applicability for other facets of their lives and show what "good" youth community practice programs can accomplish.

ASSETS-FIRST

An embrace of an assets-first value introduces a significant shift in the paradigm concerning youth and their communities from a commonly accepted deficit or charity ("at-risk") perspective to one that emphasizes capabilities and indigenous resources (Delgado & Humm-Delgado, 2013; Green & Haines, 2015; Mohammadzadeh, 2015). This shift brings new ways of looking at conditions and behaviors, corresponding excitement, and a new vocabulary that helps capture an affirmative form of thinking.

Applying an assets-first approach to performing arts introduces language and concepts that identify the knowledge and skill sets (tools) that youth bring and wish to enhance through participating in and staging a performance (Wrentschur & Moser, 2014). The performing arts can accommodate youth with varying abilities and interests when programs place a high value on being inclusive.

No community, regardless of how stressed, underresourced, or challenged, is absent of assets. This value is at the core of an assets-first social intervention and challenges conventional wisdom that these communities can be mobilized to help themselves only with external support. This stance takes on greater significance when the intervention is focused on youth who are often thought of as second-class citizens with all of the negative attributes associated with being second in a society that values winning and being first. Furthermore, this stance translates into youth not having assets they can draw upon. It is no wonder that a "rescue" stance can permeate a program's philosophy and actions.

All forms of capital can be enhanced when this value is used and there is a willingness to use innovative methods to maximize capital. Acknowledgment of cultural assets helps shape the central themes that a performance wishes to highlight. It can promote—if performers obtain a stipend—economic capital, and human capital is enhanced in the case of talented youth and the desire to enhance it or even possibly seek a career in the performing arts. Social capital, which is critical in important relationships, expands peer networks across new groups and strengthens cultural capital (Dixon-Román, 2013; Kapucu, 2011).

INDIGENOUS KNOWLEDGE

Knowledge greatly depends on how it is defined, collected, and disseminated (Vadeboncoeur, 2006). A profound insight into a particular phenomenon is only as significant as the number individuals who know about it and can translate this knowledge into action. In a society that values formal educational credentials (educational expertise legitimacy), this effectively translates into a valuing of formal educational courses (degrees), formal research, and publication in highly respected journals with high impact scores. Knowledge formation is in the hands of an elite group who have many initials after their surnames.

A revolutionary call has been heard to broaden (democratize) the production of knowledge beyond the academy. Democratization of knowledge production has consequences for all groups, but youth stand to gain the most as an age group (Baker, 2016; Mitchell, 2009). Indigenous knowledge goes by different names, but the basic premise remain the same. Informal learning and knowledge is one example (Monchalin et al., 2016; Thompson, 2012).

A view of youth as knowledge producers is facilitated when they can engage in critical thinking (Erstad & Sefton-Green, 2013; Stuart, 2010). Increased interest in the "knowledge economy" has fostered searches for new sources of knowledge, and, in the process, rediscovered informal knowledge and out-of-school settings as knowledge sources (Sefton-Green, 2006).

Indigenous knowledge can be defined as the life experiences, insights, and wisdom that community residents possess and that were obtained through lived experiences rather than through conventional educational sources. Indigenous knowledge does not have any age or abilities restrictions. This knowledge often goes unrecognized and invalidated in a world that is increasingly reliant on formal educational credentials to validate the acquisition of knowledge and competencies.

This position effectively distances those who are marginalized through low formal education levels from having their experiences validated. When examined from a youth perspective, it translates into adults being experts of youth. I admit that I am not an expert on youth of any kind. The more I learn about youth, the greater my realization of how little I really know and how ludicrous it would be to call myself an expert!

The fundamental question of deciding what knowledge is considered important enough to warrant attention and resources also must be considered, with the answer depending on where the individual answering it stands within society. Knowledge of what youth think is important is greatly shaped by their surrounding socio-economic circumstances. When place-based performance is founded on an attempt at eliciting narratives (local knowledge), it creates a dynamic relationship among performers, performance, and audience (Jones, Hall, Thomson, Barrett, & Hanby, 2013).

If you are of color, have low income/low wealth, and are young, the subjects you consider important enough to learn more about will differ from those of adults of middle or high income and wealth. Knowledge must first serve to help youth socially navigate their lived world (Dill & Ozer, 2016; Ungar, 2014). If their world is unpredictable, hostile, and focused on survival, interest in topics that have particular relevance for some future period will not resonate (Brown, 2016).

Co-production of knowledge can have numerous manifestations and benefits for youth (Baker, 2016). Pente et al. (Pente, Ward, Brown, & Sahota, 2015, p. 33) tie co-production of knowledge to self-identity and describe the potential mutual benefits of universities entering into partnerships with communities:

[C]o-production of historical knowledge' provides an approach or methodology that allows for a deeper comprehension of people's self-identities by encouraging a diverse range of people to participate in the research process. We argue that many academic historians have maintained an intellectual detachment between university history and public and community history, to the detriment of furthering historical knowledge. We argue for a blurring of the boundaries between university and communities in exploring modern British history, and especially the history of national identities. It includes extracts of writing from community partners and a brief photographic essay of projects related to exploring identities.

Indigenous knowledge, when combined with outsiders and their knowledge, results in co-produced knowledge, which expands the potential reach of these new insights beyond the immediate community to a broader and more global audience (Baker, 2016).

Knowledge related to survival, such as creative thinking, making quick decisions, social navigational skills, self-assessment, and confidence, must support competencies that facilitate that survival. This statement may seem harsh but it does capture the saliency of knowledge being relevant to current circumstances and based on operative realities. Homeless LGTBQ youth face a daily struggle for survival, and this reality will dictate the type of knowledge that they value and that aids them in navigating daily challenges and even life-and-death situations (Keuroghlian, Shtasel, & Bassuk, 2014).

Youth are best positioned to assess their own lives and needs, and we as adults can facilitate this knowledge acquisition and skill development. Youth are the best experts of their lives (Berihun et al., 2015). This may seem trite or provocative, but adults often lose sight of this point. Library-based research skills can be enhanced if the information that youth are seeking has immediate relevance in their lives (Hamada & Stavridi, 2014). The skills acquired in this arena can be transferred to other arenas and address other issues.

Libraries can also be considered physical, social, and psychological sanctuaries within their communities and can afford a place that can physically protect individuals from harm (McLaughlin, Irby, & Langman, 1994). For this to occur, these institutions must embrace social justice to ensure that all youth are welcomed. Kumasi (2012) draws on Critical Race Theory to examine how school librarians can create programs that are supportive and affirming of urban youth of color by stressing four perspectives that have high applicability for youth programs: (1) challenging cultural deficit views, (2) actively seeking to listen to student voices and life experiences, (3) recognizing structural inequalities, and (4) understanding the meaning and privileges associated with whiteness. Libraries are a community asset with the potential for engaging in collaboration projects with a social mission (Moxley & Abbas, 2016).

If ethnic/racial identity fulfills a protective role among urban youth, as in the case of males, then efforts at reaching these youth through youth practice must enhance their knowledge about their ethnic/cultural backgrounds and provide skill sets that aid them in confronting oppressive forces that undervalue them (Williams, Aiyer, Durkee, & Tolan, 2014). Tello et al. (Tello, Cervantes, Cordova, & Santos, 2010) report on the success of a culturally focused Latino youth development program that helped youth learn about their culture and have it shape positive behaviors, such as reducing the chances of engaging in risky sexual behaviors.

PARTICIPATORY DEMOCRACY

It can be argued that meaningful (co-intentional) opportunities for youth to engage in out-of-school activities permeate all of the values addressed in this section (Gal

& Duramy, 2015; Read, Fitton, & Hortton, 2014). Their integration into the social fabric of their communities and institutions bodes well for future participation because it serves as a countermeasure to hegemony. Terms such as "about," "by," or "with" stand out in separating standard participatory and social justice–focused performing arts from conventional approaches (Preston, 2009a).

Ergler and Wood (2014) call for a reconceptualization of participation through an emphasis on place-based identity development and practice as a means of encouraging meaningful versus token engagement. Wembe (2013) provides an example of theater participation (popular, dialogical, extrinsic, peripheral, and integral) in New Zealand's interactive Themba Theatre (ITT) Company and conceptualizes participation broadly and inclusively.

The question of why a participatory value should be embraced strikes at the heart of a well-functioning democratic society and raises critical elements for analysis when it is restricted to select groups. Beck and Purcell (2010, p. 76) provide a succinct answer that stresses the importance of local knowledge and priorities shaping conceptualization:

> The main rationale for participative methods is based on the belief that people themselves are best placed to know what their problems are and, with the right support, can develop the most appropriate solutions to those problems. It is therefore incumbent on workers to develop approaches which tap into the local knowledge and capacity for change. To do anything else is to impose external culture and values and, even for the best of reasons, further disempower the communities we work with.

Valuing participation connects well with other values. Participation does not have to be problem-focused and can be in response to a desire to enhance community assets, with theater being successfully tapped in policy-making (Guhrs, Rihoy, & Guhrs, 2006).

Gallagher (2014) poses the provocative question of when youth disengagement can be an act of resistance as well as a strategic decision for self-protection that cannot be ignored. Not joining because of a perception of an unhealthy situation may be a wise decision on the part of youth. This question can be answered when youth views are solicited and acted upon by adults (Smyth, Down, & McInerney, 2014; Westheimer & Kahne, 2000).

Ife (2004, p. 4) ties human rights and community development together, and this concept can also be applied to youth practice, bringing a new dimension to discussions on participatory democracy and youth programs:

> A society that respects and values human rights is one where people are encouraged to exercise their rights, and accept a responsibility to do so where they can. This is an active participatory society, that requires citizens to be active contributors rather than passive consumers; and the promotion

of such a participatory society has long been the agenda of community development.

A human rights stance permeates all values either explicitly or implicitly and resonates across all age groups; youth understand that they do not share the same rights as their adult counterparts.

Beck and Purcell (2010, p. 93), in discussing Foucault's views on the role and influence of discourse on power, highlight how a dialogue focused on participation can become the norm rather than the exception and, in the case of youth, an essential process to achieve agency:

> Michel Foucault said that power comes from discourse. By this he means that, if all we talk about is participation and partnerships, they then become the new orthodoxy, and alternative ways of working begin to be seen as strange, out of date, unfashionable, or unacceptable, in effect the world changes because the way we talk about it changes.

Youth participation is at the root of significant changes in attitudes and behaviors concerning programming (Hart, 2009). Social justice programming is not possible without active participation and engagement in partnerships. Civic engagement is closely related to democracy; it is part of the "great American experiment" (Braun & Williams, 2002), and is never meant to exclude individuals who share similar demographic profiles—and that goes for youth, too.

Participatory democracy is associated with formal engagement in a nation's civic processes associated with elections and voting (Allen, 2012). Although this is an important perspective, it is too narrow a view because youth participation can occur in a variety of settings, including out-of-school organizations and social actions that emerge without institutional affiliation sponsorship (Bermudez, 2012; Mitra, Serriere, & Kirshner, 2014). Participatory principles can be taught and find expression through theater performance and, we can argue, other performing arts as youth deliberate and make decisions about how performances should unfold (Neelands, 2009).

Youth community-based organizations represent ideal settings to engage in civic engagement or participatory democracy because of their centrality within the confines of where youth live (Shiller, 2013). These settings are geographically located within the neighborhoods where youth live and are likely to hire staff representing the backgrounds that youth come from, thus minimizing a lacunae in communication and relationships and enhancing program outcomes. These organization are positioned to identify the barriers youth face in civically participating in their community (Balsano, 2005).

Youth's sense of community and willingness to assume a civic position are closely tied, but they must be heard by adults for them to actively engage (Evans, 2007, p. 700): "For young people to fully experience voice, it requires resonance—some signal that their contributions are being heard and actively considered." This "resonance" can go by many different terms.

Evans (2007, p. 705) summarizes the situation of marginalized youth within their community and a fundamental decision adult residents must make concerning them:

> Unfortunately, the influence that young people feel in community contexts, and families, is seldom reciprocal. They are the recipients or objects of the influence and power of adults, but the opportunity to return the influence is too often nonexistent. Described more dramatically, young people experience oppression in community settings and this is especially true for disadvantaged youth. They are often silent and invisible unless they are perceived to be causing trouble. They are excluded from many of the decision making processes that affect their lives. As they are developing the capacity and the need to contribute in the world, the opportunities to develop skills and play meaningful roles are less than plentiful. The reality is, there is always going to be a limit on how connected to these contexts teenagers feel as long as their voice, influence, and support is limited.

Connecting marginalized youth is a goal of youth practice regardless of geographical settings. To accomplish this goal requires active soul searching on whether adults wish to have these youth be a significant part of their surroundings.

Participatory avenues provide youth with an opportunity to engage in activities that best meet their immediate and long-term needs, as determined by the participants themselves (Checkoway & Aldana, 2013; Checkoway & Richards-Schuster, 2006; Fine & Torre, 2004; Torre & Fine, 2006). Meaningful participation and empowerment go together hand in glove (Jupp, 2007). Increased youth participatory democracy cannot be realized without addressing the barriers that must be overcome to achieve this goal from both institutional and community-level standpoints (Bessant, 2004; Childers, 2012; Lansprey & Hughes, 2015).

Formal education plays an influential role in shaping and maintaining democracies when engaging in critical thinking is encouraged as part of the pedagogy. Hytten (2006, p. 22) describes the central purpose of education in a democratic society, as in the United States, and the role and importance of participation:

> Arguably one of the central purposes, if not the central purpose, of education in the United States is to help students develop the knowledge, habits, skills, and dispositions necessary for democratic citizenship. These include learning to think critically, to participate in public dialogue, to consider the rights and needs of others, to live in harmony with diverse groups of people, to act on important social issues, to be accountable for one's choices and decisions, and to work to bring about the conditions in which all individuals can develop to their fullest capacities and potential.

Democracy, to be successful in achieving its lofty goals, requires its principles being supported throughout all segments and age groups, with educational institutions fulfilling this role but not exclusively so. Democracy, after all, encompasses all groups regardless of their demographic composition.

Enhancement and validation of this value must not be left to chance in social justice youth practice involving the performing arts. The introduction of "meaningful" as a prefix to participatory democracy brings an added dimension of "tokenism," which is counter to the purpose of enhancing participation, as in the case of advisory committees that only give the illusion of "meaningful" decision-making (Taft & Gordon, 2013).

EMPOWERMENT

The identification of empowerment is a critical value in social justice youth practice. Empowerment is a construct that has been around since the early 1970s, and it has evolved during this time period to take into account various disempowered groups. It is also a construct that can be found in virtually all forms of youth practice and is an essential or core element in social justice–focused youth practice because of its power for transformation. Empowerment must be addressed in the performing arts (Wijnendaele, 2014).

Empowerment has achieved a central place in youth practice, including the performing arts (Morrel-Samuels, Hutchison, Perkinson, Bostic, & Zimmerman, 2015; Wernick, Kulick, & Woodford, 2014). Levy (2011) describes using eco-drama as a means of empowering youth in a participatory process. Youth practice without corresponding reflection on values will be counterproductive to the central goals of this practice (Beck & Purcell, 2010, p. 29): "Education, whether formal, informal or community-based is a potentially dangerous process. As youth and community workers, we bring our cultural values into the communities we work with; this is inevitable. The danger is, if we do without reflection or criticism we will unwittingly impose our culture, thereby disempowering the very people we want to empower."

French's (2015) literature review of youth empowerment theories and models identified five critical themes in creating a comprehensive understanding of youth empowerment programs: (1) a youth–adult sharing of power, (2) an individual and community-focused orientation, (3) a safe and supportive/affirming environment, (4) a valuing of peer collaboration, and (5) an opportunity to engage in reflection. Morton and Montgomery (2013) also reviewed the literature to assess the state of evidence of youth empowerment programs (YEPs) on adolescents' (aged 10–19) self-efficacy, self-esteem, and other social, emotional, and behavioral outcomes and found insufficient evidence to support YEP impact. Values shaped how these themes were operationalized and researched with social change outcomes (Harvey, Roberts, & Dillabough, 2016).

Participatory theater is a powerful mechanism for empowering oppressed groups (Singhal, 2004). Melbourne, Australia, hosts an example (Western Edge Youth Arts) of how participatory theater provided youth with the space and place to share their stories and reflect on their lived experiences, as well as allowing them re-present themselves and gain skills to respond to racialized situations (Sonn, Quayle, Belanji, & Baker, 2015).

Pearrow (2008) identified six critical elements to urban-based youth empowerment that mirror those raised by French (2015), and these elements must be integral to any social justice youth practice using the performing arts: (1) having an environment that is perceived as welcoming and safe, (2) engagement in meaningful activities, (3) power-sharing between youth and significant adults, (4) an opportunity to engage in critical reflection (praxis), (5) engagement in sociopolitically motivated social change, and (6) the integration of individual with community-level empowerment. One can discern how and why these elements are essential for helping youth performing arts embrace the other values addressed in this section, making them more relevant in youth lives and communities.

Key Ethical Challenges

All micro- and macro-focused social interventions bring inherent ethical tensions and potential conflicts, and this is endemic to this type of work. Interventions that address power imbalances and strive for significant social change bring additional challenges not found in social interventions that do not seek to upset the status quo (Beck & Purcell, 2010).

Larson and Walker (2010, p. 339) argue the importance of understanding challenges in youth programming: "Examination of the dilemmas of practice provides a window for understanding the challenges to achieving program quality in the daily life of programs. By analyzing the types of problems, situations, and dilemmas that practitioners encounter, we can better understand how to create and sustain quality." Understanding these challenges is an essential step in solving them.

Addressing ethics and youth performing arts is further complicated because social justice youth community practice is an ever-expanding field. Kelman and Warwick (1978), almost 40 years ago, addressed ethics and social interventions, and their approach lends itself well to youth performing arts practice. They identified four ethical realms: (1) the ends achieved by an intervention (so what), (2) an understanding of who is to benefit (who), (3) how these changes are to be accomplished (means), and (4) accounting of the intended and unintended consequences (actual outcomes). Each realm manifests itself at various intervention stages and in subtle and nonsubtle ways.

Ethics is interwoven into all aspects of social interventions and take on even greater importance in social justice youth practice. Discussions of ethical dilemmas are many and thorny, representing significant challenges for practitioners and academics, and embedded in potentially all social interactions (Banks, 2012; Nybell, Shook, & Finn, 2013). This statement is not intended to scare off practitioners, but rather to normalize the subject so that we can successfully minimize the social consequences of these dilemmas. Identifying potential dilemmas increases the chances of success in addressing them in a manner that is affirming, empowering, and syntonic with an explicit value system. Capturing these situations provides insights and lessons that will influence the education and training of youth practitioners in the classroom and the field.

Ethical Dilemmas

Ethics is a topic that is bound to elicit far-ranging debates; it is the nature of the subject matter. Ethical dilemmas are integral to any social practice and more so when that practice is based within communities. It becomes a question of determining how they are expressed and addressed rather than deciding if they exist. Adding a focus on urban marginalized populations raises more potential ethical dilemmas, as in the case of youth performing arts practice.

Although an entire book can be written on this topic, only three ethical dilemmas were selected for discussion here because these rarely receive attention from research on and with youth: (1) challenges of representation, (2) agents of control or liberation, and (3) organizational barriers. These dilemmas touch core issues of social youth community practice. Although these dilemmas are addressed as separate entities, in reality, like values, they overlap, representing the difficulty facing youth practitioners and researchers.

1. The Challenges of Representation. Moletsane et al. (Moletsane, Mitchell, Stuart, Walsh, & Taylor, 2008) raise ethical issues of representation in participatory video that are also applicable to the performing arts. The "legitimacy" of this narrative takes on significance when it seeks to capture a social injustice. Simply accepting responsibility and doing so with the express intent of "least harm" is unacceptable (Moletsane et al., 2008):

> Clearly the ethical issues surrounding "least harm" must also contribute to "most good." For Ethical Review Boards in universities and research units, too often the principle of least harm, we would argue, is not balanced with "most good," and even least harm is defined only in relation to perceived immediate dangers but not in relation, say, to long-term disillusionment.

Destroying dreams is a serious offense, and the use of false narratives makes it that much more unethical. It is a serious ethical issue with long-term implications when those dreams are those of youth. Minimizing or underestimating youth potential is one way of destroying a dream.

2. Agents of Control or Liberation. The increasing concern of adults in authority, as manifested in surveillance and punishment policies, raises the potential of youth practitioners emphasizing control rather than social justice roles (Jeffs & Smith, 2010b). Scrutiny of funding sources and their influence on shaping expectations and behavior takes on greater significance when focusing on youth. It is impossible to discuss ethical dilemmas and challenges by separating out youth performing arts from the organizational settings in which they transpire (Conrad, 2006).

How participatory and empowering can the performing arts be when settings severely restrict the power youth have to shape the performance? Settings can either provide the space for youth to exercise control over the performance or relegate them to secondary status. Sometimes it is easier to take a shortcut and compromise youth positions; this ethical tension requires a daily check-in with youth as part of an ongoing evaluation effort.

Labeling activities with the prefix "social justice" only increases the disservice of an intervention that has no intention of achieving this goal and betrays the trust of youth. This results in a continuation of distrust and makes it difficult for youth to commit to a program that embraces social justice because of a history of betrayal.

3. Organizational Barriers. Ethical challenges associated with competing organizational demands are not unique to youth programs. Organizational barriers are never minimal because of how profoundly they shape culture and operations. Disenfranchised youth, unlike their adult counterparts, cannot vote and therefore do not wield the influence associated with adults, making this challenge particularly significant and not uncommon. Larson and Walker (2010, p. 344) address this among many other challenges:

> Programs for youth are typically embedded within a larger organization, such as a community agency or school, and what happens at the organizational level can influence what happens with the youth. Behind the scenes administrators and staff make decisions, set policies, develop relationships, and attempt to sustain the organization.

How practitioners handle this balancing act has short- and long-term implications. Youth, too, must learn to balance competing personal and employment demands in their lives and to do so in a manner that increases their chances of succeeding.

Sanderson and Richards (2010) found four ethical barriers for after-school activities: (1) concerns about personal safety, (2) lack of transportation, (3) carrying out of family responsibilities (e.g., care for siblings, household chores), and (4) lack of information about available programs. Why should these barriers fall within the ambit of ethical dilemmas? The answer is quite simple: they are basic to organizational culture and fabric, and allowing these barriers to exist is unethical.

Conclusion

Performing arts youth practice cannot be accomplished without encountering a potential minefield of conflicting values and ethical dilemmas, and that is so even when practice unfolds in a youth-focused and respectful manner. There is no such thing as a value-free and ethical conflict-free intervention. Making values explicit and understanding that ethical challenges are part of the journey helps clarify goals and the methods that will help us achieve them.

Values and ethical dilemmas covered in this chapter were addressed briefly due to limited space and not because of their lack of importance. Yet this chapter has hopefully helped create an appreciation of the challenges faced by social justice youth community practice involving the performing arts. The following chapter uplifts the importance of social justice programming and the role that out-of-school settings can play in moving this agenda forward with youth in prominent roles.

5

Social Justice Youth Community Practice and Out-of-School Settings

Introduction

Youth practice is firmly placed within communities and organizations, and when the prefix of social justice is added, it politicizes work with marginalized youth. Out-of-school settings target youth during periods when they can function where they choose and feel safe psychologically and physically. In-school participation is often highly structured and counter to social justice values and personal interests, so the value of out-of-school settings can be considerable among youth facing constant social and physical threats to their well-being (Bean, Whitley, & Gould, 2014; Vandell, Pierce, & Dadisman, 2005).

These settings are attractive because they offer youth a set of activities that have special appeal to them. These settings also provide a climate that is conducive for youth to interact with each other and affirming adults and to explore interests in a manner that is conducive to both having fun and learning. Urban settings wishing to keep youth engaged must understand how they perceive space (Fusco, 2007) and offer the possibility that youth can just "hang out" without engaging in highly organized activities or being under constant surveillance (Giroux, 2015).

Time is a challenging construct, and every generation contends with defining it. Teitle (2012, p. 1) addresses the importance of unstructured time or what is often referred to as "hanging-out" or "free-time" within and outside of youth programs. He raises concerns about how this time has slowly disappeared, even within after-school settings, which are increasingly becoming very structured and not allowing for spontaneity and exploration of interests:

> While many adolescents list unstructured "hangout" spaces as central to their social lives and activities, the availability of such spaces has dramatically declined in the last two decades, and attendance at afterschool programs has increased. Concurrently, these programs have drawn new scrutiny: from researchers eager to show their educational value, and from funders and

policy makers seeking measureable evidence of that value. Even youth centers that were deliberately designed to give young people a space to "hang out" have been forced to reorganize due to the pressure to demonstrate program results.

Understanding how youth perceive and use time is a critical aspect in any effort to research time itself (Wolf, Aber, & Morris, 2015). Time is viewed as a commodity in our society, and everyone has an opinion of its importance. We are urged not to "waste" it because of its preciousness. But time does not have the same meaning across the lifecycle.

The stagnation and even decline in theatre attendance must be viewed against a backdrop of competing mediums for time and attention to understand its place within the arts constellation (Martin, 2006, p. 26):

> While it is important to refuse the notion that people have stopped going to the theatre or that attendance is in decline, surely theatre has always been a minor cultural form compared to radio, cinema, television, or computers, at least in terms of percentage of a given population that it can claim as its actual public at any given moment. Although half the US adult population has seen theatre of some kind in the past year, most will have watched television daily.

The percentage of youth who have attended theatre can be expected to be much lower than their adult counterparts, and theatre has faced stiff competition from other media for attention.

"Hanging-out" is often thought of as a time that increases the chances of youth getting into trouble, rather than as a time to de-stress and sharpen interpersonal skills. This belief is predicated on the importance of providing structure and activities to keep youth busy and control interpersonal relationships. A recasting of this time is necessary because socialization, learning, and reflection can transpire during unstructured time as well as during an "activity" in a world that is increasingly highly structured, and this is even more true for youth who are constantly being monitored and under surveillance.

Youth Participation and Engagement

Tracing a construct's origins is always hard. There is little argument that the United Nation's Convention on the Rights of the Child (1989) played an instrumental role in fostering the concept of engagement. Thomas (2012) reflects on the progress achieved since this convention was adopted by the United Nations and summarizes the rewards, tensions, and challenges in having children/youth exercise greater freedom over how their lives unfold.

The United States is the only nation that has not signed this convention, in contrast to the vast majority of the 196 nations that signed on in the early

1990s. The United States use to have the distinction of being one of two nations not having signed, but Somalia signed the treaty on October 1, 2015 (Corrarino, 2015). Mitra, Serriere, and Kirshner (2014) point out that, in this country, unlike in the United Kingdom and other nations, there are no mandates calling for meaningful participation. There are a paucity of opportunities where youth can engage in democratic participation, particularly without adults controlling this process.

The United Nations Convention on the Rights of the Child Article 12 has played an important role in uplifting and fostering the concept of youth participation, although the political motivation for encouraging participation has drawn its share of critiques (Raby, 2014). The concept of participation or engagement is universal when applied to social interventions regardless of the demographics of the group being discussed. Why has the topic of youth engagement been so popular over the past 20 to 25 years? The answer should not be surprising (Gallagher, 2014, p. 11):

> [E]ngagement has been regarded as a way to explain how low levels of academic achievement, as well as generalized boredom at school and high early-leaving rates, in urban areas. Also, because engagement is presumed to be a dynamic quality, it has been regarded as a field of potential for policy intervention aimed at increasing student success.

Gallagher's assessment, although school focused, is applicable to out-of-school settings as well and emphasizes their importance in filling gaps in the lives of youth who have high probabilities of leaving formal schooling before graduation. Participation in meaningful activities and decision-making translates into self-respect, an essential well-being factor, and enhances other indicators of well-being (Edmonds, 2013; Woodland, 2008).

Weiss, Little, and Bouffard (2005) conceptualize participation as a three-part construct (enrollment, attendance, and engagement), with each element open to further conceptualization and operationalization. Each element brings rewards and challenges as programs specifically attempt to reach marginalized youth. Borden and Serido (2009), too, identified three phases (participation, connection, and expansion) on the journey from engagement in programming.

Meaningful youth engagement discussion must begin with their fundamental decision to engage in participation in an organized activity. Helping professions can play an important role in fostering this mindset (Pritzker & Richards-Schuster, 2016). Engagement begins when youth enter a deliberation process and make a commitment to a program. This commitment represents an important step in their lives and may well represent one of the few, if any, times that they had the power to actually make a commitment on their own. How this commitment is solicited and formalized takes on significance in youth programming that is voluntary and grounded within their familial support and community context (Morrissey & Werner-Wilson, 2005).

A verbal commitment is important, but signing a document (contract) spelling out expectations and desired benefits and outcomes signifies an "official" decision that they have control over. When this contract has been developed by youth or had significant youth input, it takes on added meaning because they have ownership of its contents, including rules, which is highly unusual in adult-led organized activities.

Meaningful engagement can have at least three significant benefits: (1) youth participation is a right that must be protected and fostered if youth are to be treated with respect, (2) efforts to reach and meet the needs of youth are enhanced when their perspective is actively sought and acted upon, and (3) youth derive instrumental and expressive benefits when they participate, and society also benefits from active engagement (Head, 2011).

Youth engagement may entail participation in various circles beyond an immediate familial group and geographically bound neighborhood (Nenga, 2012). This expansion brings youth into a broader social fabric, benefiting society as a whole. Social media broadens this reach beyond narrow place-based boundaries.

Another way of conceptualizing participation is to break this construct down into stages. Thinking of youth performing arts as consisting of distinct stages provides a framework for inclusion of local talent and stories to shape a performance. Various frameworks have been proposed and are available. For example, Vasudevan et al. (2010)provided a seven-stage framework that illustrates participation/inclusion in shaping a performance: (1) training, (2) workshop, (3) rehearsal, (4) warmup, (5) performance, (6) cool down, and (7) aftermath. I suggest adding another important stage: the recruitment/try-outs phase.

Vasudevan et al. (Vasudevan, Stageman, Rodriguez, Fernandez, & Dattatreyan, 2010) identified six stages in which youth can engage in narratives related to social justice in theatre: (1) improvisation, (2) focused storytelling sessions, (3) composing scripts, (4) rehearsals, (5) performances, and (6) talk-backs. Each stage taps a different narrative aspect that builds on the preceding stage as well as on collective efficacy.

Youth engagement in out-of-school activities has also been conceptualized as "the simultaneous experience of concentration, interest, and enjoyment" (Shernoff & Vandell, 2007). Practitioners have multiple frameworks to select from to guide their engagement once they embrace a set of values that are participatory and empowering.

Each framework stage brings its own set of goals and activities, including rewards and challenges, and necessitates paying particular attention to youth engagement, motivation, and the potential ways in which they can be pulled to or pushed away from a program. Each stage must take into account youth characteristics, experiences, and social circumstances, including newcomer youth acculturation levels. Metzger et al. (Metzger, Crean, & Forbes-Jones, 2009) advance a person-centered approach for understanding the role and importance of organized activities in the lives of youth.

Our understanding of youth motivation and the benefits they derive when engaging in activities that enhance social and cognitive competencies is better appreciated due to scholarship conducted over the past decade (Caldwell & Witt, 2011; Sou, DeAngelo, Jones, & Veth, 2012). There is relatively little support for understanding that increased time and degree of participation in afterschool programs does not result in increased academic, behavioral, or socioemotional indicators (Roth, Malone, & Brooks-Gunn, 2010).

The performing arts have relevance for all social groups, with their appeal differing considerably based on youth experiences in growing up. Not having access to attend and participate in performances is an obvious factor. Youth interest in participating and attending theatre also is greatly influenced by familial attitudes toward this performing art (Anderson, Ewing, & Fleming, 2014).

Family attitudes and behavior need to be addressed when working with youth without a background in the performing arts. Youth engagement in a performing arts programs will, in all likelihood, be influenced by their friends and peers and the assessment of their artistic talent (Freer & Tan, 2014). Peer relationships have received increased attention in youth practice and scholarship because of how attendance at these events are rarely an individual phenomenon (Delgado, 2017; Donlan, Lynch, & Lerner, 2015).

There still remains a need to view participation/engagement in a more nuanced and less formulaic fashion that is sensitive to the interplay of personal (sociocultural) and environmental factors, particularly in the case of low-income urban youth of color who are facing incredible social forces that only promise to continue a marginalization and stigmatizing process with substantial lifetime consequences (Hoang (2012; Lawson & Lawson, 2013; Williams, Aiyer, Durkee, & Tolan, 2014).

This nuanced view acknowledges that there is no standard "formula" for understanding the reasoning youth use to decide on whether to engage in youth programs. This is not to say that there may not be core elements that apply across youth groups. It does mean, however, that how these core elements are manifested may differ according to a host of social-cultural and locality factors.

Engagement can also be facilitated through various actions. Providing stipends in addition to food and snacks is a viable way of demonstrating commitment and caring for youth participants, and more so in cases where they may have difficulty in getting proper nutrition at home (Flicker, 2008). A group process and solidarity development can be enhanced when youth shop for food and help prepare meals, as well as doing cleanup after a meal. When the participants represent different cultural backgrounds, native meals can be cooked, and youth can learn about cultural traditions through food.

Youth practitioners and scholars must be open to these and other factors in shaping the decision-making process. Formulaic approaches do a disservice to these youth and their respective communities, and formulaic approaches must be captured in any evaluation or research. Youth programs can provide apprenticeships to encourage retention and open up new avenues for skill development (Halpern, 2006).

Kirshner (2015, p. 25) addresses the importance of an organizational climate that encourages praxis, which is not possible in out-of-school settings that emphasize conventional mentoring and academic skill building: "Young people experiencing oppression need more than just mentors or academic skills; they need opportunities to talk about challenges in their everyday lives, examine root causes of inequality, and take action, broadly defined, about issues that affect them." Teaching and learning are not apolitical activities, and this must be acknowledged to maximize the process of discovery and reflection in praxis.

Practitioners and educators may argue that accomplishing this goal is arduous. The teaching of academic skills can be accomplished at the same time that social justice issues in youth lives are integrated into lesson plans (Delgado, 2016a). Teaching and social justice are not mutually exclusive of each other, but staff/educators must understand the possible connection between them and possess the values, competencies, and relationships to achieve social justice–inspired learning. We can argue that bringing together academic and social justice enhances learning by increasing the relevance of the learning process.

Nolas (2014) puts forth a compelling argument that adults must embrace a more contextual and nuanced understanding of how youth benefit from having their own spaces that they control, and this necessitates an epistemological approach to youth praxis that takes into account the vicissitudes of their operative life and the forces that undermine agency. Any meaningful discussion of place-making necessitates a discussion of the spatiality of place. Lefebvre (1991), a leading social theorist, posits that space can be conceptualized as a product that is manufactured.

Space and place are constructs that are closely interrelated and must receive serious consideration in any youth programming (Rios, Vazquez, & Miranda, 2012). Such a stance influences how, where, and why youth performing arts have a place and space within performing arts—and not just any youth practice, but more specifically one that is social justice– and youth-driven and represents the ultimate youth empowerment.

Adults often argue that youth-driven initiatives increase the chances of youth failing to achieve their goals. Adults fail, too, yet that does not prevent us from continuing to engage in creating activities and initiatives. Why shouldn't youth have the same option? After all, adults like to say we learn from our mistakes; youth, too, can learn from their mistakes.

A nuanced view brings potential tension and even conflict when youth organizations and funders ignore youth backgrounds and interests and further oppress them in the process of trying to aid them. Youth who normally would not consider participating in the performing arts can be reached if careful attention is paid to the message and to the purpose of these arts initiatives (Hoxie & Debellis, 2014; Salmon & Rickaby, 2014).

Program attrition is a critical factor in any community programming and is in need of close examination, as in the case of youth and sports (Balish, McLaren, Rainham, & Blanchard, 2014). Very often, a considerable amount of time and resources are devoted to doing outreach and engagement; similar attention must be devoted to understanding program attrition. There are organizational factors that wield considerable influence on participation (e.g., enjoyment), and having significant responsibilities has been shown to be positively associated with engagement and achievement of outcomes (Hansen & Larson, 2007). This conclusion makes intuitive sense.

Group composition is part of a nuanced approach. It received increased attention in PYD programs and raises considerations, such as in girl sports, that can enhance the benefits from participation, as in the case of those participants from "non-intact" families when compared to those from "intact" families, although this subject is bound to prove controversial in determining what constitutes intact (Schaillée, Theeboom, & Van Cauwenberg, 2015). Delgado (2017) addresses the importance of urban youth friendships as key motivators for engaging youth but also for broadening their social networks in the process of participation, thereby grounding them within a more expansive and potentially supportive system.

Youth do not wish to be passive; they prefer action and engagement in activities that challenge them. Adults worry when youth are not active. Music makes youth physically active. However, engagement goes beyond physical activity and must also entail engagement in decision-making (Agans et al., 2014; Blomfield & Barber, 2009; Campbell, 2010; Taylor, 2008). Jennings et al. (Jennings, Parrar-Medina, Hilfinger-Messias, & McLoughlin, 2006) found that meaningful participation and engagement resulted in youth empowerment. Is it possible to be empowered without meaningful participation? The answer is quite simple—no! Youth programming must systematically increase youth decision-making to achieve the maximum possible results, and this means adults sharing power.

The saying "If it is about us, without us, it isn't for us" resonates in youth practice. Participation motivation is enhanced when youth feel that their efforts can lead to the betterment of their lives and that of their community (Ballard, Malin, Porter, Colby, & Damon, 2015; Thomas, 2013). If their community is pushed to the fringes of society, "betterment" cannot be achieved without a strong embrace of social justice values and actions (Christens, 2012; Rogers, Mediratta, & Shah, S. (2012). Youth who embrace a collectivistic value place greater importance on their family's and community's well-being and on social justice ideals and goals.

Context and community issues can be key motivators for youth engagement in the civic life of their community because they sense the urgency of these issues for their families and community. Immigrant youth, in this case Mexican, are highly motivated to participate in civic life through involvement in immigrant-reform issues because of how these issues impact all facets of their community (Ballard et al., 2015; Santos, 2013).

There is a relationship between engagement and neighborhood assets when taking gender into account. Girls achieve better results when assessed on the outcomes of positive youth development, risk behavior, and depression when compared to boys (Urban, Lewin-Bizan, & Lerner, 2009). This reinforces the importance of taking contextual influences into account when promoting PYD. Some activities have particular relevance to gender, thus necessitating use of creative activities to increase appeal across different group characteristics.

An individualistic view of benefits is much too narrow a conceptualization for youth who may culturally subscribe to collectivistic values, as is the case of those who are newcomers to the United States and who have not been acculturated to the dominant (individualistic and competitive) values of this country (Silver, 2012; Updegraff, Umaña-Taylor, McHale, Wheeler, & Perez-Brena, 2012). A shift away from a focus on individuals toward groups/collectives highlights a worldview that is antithetical to prevailing individualistic value orientations.

Collectivistic values emphasize the importance of the group (family and friends, for example) and is counter to prevailing views in this society that focus on individuals at the cost of family and others. It is not unusual to find collectivistic values alongside cooperative values, as opposed to the more popular emphasis on competition in this society. A collectivist value necessitates use of planned activities that introduce this stance into PYD goals and programming (Shek & Sun, 2014).

An emphasis on teamwork or group activities is a direct manifestation of this value. The ability to work within groups can be translated into teamwork competencies. This shift needs to be captured through evaluation, particularly its nuanced manifestations (Cater & Jones, 2014). Teamwork life skills must be addressed in youth practice in any evaluation of programming (Lower, Newman, & Anderson-Butcher, 2015). Dutton (2001) stressed the importance of groups in the youth performing arts and community practice field more than 15 years ago, and the importance has not changed since then. Staff abilities to work with groups and individuals is a competency that must be covered in formal education and training endeavors.

Marginalized youth engagement in out-of-school programs takes on even greater significance because of how school systems are failing them and the paucity of institutions capable of filling the gap of intellectual and emotional fulfillment normally met by being intellectually stimulated (Anaby, Komer-Bitensky, Law, & Cormier, 2015; Gerber & Horoschak, 2012). Youth participation in out-of-school programs can encompass multiple activities (Balsano, Phelps, Theokas, Lerner, & Lerner, 2009; Wilson, Gottfredson, Cross, Rorie, & Connell, 2010), and participation transpires in a range of organizations, too (Barton & Butts, 2008; Delgado, 2000, 2002; Zarrett & Lerner, 2008).

Although Cohen-Cruz's (2006, p. 4) observations relate to grassroots theatre, they also can be applied to all performing arts and youth-focused organizations: "I have identified the linked characteristics of these theatres as: primary of place, deep interaction with constituents and commitment to goals including and exceeding the creation of great theatre. These characteristics are not just linked, they are inseparable from each other." The power of narrative is best appreciated within settings with deep community and organizational roots.

Great performances are not "great" because critics say that they are; performances are great because they deliver a meaningful message in a manner that does not underestimate the capacity of an audience to receive the message and they leave a long-lasting impression. Great performances never speak down to an audience; they speak with an audience to create an engaging and meaningful dialogue.

Youth out-of-school participation does not preclude in-school participation in activities that are appealing to them, as in the case of sports, art, and the performing arts. Youth can engage in a wider range of activities for enhancing their competencies and structuring their out-of-school time in a productive and potentially culturally affirming manner when these activities specifically focus on culture (Goldman, Booker, & McDermott, 2008; Wood, Larson, & Brown, 2009). Out-of-school activities are attractive because in-school extracurricular activities may not meet youth of color needs; research outcomes are mixed, and this calls for further advances in measurement, analysis, and causal models (Farb & Matjasko, 2012).

Individual efficacy has grown in tremendous appeal within the youth practice literature. Collective agency, which is predicated upon the power of the group without losing sight of individual agency, creates opportunities for change but has not benefitted from comparable attention (Kirshner, 2015). Structural barriers often require collective responses and are best addressed when praxis and corresponding social change involves groups coming together.

Collective efficacy (connectedness and willingness to intervene) and camraderie can be the primary benefits of efforts in a supportive environment (Flanagan, Martínez, Cumsille, & Ngomane, 2011; Siapno, 2012; Smith, Osgood, Caldwell, Hynes, & Perkins, 2013). Wernick, Kulick, and Woodford (2014), in this instance related to LBGTQ youth, note that theatre makes unique contributions to individual and collective empowerment by using an iterative process of creating community and support systems. Afterschool settings create unique bridges between schools and neighborhoods.

Bohnert, Fredricks, and Randall (2010) see the importance of more clearly understanding the socioenvironmental and personal factors that facilitate engagement in activities, which has been limited by a lack of consensus on how best to assess involvement. They identified critical four dimensions: (1) breadth, (2) intensity, (3) duration/consistency, and (4) engagement. Strobel et al. (Strobel, Kirshner, O'Donoghue, & Wallin McLaughlin, 2008) examined afterschool settings and participation and identified three crucial elements that increased youth commitment: (1) supportive relationships with adults and peers, (2) safety, and (3) opportunities to learn. These elements are closely associated, yet bring unique dimensions to the discussion.

Stodolska et al. (Stodolska, Sharaievska, Tainsky, & Ryan, 2014) specifically addressed youth of color in sporting activities and developed a three-stage framework for assessing motivation: (1) the impact of innate psychological needs, (2) motivation for participating in an organized program, and (3) the role of facilitators/staff in promoting youth participation. These and other efforts have helped academics and practitioners develop a better understanding of the multidimensional factors influencing and sustaining youth participation in programs (Durlak, Weissberg, & Pachan, 2010; Hart, 2013; Mitra et al., 2014).

There are numerous ways to think about youth practice, and this is both exciting and terribly frustrating. I like to use a restaurant menu as a metaphor for this field. It is best to conceptualize youth practice as an extensive menu at a well-known restaurant. There are many different entrees to select from depending upon the mood and budget of the diner. In youth practice, there is no one community organization that can offer an all-encompassing menu of all the programs covering an extensive field and budgets.

Being able to direct youth (diners) to other organizations (restaurants) that offer the type of programming (food) these youth want becomes an important function for youth practice organizations. Developing a comprehensive listing of options and fostering new programs to fill gaps becomes an important function of practitioners. Youth should not be forced to choose from a very limited list of foods that they are not interested in. Providing an array of activities that can encompass sports, computers, civic engagement, academics, and the performing arts taps into youth interests and strengths, thus increasing the chances of success (Cox, 2008).

PYD and other programs open up post school career options that can be maximized through participation in the performing arts (Bakshi & Joshi, 2014). As in any youth activity, a small percentage of youth may have the desire and competencies to make their chosen activity a career choice, as with elite athletes and artists. Not every youth may elect to do so even when they have the competencies to continue, and there must be a place and space for them, too.

No two communities are the same, regardless of how similar they may appear to be (McHale, Dotterer, & Kim, 2009). They may differ according to assets, needs, and history, and this influences how a music, song, dance, or theatre program would be received and if it would have a high probability of succeeding (Ungar, 2011). A community that has a history of offering these youth activities will be in a different position when compared to a community that historically relied upon sporting programing; one with a history of youth programming failures may be reluctant to initiate new programs, while a community with a history of successfully launching innovative programs may not be hesitant to do so once again.

A comprehensive assessment, along with a detailed inventory of past and current efforts using the performing arts, is needed if we are to increase the odds of a performing art program achieving success. This type of assessment, although quite logical, is rare in the field because such assessment is difficult; but just because it is difficult to undertake should not be an excuse for not doing it because it has practical and everyday implications that take into account various budgets and local goals (Delgado & Humm-Delgado, 2013).

Finding the "secret" to meaningfully engaging youth in programming remains a goal of youth practice, but there is no denying that we are getting closer to finding the answers to this puzzle (Hirsch, Deutsch, & DuBois, 2011; Sullivan, 2016). There is no one simple answer to this quest. Dawes and Larson (2011) found that the presence of three youth goals play influential roles in shaping increased expectations: (1) learning for the future, (2) developing competence, and (3) pursuing a purpose. These goals necessitates a social-cultural grounding to meet youth needs in an affirming manner. This grounding takes on greater significance when geographical setting is taken into account.

Dawes and Larson's findings emphasize the importance of youth learning and having a noble purpose to motivate them to do so. Education, when relevant to their lives, is possible. Bronk (2011) notes that having a noble purpose is an important component of PYD, yet the field is in desperate need of an in-depth understanding of how this is initiated, sustained, increased, and changed over time for different subgroups, with particular relevance for urban youth of color.

An evolutionary grasp of this concept provides a window into how to enhance purpose at various stages, including barriers and forces operative in undermining hope and purpose. Positive experiences and constructive feedback shape how having a noble purpose can be enhanced for youth, translating these experiences into gains in multiple social arenas (Bundick, 2011).

Civic purpose, which is defined as a "sustained intention to contribute to the world beyond the self through civic or political action," too, has emerged to capture the complexity and multifaceted nature of caring (Malin, Ballard, & Damon, 2015, p. 103). Moran (2014) introduces the concept of purpose (Supported, Strivers, Givers, and Disciples) and its role and influence in shaping youth motivation to participate in activities. Purposefully bringing social justice into activities serves to engender or enhance a social purpose for youth who are marginalized and has a ripple effect throughout their peer network and community.

Segal (2011) discusses how social empathy and caring about social justice is a manifestation of a humanistic stance resulting in a noble purpose. Youth empowerment is not possible without social empathy and social connections (Modirzadeh, 2013; Stanton-Salazar, 2011; Wagaman, 2011). Increased connectedness facilitates the development of a noble purpose that is reinforced, encompassing, social justice–driven, and much more powerful.

A desire to address White privilege is one way that caring can be expressed when there are differences regarding race and ethnicity (Pennington, Brock, & Ndura, 2012; Young-Law, 2012). Embracing this stance necessitates that we, as adults, and particularly those of us in authority, be willing to question our assumptions about who youth are but also about what constitutes race (Mayor, 2012). An embrace of intersectionality theory necessitates that this questioning be done in a manner that captures and gives voice to the lived experiences of youth.

Activities that can successfully tap youth interests and agency, and seek to find or enhance a noble purpose in the process, represent a potential growth area for a field that is seeking to widen its appeal nationally and internationally (Forkby & Kiilakoski, 2014; Guèvremont, Findlay, & Kohen, 2008; McBride, Johnson, Olate, & O'Hara, 2011; Whittaker, 2014). Seeking a noble purpose lends itself to embracing social justice goals with marginalized youth and introduces the potential of critical civic engagement into youth practice, including the performing arts, as an act of service and a mechanism for achieving social change (Delgado, 2016a).

Music, song, dance, and theatre can tap into interests in the performing arts that may exist in youth not interested in sports or other conventional activities. And there are other activities that can be tapped: poetry has been proposed as an arts-based approach to social justice (Dill, 2015; Foster, 2012; Thomas & León, 2012; Weinstein, 2010), even though urban youth are not usually associated with writing poetry because of its heavy social class and racial associations.

However, *slam poetry*, probably more so than any other form of poetry, has found a home with urban youth and embraces social justice (Fields, Snapp, Russell, Licona, & Tilley, 2014; Garcia, 2014; Pellegrino, Zenkov, & Aponte-Martinez, 2014; Waite, 2015). Camangian (2008) extols the virtues of "spoken word poetry" as an effective vehicle for engaging urban youth in literacy and found that poetry assisted youth in self-expression, provided a counter-narrative to the deficit view imposed on them, and was a means of positively managing their temperaments, which if not done, can result in dire consequences.

The thought of engaging in the performing arts will elicit a smile from anyone who is approached about participating because they are often associated with fun, laughter, high energy, and putting oneself out there. To say it would be exciting is a serious understatement. Capturing these sentiments and translating them into programs should not be a hard sell, and this will practitioners recruit and maintain youth in these programs–which in some instances can be quite challenging due to the competing demands youth face on a daily basis.

Ferreira, Coimbra, and Menezes (2012, p. 126) stress the importance and interconnectedness of participation for undervalued groups and why engagement cannot be viewed as a token effort but as a meaningful and sustainable process because of its importance in the lives of these youth:

> Since one's well-being depends on positive community integration, meaningful participation and the amount of power enjoyed for self-determination in one's community become essential elements. . . . A social climate favoring fairness, participation and expression is also related to sense of community . . . and integration. Opportunities to participate—particularly in contexts open to others and diversity—in addition contribute to gains in social capital and to relationships of mutual recognition. Yet mutual recognition must lead

to integration beyond adaptation. That means going beyond removing differences and erasing diversity, and creating the conditions for different groups—especially those in most vulnerable positions—to affirm their difference in a plural context and exercise civic and political rights.

Mutual participatory recognition and benefits derived from this stance on fairness recognize the power of being a meaningful member of a community and society, providing much needed grounding.

Youth cannot be considered second-class citizens if they are to make significant contributions in society. Such a position is inherently unfair and borders on "blaming the victim." We do not give youth an opportunity to enhance their competencies and then turn around and ask them why they do not have more to offer their communities and society.

This section on youth participation/engagement would not be complete without touching on youth who have negative experiences in programs. Dworkin and Larson (2006) address an often overlooked aspect of participation: negative experiences that can create situations that anger youth, making it harder for them to engage and benefit from participation.

Furthermore, negative experiences can disrupt critical developmental relationships among youth with few positive attachments in their lives. Learning requires a climate that is safe and affirming, and negative emotional experiences will interfere with the acquisition of new knowledge and competencies. In situations where youth are in a particularly stressful period in their lives, this sort of experience further compounds their situation and may push them to engage in unwise behaviors that can compromise their participation in a program.

Undocumented and Newcomer Youth

Undocumented immigrants have become a hot political issue in national politics (Passell & Lope, 2012), even though undocumented immigration has slowed dramatically in the past few years (Lopez & Patten, 2015). Is it possible to view youth who are undocumented as separate both from their parents and from this issue in this country? It should be noted that US youth under the age of 18 can hold a variety of legal statuses, with being undocumented being but one. One prominent way to understand documented status is to define these youth as either foreign-born or US-born to immigrant parents, which accounted for 25% of the country's 75 million youth (Passell, 2011).

Undocumented immigrants number 11.3 million, or 3.5% of the total population, with Mexicans representing the largest group at 52% (Krogstad & Passel, 2015). Certain states and regions of the country are home to the majority of these individuals, with Texas, Florida, New York, New Jersey, and Illinois leading the country. This distribution is starting to change, and undocumented immigrants are demographically projected to impact the nation's racial and ethnic composition for the next 50 years, barring major international social changes (Pew Hispanic Research Center, 2015).

Marginalized youth are not monolithic in composition, and a number of subgroups stand out for attention, with one being those who are undocumented. Undocumented/newcomers youth take on greater significance because of their increasing percentage of the population, particularly among certain groups such as Latinos. The performing arts and other youth practice interventions have a role to play among these youth and their communities. Before using the performing arts or any other youth programming, they cannot remain invisible or viewed from a very narrow perspective because they, too, are not monolithic in composition and aspirations.

Diaz-Strong et al. (Diaz-Strong, Gomez, Lance-Duarte, & Meiners, 2014) detail how undocumented youth are facing incredible social forces, are resisting, and are determined in their quest for social justice. Finding context-driven mechanisms for these voices and actions that are attractive for these youth must be a central goal of social justice youth community practice, with the performing arts assuming an increasingly important potential among these youth.

Garzon (2014) describes using Boal's *Theater of the Oppressed* to reach immigrant youth by tapping their own voices for self-reflection and achieving personal growth. This was then translated into life skills to help them navigate their social reality, which is often grounded in fighting against racism, discrimination, and internalized oppression. *Theatre of the Oppressed* has also been used to uncover representations of girls' subjectivity and social relations and the sexual violence they have experienced (Clark, 2009), and it even has been used in houses of worship and in theology education (Heltzel, 2015).

Demographics provides a picture, although unidimensional, that can be supplemented through qualitative research methods that capture voices and stories. Marks, Ejesi, and García Coll's (2014, p. 59) demographic profile of newcomer youth and their corresponding challenges shows that they have a powerful story to share with the nation and the world, one that can be inspirational and transformative:

> A full 25% of the US population under age 10 is either a first- (foreign-born) or second- (U.S.-born to foreign-born parents) generation immigrant. . . . Most of today's immigrant youth are Hispanic or Asian, with many recent refugees also from Eastern Europe, Africa, and the Middle East. Most of these children are US citizens, but nearly 5 million have at least one undocumented parent. . . . Approximately 1.7 million children are themselves undocumented, yet have lived in this country for most of their lives and do not know another country of origin.

Their young age and their place within the life of their communities throughout the country makes them attractive for engagement in youth practice initiatives.

The narratives that undocumented immigrant youth have to share have implications for the nation, but particularly for those states and regions where their presence is increasing and, in the process, generating fears, as is the case with Latinos and Muslim refugee youth. The performing arts tap their cultural traditions of storytelling, and these stories can act as a bridge.

Youth–Adult Relationships

Youth–adult relationships are best understood from an evolutionary viewpoint to appreciate why they have achieved their particular manifestations in the present. Zeldin, Camino, and Calvert (2012, pp. 77–78) provide an important grounding for how youth and adults enjoyed a close working relationship in the early founding of the nation and how it changed:

> Youth were critical to the economic and social vitality of their communities from the days of the early settlement of the United States to the second half of the nineteenth century. They worked with their parents and other adult laborers on farms and in mills, and interacted with them during local celebrations and rituals. This community context changed with the onset of the industrial revolution. As the need for youth labor diminished, and formal schooling became necessary for occupational success, youth became increasingly separated from adults and from the day-to-day lives of their communities.

As opportunities for youth–adult working relationships have evolved, this has caused a power differentiation that translates into adults having decision-making roles and youth suffering a power loss in the process. The fact that the situation has evolved in a way that is not to the benefit of youth, bodes well for its potential to evolve to benefit youth.

The quality and nature of the interactions between staff and youth provide a critical window into the types of relationships that foster engagement and growth and can be used in other settings (Kirshner, 2015, p. 29):

> What is less well articulated in youth development practice of theory, however, is how these caring adults should engage in conversations with youth—who are marginalized because of their race, class, or sexual identities—about the political context in their lives, particularly in ways that don't further anthologize their neighborhoods or peer groups. Put another way, early work on youth programs tended to frame them as safe spaces or sanctuaries from difficult environments.

These interactions are far more important than the activities youth typically engage in, representing an organic dimension to youth–adult relationships that is difficult to predict and/or generalize beyond general themes. These interactions and conversations, when involving racism, can have a profound impact on youth–adult relationships.

Mentoring is a popular method often used in youth–adult relationships within and outside of formalized youth programs, and it can be an effective in helping Latino/as in understanding and negotiating the influence of acculturation when mutual respect and trust are present in the relationship (Liao & Sánchez, 2015). Mentors, particularly those who are natural, community-based, and of similar ethnic and racial backgrounds to youth mentees, can help youth of color achieve economic and socially related benefits (Timpe & Lunkenheimer, 2015).

Mitra (2006) identified three youth–adults approaches: (1) at a systems level through a focus on issues related to intolerance and injustice, (2) at an organizational level, and (3) at the individual level by fostering youth leadership and the helping of peers. How youth leadership is conceptualized depends greatly on how programs foster youth in assuming these positions (Klau, 2006). Out-of-school settings must embrace youth as leaders and need to do so from a nontraditional viewpoint, calling for youth leadership models that are responsive to youth needs and their own definition of leadership (Sullivan, 2015).

Youth–adult relationships share importance with youth-to-youth relationships, including friendships (Delgado, 2017), although I considers youth-to-youth interrelationships as being in need of far greater understanding and scholarship. An adult-centric perspective is too narrow a view and misses other critical dimensions related to age as a bridge in establishing connections, including the role of youth culture and language.

Zeldin, Christens, and Powers (2013) point out that although much attention and corresponding research has been paid to youth–adult relationships and their importance for youth development, this relationship construct has remained vague and has not benefitted from sufficient grounding in developmental theory and practice. This observation takes on even greater significance when introducing intersectionality into these relationships to identify the social forces that are operative in pushing these youth into a marginalized status.

This is not to say that intense attention has not been paid to youth–adult relationships. Program staff abilities to effectively work with the parents and official guardians of youth engaged in programming brings an added and often missing dimension in youth–adult relationships, and one requiring considerable attention (Evans et al., 2012; Vincent & Christensen, 2015; Wallace, Waybright, Rohner, & Crawford, 2015). My years in the youth practice field have led me to conclude that it is rare to find staff capable and willing to interact with parents.

An ability to relate to multiple age groups requires a skill set that often goes unrecognized and is not taught in school. For instance, African-American youth engagement and outcomes are increased when parents also participate when called upon to do so (Hanlon, Simon, O'Grady, Carswell, & Callaman, 2009). Having competencies to engage parents translates into increasing the likelihood that their children gain increased benefits from participating.

Non-school teachers, too, can have a prominent role to play in helping youth, although they rarely are thought of as being in a position to exert influence (Noam & Bernstein-Yamashiro, 2013). Supporting them expands the scope of potential adults who can establish positive relationships with youth by carrying out different roles, most notably as educator, mentor, connector, and even friend. Nonprofessional support staff also can play a role beyond their immediate responsibilities.

Deutsch and Jones (2008) advance the argument that the concept of authority has generally been overlooked in the research literature, with the exceptions of school and family. Out-of-school settings provide youth and adults with an opportunity to create a relational climate that can foster mutual respect, which encompasses bidirectional respect as opposed to respecting rules. Creating an important balance between the needs of youth for autonomy and adult needs to exercise authority is a goal that must be explicitly sought if these settings are to achieve maximum results.

Larson et al. (Larson, Walker, Rusk, & Diaz, 2015) note that systematically tapping youth practitioner perspectives is essential if we are to understand their challenges and if this field is to continue to make substantive progress in the immediate future. Youth programming is only as good as its staffing. This observation does not take away from "good" leadership: frontline staff are the heart and soul of youth programming and are in the best position to know youth, their families, and their daily struggles and joys.

Informal time and space present the potential for significantly influencing the shaping of youth practice, yet it also brings its share of potential ethical challenges (Banks, 2010, p. 84): "In the informal contexts in which youth work occurs, youth workers need to be clear about the nature of their relationship, and especially the limits of that relationship. It is the limits of the relationship that define it, that create its quality, and that channel its energy." This space opens up opportunities for positive engagement and intergenerational sharing, representing a unique opportunity for youth to meaningfully engage with adults.

Successful youth–adult partnerships do not simply occur organically, although that is possible and does occur in the community. Even when these relationships occur organically in programs, they still need to be fostered by ongoing training and built-in support (Zeldin & Leidheiser, 2014). Instrumental projects can serve as a basis for structuring and establishing affirming and constructive youth–adult interpersonal relationships (Halpern, 2005). Staff ability to grow professionally cannot be an afterthought, just as youth ability to grow personally cannot be an afterthought.

Respect, friendship, hope (intentional self-regulation, positive future expectations, and connectedness), trust, joy, and fun are all tied together through the construct of caring, which can be manifested in countless ways that have implications for youth community practice (Callina, Johnson, Buckingham, & Lerner, 2014; Callina, Mueller, Buckingham, & Gutierrez, 2015; Ginwright, 2011; Kirschman,

Roberts, Shadlow, & Pelley, 2010; Ross, Capra, Carpenter, Hubbell, & Walker, 2015; Sevdalis & Raab, 2014; Walker, 2011). The saliency of caring or empathy as a guiding construct offers great potential for youth–adult relationships and for youth–youth relationships, which play an even more critical role in their school and leisure time.

Ginwright's (2015) book *Hope and Healing in Urban Education* places emphasis and importance on the role of hope in counteracting the consequences of a long history of structural oppression. Ginwright identified three concepts that shaped this book: (1) how structural oppression systematically diminishes and harms hope, (2) that healing must transpire in a significant way in building hope, and (3) that it is best to conceptualize hope as a political activity. These perspectives attest to their importance in the assessment and development of youth interventions that are social change–oriented and have relevance for using the performing arts when tapping hope as a change motivator (Ginwright, 2015, p. 4):

> Hope, healing, and well-being, however, are not fixed to social conditions and therefore can be strengthened through practices, programs, and policies. Research suggests that hopefulness is the function of agency, the belief that one can changes things, and pathways, opportunities to act to achieve a desired goal. . . . The fact that we can foster hope and healing allows us to consider how community power, public policy, and educational strategies can support this process in schools and communities.

Fostering hope has far greater implications beyond psychology, crossing over into the social and political realms. Hope is tied to passion, and passion is tied to channeling energy and commitment, all critical elements in youth social agency. Creativity, too, can be included in this discussion.

Co-learning between adults and youth also introduces a power-sharing relationship that can foster these relationships in a manner that promotes long-term benefits for all parties and introduces the potential for innovative situations where learning actively involves youth and adults together (Kinloch, 2012; Shaw-Raudoy & McGregor, 2013). The concept of reciprocal mentoring or co-mentoring has emerged as a mechanism for capturing and fostering relationships where learning is not restricted to one party but is a result of adults and youth sharing activities and trusting relationships that are mutually beneficial (Armon & Grassi, 2012).

Noddings (1995), as quoted in Cohen et al. (Cohen, Silber, Sangiorgio, & Iadeluca, 2012, p. 188), identified four benefits of caring for teaching but with equal applicability to youth practice and the performing arts: "(1) It expands children's cultural literacy, (2) it helps children perceive transfers across standard school subjects, (3) it addresses existential questions, such as how one should live and the meaning of life, and (4) it helps children connect with one another and demonstrate respect for all human talent." Youth practice performing arts is, first and foremost, about shaping lives in the moment and in the future. When integrating social justice, it is also about living in a future that is just and affirming. The two time periods are not mutually exclusive.

Community practitioners who are willing and able to share that they care about youth will translate their caring into having youth be more willing to commit to a program and to develop trusting and respectful relationships with adults (Rauner, 2013). This outcome will not be accomplished without tensions, testing, potential conflict, and ethical as well as political challenges. These are often key elements in meaningful relationships. This process and goal are noteworthy.

A socioecological view of youth stresses the presence and interactions of communities and organizations. Rimmer (2012) examined the role of participation and decision-making in three urban-focused music projects (school, community center, and youth center in an inner-city community) and illustrated the importance of an organizational setting in shaping how "music-making with social goals"is manifested. Where performing arts projects originate can be expected to play an influential role in how they are manifested and the degree to which youth can have project-shaping influence that dictates youth–adult relationships.

In-school performing arts generally have a heavy emphasis on conventional teaching methods, Eurocentric biases, limited time periods, academic goals, educational policies, and rigid roles for participants as students and teachers as teachers. In-school projects limit the ability for youth to take charge (decision-making), and their embrace of social justice messages can be considered "too political." This perspective should not be surprising, particularly for those of us working in schools that are not considered to be hotbeds of high achievers and are known more for expulsion and arrest records rather than for graduation and college placement records.

Socially mainstream arguments are often heard to depoliticize education and curriculum because it does a disservice to youth of color and other youth groups by not preparing them to occupy positions in the "real world." To be marginalized is to be in a social situation that *is* political, and this must be acknowledged as such. When we elect to ignore this, we do a disservice to youth and those who educate them (Checkoway, 2011).

All formal education is predicated upon political assumptions concerning the value of the material being taught, and these assumptions are often implicit. Making these assumptions explicit facilitates learning by creating an atmosphere that is conducive for praxis to occur. How can youth be expected to change the world if we are not giving them the proper space and tools with which to accomplish this goal?

Zeldin, Camino, and Calvert (2012, p. 77) note that youth in PYD programs are present in decision-making roles, further increasing the impact of this approach to youth practice:

> For more than a decade, many researchers and practitioners have endorsed a "positive youth development" approach, which views adolescents as active

contributors to their own development and as assets to their communities. As part of this shift, youth are increasingly being invited to engage in community governance. In youth organizations, schools, community organizations, and public policy arenas, youth are making strong contributions to advisory boards and planning councils, and integrally involved in key day-to-day functions such as program design, budgeting, outreach, public relations, training, and evaluation.

In any program, we must determine whether the youth role is advisory or is actually decision-making. Participation can mean many different things. Youth decision-making in the performing arts will be addressed, emphasized, and highlighted in this section because of how it shapes youth–adult relationships.

Youth participatory research builds on a common set of values and approaches. It is civic engagement, lending itself to use in gaining greater understanding of youth and the performing arts. Wernick, Woodford, and Kulick (2014) advance the close relationship between youth participatory action research (YPAR) and theatre in achieving change by empowering LGBTQ youth to engage in decision-making roles and develop adult allies in their quest for social justice.

Jacquez, Vaughn, and Wagner (2013) undertook an extensive review of the literature on community based participatory research (CBPR) and participation and found that almost one-quarter of all studies were community-based but did not have a community partnership and/or participatory dimension. Fifty-six did have an explicit partnership with youth and involved them in various phases of the research process. Limiting youth and decision-making to select phases is not tapping into the spirit of CBPR, and, it can be argued, it is disempowering in a process that ostensibly is supposed to be empowering (Sprague-Martinez et al., in press).

It is appropriate to end this section by noting that successful youth engagement is multifaceted (emotionally, socially, and cognitively) and it would be foolhardy to narrow it to just relationships between youth and adults and parental willingness to allow them to engage in activities outside of the home (Bruening, Clark, & Mudrick, 2015). We must also take into account neighborhood characteristics in determining the probability of success for youth engagement that has meaning beyond occupying time (Duke, Borowsky, & Pettingell, 2012, p. 422):

> By facilitating a sense of community, parental social networks, informal emotional and psychological support, and interpersonal ties for mutual exchange, parents perceiving greater neighborhood social capital may be more willing to allow youth to participate in activities outside of the home environment. Informal mechanisms of support perceived by parents that directly and indirectly relate to aid or assistance, protection, and supervision of their child may translate into a youth's sense of safety and well-being, which may affect a youth's likelihood of engaging in activities beyond home and family, the most proximal developmental context.

The interplay of community context, parental/legal guardian influence, and youth willingness to engage in activities all come into play in shaping engagement. The interrelationships are complex and difficult to untangle but must not dissuade scholars from seeking to identify important trigger points in the decision-making process.

Outreach must extend beyond youth themselves to be successful, and this require specific skill sets that include the engagement of adults (family, legal guardians, natural mentors). We can argue that these practitioners possess "people skills." These relationships must be age-group responsive and carry a corresponding message about how we engage youth.

Walsh (2012) advocates for greater attention to youth family bonds in youth programs to strengthen multigenerational relationship networks that can enhance youth participant resilience. Such a broad participatory stance and its reach beyond youth themselves necessitating changes in how information and data are gathered in assessing the impact of participation in programs.

What Are Out-of-School Settings?

We can answer this question in a short sentence: Out-of-school settings represent a fundamental element in how this nation addresses its youth, and, in some if not many communities, they are vital sanctuaries in youth lives and part of a community's social fabric. Modern-day out-of-school settings have deep historical roots in this society. Yet their proliferation has generally not gone without critique because of a tendency for some to view them as societal efforts to domesticate and professionalize social activism (Kwon, 2013). Managing or controlling youth is the guiding philosophy on this stance.

Some of the most popular out-of-school activities that take place in these settings cover a range of afterschool programs, extracurricular activities, sports, community service, and summer day and away camps (Vandell, Larson, Mahoney, & Watts, 2015). Historically, afterschool settings targeted youth with high probabilities of not succeeding in society, particularly newcomers; those from low-income households; those with various intellectual, physical, and emotional challenges; and youth of color (Durlak, Mahoney, Bohnert, & Parente, 2010). Kwon (2013, p. 8) raises the provocative question about present-day institutional efforts to accomplish central political goals:

> Participation in wholesome community-based programs continues to be offered today with this implicit, if not explicit, purpose as this story goes, involvement in such programs will steer poor youth of color onto an alternative path of responsible citizenship away from those dangers (drugs, gangs, prisons, sexual disease, and pregnancy) assumed to otherwise loom close at hand for these youth. Too often such prevention measures are offered as ways

to control male criminality and female sexuality, through which youth of color are already marked as deviant.

It is easy to see an "at-risk" label being attached to these youth and the programs targeting them. Staff, too, bring the label of "at-risk" youth specialists and assume the stigma attached to the youth they serve. Righting these labels becomes arduous when program funding specifically targets youth from this deficit perspective.

The National Research Council's Institute of Medicine (Eccles & Gootman, 2002, p. 31) addressed how best to define a community program, and this definition is intrinsically related to out-of-school settings in a variety of ways, but also arduous to arrive at without debate:

> One hurdle faced by the committee was developing a common understanding of what constitutes a community program for youth. The characterization of these programs is complicated, and the landscape is vast. They may be called after-school programs, youth programs, youth activities, youth development programs, community programs, extracurricular activities, or programs during out-of-school time or non-school hours. In addition, we debated whether school programs should be included, since schools in the United States are, for the most part, locally controlled. We also debated what constitutes a community.

A consensus youth community setting definition is no easier to answer almost 15 years later, although the expansion of youth programs has been exponential. Eventually arriving at such a definition will prove monumental for the field.

Out-of-school settings cover a range of community organizational types and programming, and this complicates compiling a comprehensive inventory and understanding of their roles in the lives of youth, particularly those who are facing daily challenges to their health and well-being. An expansive view of community settings opens up the performing arts to innovative thinking about to where they can transpire to best meet local needs.

Houses of worship can have a prominent place within the out-of-school world, depending on whether they host community-based youth programming or ministries (Kim, 2014; Strommen, Jones, & Rahn, 2011). Performing arts conducted within houses of worship can foster greater awareness and opportunities for youth to participate in civic engagement (Beyerlein & Hipp, 2006). These opportunities can transpire outside of these institutions, but also within an ample number of activities that cover an entire age range of youth. Houses of worship also can serve as excellent settings for outreach to newcomers to the country (Numrich & Kniss, 2007).

When discussing marginalized populations, youth practice efforts do not have the luxury of dismissing any community setting as being "exempt" from undertaking an intervention. Heinze (2013), in a rare article, discusses how PYD can be instituted in community emergency shelters. Some may argue that emergency shelters must not be categorized as out-of-school setting because they do not fall within the conventional thinking on this topic. But conventional thinking must go out of the window, and, when it does, it facilitates a more expansive view and the introduction of innovative strategies that take into account key organizational factors.

Summer camps, either sleep-away or day camps, are out-of-school settings with a seasonal cycle, and youth practice goals also can be integrated into this type of experience (Garst, Browne, & Bialeschki, (2011). Summer camps are often guided by themes, and camps devoted to the performing arts represent one viable way of introducing these types of activities to youth, particularly in communities where there are no established organizational efforts incorporating the performing arts.

Even universities and colleges can be thought of as out-of-school venues, and this is particularly the case with community or junior colleges. Institutions of higher learning derive benefits for their faculty and students in internships, research, and, in some cases, in efforts to expand physically within their respective communities. There are excellent university/college-provided program models that practitioners can select from when developing their own programs. Just because they may be located within a community does not automatically make them out-of-school settings.

Kane (2014, p. 224) discusses a successful performing arts model that has applicability for university–community out-of-school partnerships seeking to engage youth and that lends itself to being modified to take into account local circumstances and different demographic youth groups:

> A summer performing arts program set at a university site is an ideal opportunity to implement a sequence of strategic creative and social activities that offer high school youth daily activities that can establish a foundation for these significant relationships to emerge. By including college-aged program counselors who attended the program when they were in high school, acting as "step-ahead" peers, a program model such as this one provides potent possibilities for burgeoning leaders and mentors to emerge and meaningful relationships to take hold. Furthermore, the performance material generated in such a program can directly represent the personal evolutions of the students and the developmental relationships that are originated throughout the program's creative and social processes . . . uses the UCLA Summer High School Dance Theater Intensive program as a case study of a progressive, multidisciplinary, summer performing arts program that positions the initiation of developmental relationships as one of its core values.

Universities and colleges are positioned to foster these collaborations because of the tangible and intangible resources they possess, particularly during the summer when institutions have space available and youth have time to engage (McDonald,

2006). Time and availability match in a rare moment, and many institutions of higher learning do take advantage of this opportunity.

Pryor and Outley (2014) advance the notion of "urban recreational centers" as out-of-school settings that are potential sites for social justice youth development if they are to be relevant in the lives of youth from those communities. These sites are accessible (geographically, physically, psychologically, culturally, and operationally) and can be destigmatizing while reaching out to youth. These settings can incorporate the performing arts as youth-centered activities for explicitly achieving social justice goals.

There are numerous examples of community-grounded performing arts centers throughout the country, reflecting on the popularity and viability of these organizations using the performing arts to reach marginalized youth and their communities. The performing arts can transpire in non–community performing arts centers as part of general programming, taking into consideration the space and supports available. There is great potential for the performing arts as an activity that can reach countless youth and corresponding non–youth serving organizations, thus expanding the reach of programs beyond traditional settings devoted to the performing arts.

A few examples of these types of centers from across the country include the Boston's ZUMIIX; Denver's Creative Strategies for Change; Richmond, California's East Bay Center for the Performing Arts (Engdahl, 2012); Hartford, Connecticut's Artists Collective (Rhodes & Schechter, 2014); Los Angeles's Unusual Suspects Theatre Company (Mohler, 2012a, 2012b) and Peace and Justice Center (Viesca, 2012); and New York City's Creative Arts Team. This brief list illustrates the nationwide appeal of youth performing arts organizations that cover various performing arts manifestations.

This popularity does not mean, however, that when these organizations embrace social justice principles funding is free-flowing and without sociopolitical challenges (Heppner & Jung, 2012). An increased narrowing of governmental funding focus will work to the detriment of programs embracing social justice and highly creative approaches toward youth programming (Lenette & Ingamells, 2015). The support of youth, their families, and communities is essential in these situations as a means of counteracting the potentially negative influences of funding on programming.

Budget flexibility, particularly regarding in-kind donations and civic engagement that can be sought from conventional and no-traditional sources, makes performing arts possible regardless of funding levels. Obtaining local in-kind donations increases ownership of the performance by the community, increases the potential for social changes at the local level, and creates important collective community memories. The sites where these performances occur are not restricted to auditoriums, which low-income communities rarely control; these performances can occur in houses of worship, parks, and other community venues.

Why Are They Important?

Why are community organizations that sponsor youth performing arts so important? The answer may seem rather obvious at first sight. These types of organizations are in need of expansion, and that is one of the reasons for writing this book. It is so much easier to find organizations that specialize in providing "therapeutic" services to youth who are troubled and considered "at-risk."

A language that uses terms such as "saving" and "rescuing" youth of color is often associated with out-of-school settings and serves to reinforce stereotypes (Baldridge, 2014). I much prefer the term "marginalized" because it takes the onus away from the individual and places it within the broader context of society. Youth do not simply marginalize themselves; they get marginalized. This observation may seem simplistic, but it sheds light on how social forces select certain groups to push to the margins, and youth fall into this type of situation.

Some readers may believe that we are arguing semantics, but that is not the case: the difference is significant from a sociopolitical perspective and has potentially devastating consequences. Marginalized youth are often viewed as victimizers rather than victims. There is no small distinction between being a victim and being a victimizer. Labeling youth as "at-risk" casts them in a negative role. Out-of-school programs must not label youth; instead these programs must seek to empower yourth to resist these efforts to marginalize them with the aid of adult allies.

For out-of-school settings to achieve youth empowerment, they must develop programming with an acute understanding of how youth use their free time and their decision-making processes. Browning and Soller (2014, p. 165) stress the importance of research on community and youth routine activities to inform out-of-school programs: "Research into the causes and consequences of urban neighborhood routine activity structures will illuminate the social processes accounting for compromised youth outcomes in disadvantaged neighborhoods and enhance the capacity for effective youth-oriented interventions."

Routine activities can be quite revealing and are profound in shaping attitudes and possible programming responses. Woodland (2016) argues that even though afterschool programs are ubiquitous, they are based on minimal attention to how theoretical models differ and how they inform the conceptualization of activities, and as such do not maximize their potential impact on African-American/Black and other youth of color. Context shapes these activities and experiences.

Self-identity was addressed earlier, and out-of-school settings can influence youth to counteract negative social forces and develop positive identities in the process. Halverson (2009, p. 4) discusses the important role that youth-based organizations (YBOs) can have in helping marginalized youth to develop positive identities, a critical dimension to any successful youth intervention:

> YBOs provide developmentally supportive experiences and have documented positive outcomes for participating youth. One key outcome of participation

is adolescents' use of these organizational experiences for identity develop-ment and exploration, including personal exploration, self-knowledge, iden-tity reflection, and a sense of belonging to a community with clearly defined identity markers.

A safe and affirming organizational climate, as manifested through youth and adult staff interactions and activities, can play an influential role within communi-ties that feel under siege and that have poor prospects for the future of their youth. Establishing organizational climates such as these is never easy because it often involves undoing many years of possible distrust on the part of youth.

Insights garnered through an understanding of the types of activities youth prefer and benefit from help focus programming by elucidating on how time is perceived and manifested in their lives, particularly the options that are availa-ble to them for engaging in activities they consider to be "worthwhile" and that may alter their living circumstances and those of their families and friends. These insights influence scholarly publications, which influence the preparation of future practitioners as well as policies and funding for youth initiatives tapping the performing arts.

Performing arts organizations embracing a range of art forms have a higher likelihood of being more community-focused and willing to engage in innova-tive undertakings, thus creating a more diverse constituency (Cohen, 2014). Their potential for youth engagement holds tremendous promise, particularly in com-munities with few performing arts organizations and school systems where there are limited or no opportunities to engage in these activities.

Grodach (2011) sees tremendous value for neighborhood arts organizations helping residents enhance their social and human capital (artist incubator). But this is not without challenges, since these organizations cannot be all things to all people, particularly in communities with high needs. Neighborhood institutions cannot accommodate all art forms because each type often requires a unique con-figuration, and, by necessity, certain types of art will be emphasized over others.

Evaluating Youth Community Practice

Evaluation and evidence-based practice has re-emphasized the importance of youth community practitioners being able to document their results in a man-ner that facilitates external scrutiny that will influence policies and the fund-ing that follows (Sullivan, 2016). The youth practice field is complex, and the introduction of new activities, particularly those that are participant-driven, has increased the challenges in developing evaluation methods that do justice to the field's impact.

PYD's popularity has garnered its share of evaluation and research articles, reports, and books, and this has fostered increased funding from governmental and private foundations as the academy has achieved greater prominence in shaping this field through research and publication of scholarly material (Campbell, Trzesniewski, Nathaniel, Enfield, & Erbstein, 2013). This increasing attention fostered the creation of a cadre of academic and practitioner advocates and the need for youth organizations to establish relationships with the academy to attract funding.

Exciting and innovative evaluation approaches have emerged to garner greater and more nuanced understanding of how this field is impacting various spheres in the lives of youth (Deane & Harré, 2014; Lopez, Yoder, Brisson, Lechuga-Pena, & Jenson., 2015; Maposa & Louw-Potgieter, 2014). Social media provided an attractive method for reaching audiences after performances (Bernstein, 2011), allowing a broader reach beyond the immediate performance and strengthening the possibility for longitudinal evaluation and research.

Performance ethnography transforms theatre from a source of entertainment to one that educates and is conducive of reflective research (Oberg, 2008). Youth have assumed a more participatory and decision-making role in helping to shape and carry out these research and evaluation efforts and have introduced much-needed innovations (Bradley, Deighton, & Selby, 2004; Fine, 2012; Flores, 2007). The authenticity of these efforts is closely tied to active participation and decision-making.

Social media plays into youth strengths concerning technology. These advances do not mean, however, that tensions and challenges have not emerged in questioning many different aspects of this field about how it has been conceptualized, its value base, and the focus of how research has been conducted. Lerner, Lerner, et al. (2015) call for multimethod integration, including ideographic and nomothetic perspectives, to fully grasp PYD scholarship.

Yohalem and Wilson-Ahlstrom (2010, p. 350) comment on the challenges that the rapid youth development expansion has caused in the field: "The rapid expansion of the field and the potential of programs to contribute to child and youth development have made defining what high quality programs look like and learning how to improve program quality key challenges facing the field." Rapid expansion reflects excitement and a desperate need for a new model or direction.

Efforts to develop a model of practice, a "unifying theory," and to standardize this practice have caused considerable concern in academic and practitioner circles regarding how this field has operationalized key factors and whether the results from one program and community are generalizable to other communities, particularly when discussing youth in highly vulnerable positions due to their racial/ethnic backgrounds.

Hamilton (2015a) is careful to remind us that youth development's origins came out of the practice field rather than the theoretical or empirical world. He highlights the questions researchers must address and that policy-makers must consider: what is important for practice, for youth, and, for that matter, the communities they live in? How can we best to foster practitioner and consumer participation in knowledge creation?

This stance has significance for how this field can unfold, expand, and evolve now and in the future, and whether it stays true to its original mission. Baldridge (2012) discusses the consequences that youth of color face in out-of-school programs that have embraced neoliberal indicators of what constitutes success, thus illustrating the importance of local circumstances dictating the measures of what is meaningful for youth in distressing situations.

Attention must also be paid to the knowledge that practitioners need to carry out their responsibilities in a manner that maximizes their time (Yohalem & Tseng, 2015). Translation, too, is a perennial challenge in youth and family practice settings (Freire, Perkinson, Morrel-Samuels, & Zimmerman, 2015) and is critical to advance the field of youth development (Hamilton, 2015*b*). There is a dramatic difference between taking a practice versus a research or academic point of view. A practice stance must have youth and practitioners setting the agenda and selecting the key questions that must be answered.

There is a prodigious political distinction: the questions asked often are different, and how one arrives at the answers is also different. The latter results in youth assuming a prominent role in how activities unfold and the key questions they want answered through an evaluation. When applied to the performing arts, youth assume an artistic direction role, which is usually an adult role.

Tensions emanating from a desire both to please funders and to meet youth on their own terms is a perennial concern in youth practice (Jones, 2014). The classic social work debate between cause and function comes to mind when addressing this tension. Can any one profession do without causing and experiencing considerable tension? The increasingly prominent role of youth in these efforts has increased these and other tensions (Conrad, Smyth, & Kendal, 2015).

Life is never a straight line; no one lives without experiencing bumps and significant detours along the road, and there are even periods when we do not make progress but actually lose ground. The trajectory of direct and indirect expressive and instrumental benefits derived from participation in PYD, too, is not a straight line with a predictable and constant upward trajectory (Larson & Tran, 2014, p. 1012), raising challenges for practitioners and evaluators to capture how and when benefits emerge and how to sustain them when they do occur:

> The papers suggest that relationships adults, hope, school engagement, participation in out-of-school programs, and intentional self-regulation can serve as mediators of positive development. Yet, a striking finding was that comparatively few youth in the study manifest a pattern of change marked by the coupling of increases in positive youth development and decreases in risk/problem behavior.

This observation should not be surprising since the same can be said about any age group. "Life is not a bowl of cherries."

The same conclusions can be made about other forms of youth practice. Youth performing arts evaluation must be sensitive to the vicissitudes of youth lives if it is to capture a realistic picture of the impact of participation. There are benefits for a participant's family and friends that often go under-researched and therefore unreported, and these must be captured.

Evaluating social justice-based interventions brings inherent social-political and methodological challenges, as one should expect. Dewhurst (2013) raises provocative and unnerving questions on how social justice is evaluated, with the answers having consequences for any youth practice seeking individual and social change as part of its mission:

> This question is closely related to the question about what constitutes social justice and is predicated on how people define social change. Is it about systemic shifts or attitudinal changes? Perhaps evaluation might best be viewed on a spectrum where social impact may fall anywhere from basic community building to codified policy change? If so, shall we base our evaluative methods on the intensions of the artists? Or on the stand-alone outcome of the work itself? Who determines when social justice has been achieved—the artists? Audience members? Policy-analysts or social workers?

These questions are not relegated to the confines of university or policy circles. The answers have social and political ramifications for social justice youth practice involving the performing arts. Having youth and practitioners debate these points has immediate and long-term consequences for youth practice.

Sherrod (2007, p. 61) offers observations concerning the fine-tuning of PYD. One point stands out as an example of progress, but much more progress is needed regarding peer/social networks because of their powerful influence on youth attitudes and behaviors:

> The diversity of assets also influences their measurement; the ease with which one can measure these different assets reliably and validly varies. The sole reliance to date on self-report to measure outcomes needs to be abandoned. There are easy objective measures for some assets and good psychometrically sound instruments for others. Youth's perception of the assets they hold and of those in their environment is quite important. However, we also need to be able to verify these perceptions, at least in some cases.

Evaluation efforts must be multifaceted and go beyond self-reports (qualitative), and this necessitates quantitative methods even though tapping youth voices and narratives is essential to evaluate PYD.

A broadening of evaluation foci and methods is required. Brooks-Gunn and Roth (2014) comment on how far advances in youth development theory have gone and set the context for future advances on measurement, evaluation, and awareness of contextual processes. Strachan and Davies (2015) provide an example of advances in youth development practice through the use of visual ethnography (photo-elicitation), PYD, and sports, thus introducing an innovative research method to youth practice and an activity not usually associated with visual ethnography.

Daykin et al. (2008) argue that performing arts and youth development research is still in its infancy and that the heterogeneity of the field makes synthesis impossible at this stage, but that this challenge should not stop local communities from embracing youth performing arts as the preferred vehicle for meeting local needs.

This book represents an attempt to assess the state of the field, with an understanding that its complexity is bound to make this task arduous. Kane (2014, p. 224) illustrates the value of dance and theatre and why they are attractive for youth practice:

> A multidisciplinary dance and theatre arts program geared for high school-aged youth can result in both short-term and the long-term outcomes for its students if it seeks to offer a life-changing peak experience as part of the arts training and performance process. By integrating a combination of dance, movement, theater, music, creative and reflective writing, as well as identity exploration and creative collaborations, performing arts programs can provide participants an experience that is truly transformative. In particular, such a program can help initiate and support meaningful mentoring and developmental relationships.

Kane's comprehensive view of the performing arts outlines ways that youth can benefit through participation. It also highlights the challenges that evaluators must face and surmount in capturing and assessing these types of ventures.

There are many different schools of thought on the "best" or most "sensitive" approach to evaluating arts intervention programs. King et al. (2015) advocate for a multifaceted qualitative approach (historical document analysis and interviews with key informants and staff members) to evaluation of the arts (Spiral Garden) and, in this case, the involvement of children with and without disabilities.

Keeney and Korza (2015) note that most arts-based organizations have limited capability to undertake evaluations. Establishing partnerships between arts and non-arts organizations to undertake evaluations may seem logical, but challenges remain (Keeney & Korza, 2015, p. 191): "Partnerships between arts and non-arts agencies may result in differing frameworks for evaluation, with divergent assumptions about success and measurement. . . . This can lead to the choice of only a few specific outcome measures."

Evaluating social justice community practice performing arts interventions must be multifaceted and must view youth and youth–adult experience from both conventional and unconventional perspectives, paying close attention to how power and autonomy are manifested in shaping perceptions and relationships (Kitchen, 2015). Engaging youth in these efforts is a signature component of social justice–based youth evaluation efforts. Youth programs are not required to have "social justice" in their titles in order to embrace a social justice stance, although this may make it easier to attract disengaged youth with strong social justice leanings.

Categorizing activities by taking into account individuals, parents, and families must also emphasize friendship characteristics and maximize the use of time and financial resources in recruiting and programming activities (Barnett, 2008). Categorizing also facilitates evaluation. This stance brings additional challenges in drawing conclusions across programs. Wright et al. (2013, p. 190) discuss the excitement and promise of participatory art and highlight the challenges for evaluating this practice and capturing the many nuances that contribute to making it exciting and meaningful:

> Experiences of participatory arts are interrelated in an ecology of practice that is iterative, relational, developmental, temporal and contextually bound. This means that questions of impact are contingent, and there is no one path that participants travel or single measure that can adequately capture the richness and diversity of experience.

A socioecological frame brings with it inherent challenges, but even more so with the performing arts, which introduce aesthetic quality as a means of judging a program's "worth" or "value," and this will refocus analysis.

The evaluation of performing arts practice focused on marginalized youth must embrace several key principles to meet their unique social and emotional needs while addressing ecological forces: (1) youth participants must play prominent roles in shaping and conducting evaluation endeavors (they must own the results), (2) cultural values and customs must be central to activities, (3) social justice must have a central role in shaping process and outcomes, (4) the impact on participants and audiences must be a part of any evaluation effort, and (5) the evaluation must seek to be inclusive of all types of youth, including youth with varying abilities and challenges, the undocumented (where applicable), and LGBTQ youth.

The arts are a vehicle for expressing creativity and addressing social justice issues, and they can also present new opportunities for innovation involving research, particularly when actively involving youth in shaping how research questions and processes unfold (Osei-Kaft, 2013). These participatory approaches are community-centered and bring sufficient flexibility into their design to capture local circumstances and nuances.

Bagley and Castro-Salazar (2012) point out the potential influential role that critical arts can play in addressing undocumented youth, as in the case of those with Mexican backgrounds. Latino histories and experiences can find a vehicle for expression through the performing arts, which have universal appeal and long histories throughout the world.

These principles are best carried out with research approaches that are based on the principles of participation, power-sharing, and mutual respect, representing a particular sociopolitical stance based on youth operative reality. Participatory and ethnographic research are particularly attractive methods for researching and evaluating social justice arts and performing arts interventions (Delgado, 2015; Mienczakowski, 2009; Paris & Winn, 2013; White, Shoffner, Johnson, Knowles, & Mills, 2012).

These research methods pay attention to ethnicity and race in shaping world-views and behavior, thus lending themselves to uncovering social injustice issues by listening to the voices of those most impacted by these social forces—in this case, marginalized urban youth. These methods also uncover the most appropriate immediate and long-range targets for social change efforts from a youth perspective.

Communities consist of different youth subgroups, and programs should target these subgroups, too. Considerations rather than principles guiding social justice youth practice, but these five are essential (Delgado, 2016b). The incorporation of cultural values and community participation take on special prominence with youth of color because they rarely can learn about their racial/ethnic history and culture within schools and are also limited in assuming leadership roles within these systems (Sy, Greaney, Nigg, & Hirose-Wong, 2015).

Strengths and assets are not all of equal importance, and environmental circumstances will need to dictate how interventions are structured to enhance select personal and community asset resources (Sherrod, 2007). Assets are not static, with some increasing or decreasing in significance over time. The tailoring of youth development activities and goals targeting participant strengths and local assets are needed (Delgado & Humm-Delgado, 2013). The dynamic nature of assets makes it hard to build initiatives to be implemented too far into the future because of the time that elapses between an assessment and delivering a social program. Human beings do not stand still; nor do communities.

Why should youth practice actively seek to involve culture, a difficult, controversial, and challenging construct to measure, as a prominent core in shaping programming? The arts are often considered an attractive vehicle through which the culture of people, their experiences, and identity can be explained and shared with those outside of the group in a manner that makes such facts easier to receive and understand (Goldbard, 2006; Semán & Vila, 2012; Sidford, 2011). Youth performing arts can be a vehicle through which culture and self-identity can play a central role in shaping its incorporation into the activities.

The emergence of "diasporic youth identities" captures the multiple identities and complex narratives of self that transplanted youth face in navigating new locales and results in different identities emerging in new places (Ní Laoire, 2016). The performing arts can help capture for audiences why and how this is done in a manner that can be more easily received than a written report. Reports are very much a staple in middle- and upper-middle class communities, but they hold very little sway in low-income and/or newcomer communities. Practitioners may find that they need to have a performance for one constituency and a report for another.

Evaluation of audience takeaways (expressive and instrumental) will find a prominent role in the youth performing arts. Edelman and Šorli (2015) examined the value system of audiences at theatre and dance performances and found that amateur theatre elicited from the audience an emphasis on loyalty and community cohesion, while professional audiences valued quality of performance. This perspective has implications for youth performing arts evaluation in determining who are attracted to these performances and what about the performance is valued. Youth performance attendees seek to engender feelings of validation and hope. However, other motivations for attending will need to be elucidated.

Conclusion

How do we reach the nation's marginalized youth in a manner that is attractive to them and respectful, as well? How do we make our programs relevant to those who are most marginalized? The answers to these questions strike at the heart of why we engage in social justice youth practice, regardless of activity or program, and why we must think of adults as allies to youth in their struggles for social justice.

There are a set of core values guiding our answers and corresponding ethical challenges that are at play every day as we seek to enter the lives of marginalized youth within their organizations and communities. An explicit understanding of how values and ethics shape our involvement helps increase the likelihood that available resources are put to efficient and effective use. Section II of this book pays specific attention to the use of music, song, dance, and theatre.

SECTION II

Music, Song, Dance, and Theatre

Each of the following four chapters will consist of eight sections of varying lengths: (1) an introduction; (2) definitions; (3) a review of relevant literature, particularly as it relates to marginalized youth; (4) a summary of rewards or benefits; (5) a summary of challenges; (6) key research findings with implications for youth community practice; (7) implications for youth community practice; and (8) a conclusion. Although each section will be addressed as an individual unit, in reality there is a tremendous amount of overlap among them. Every effort will be made to highlight information relevant to each category as a way of minimizing overlap.

Each of the chapters has a section titled "Rewards and Benefits," and extra effort will be made to identify different and complementary material even though it is acknowledged that the performing arts share much in common. For instance, each performing art facilitates the exploration of identity and seeks to have youth further enhance their abilities to communicate both verbally and nonverbally. The chapters of Section II have a focused view on the performing arts, although other art forms can be interjected and often are.

6

Music

Introduction

Music permeates our entire lives; we rarely think twice about its presence and how it shapes our attitudes and feelings. We often make fun of "elevator music" but rarely question why it is there in the first place. Those who are poetically inclined can say a "life without music is life that is simply dull." The life stories of those who create music reflects how it shapes their lives and reverberates across their communities.

Music's impact is obvious when addressing youth-focused goals; music has a broad reach and can bring together disparate youth groups. Can we possibly separate youth from music? The answer is obviously "no," and using music as a central focus in youth practice fulfills this promise. Music is often referred to as a "lived" experience because of how it captures significant moments and a range of senses in dramatic and engaging fashion (Cohen, Silber, Sangiorgio, & Iadeluca, 2012).

Music's history and position within the pantheon of the performing arts is well established and offers youth of all backgrounds and abilities a range of choices on their primary instrument and type of music. Music appeals to youth of all ages and can accommodate any budget, making this performing art very attractive from a youth programming perspective and for its ability to bridge age spans (Hodkinson & Bennett, 2013). Few adults would not attest to the value of music in the lives of individuals and communities. The cultural roots of music, too, are well recognized and considered to be an instrumental part of ethnic and racially based cultures, with heavy nationalistic traditions reinforcing identity.

Youth culture always seems limited to latency and adolescence, and young children are simply overlooked, as if "culture" starts at a magical age point somewhere between latency and early adolescence. Campbell's (2010, p. 4) book *Songs in Their Hearts: Music and Its Meaning in Children's Lives* taps children's voices and provides comprehensive coverage on how music permeates children's expressive culture and lives:

> Clearly, music *happens* to children. Some of it may be hidden, untapped, and yet spinning within them. Yet much of it is "visible" and surely audible. It shows itself in songs they sing and in rhythms and pitched inflections of their play—on swings and slides; in the toy cars, wagons, and bicycles the ride; through the stories they enact with stuffed bears, dolls, and the imaginary drivers of their tiny cars; while engaged in video-gaming or at their Wii systems; and in the jump rope chants, hand-clapping rhymes, ball games and stick games, and ring and line games they play. Children think aloud through music.

Music permeates the lives of youth in countless ways (Laughey, 2006), and using music as a means of engaging youth is not a challenge for the youth practice field. The challenge is how to ground music culturally and from a social justice point of view.

Thinking of music and social justice community practice adds a much needed dimension to the work because of its appeal to school-aged youth who are marginalized and seeking relevance in their free-time activities. The concept of social justice and music can be framed from another perspective, one that seeks to understand why, in low-income and low-wealth school districts, music education is generally either not offered or is one of the first courses to get cut for budgetary reasons (Allsup & Shieh, 2012). This chapter highlights how music and social justice can be combined in urban youth practice.

Definition

Any definition of music is bound to cause scholars and practitioners great consternation. Music is not restricted to any particular setting, including youth justice settings (Daykin, De Viggiani, Pilkington, & Moriarty, 2013). Music must be contextualized for its social meaning and ramifications to be fully appreciated (Aprile, 2012). Music, simply put, is much more than just music. Fraser (2012), in discussing the spaces, politics, and cultural economies of electronic dance music, stresses how youth collaborate and work alongside each other, sharing ideas, emotions, and knowledge.

Macdonald's definition of community music (as quoted in Higgins, 2012, pp. 53–54) resonates with the way music in youth practice is viewed in this book because of its inclusiveness and emphasis on the significance on context:

> Community music involves musicians from any musical discipline working with groups of people to enable them to develop active and creative participation in Music. Community music is concerned with putting equal

opportunities into practice. Community music can happen in all types of community, whether based on place, institution, interest, age or gender group, and reflects the context in which it take place.

Macdonald does a wonderful job of placing this music within a context that invites interpretations and circumstances that introduce equal opportunity social justice without explicitly mentioning it.

It does not take a conceptual leap to associate music with urban youth. Music has been one of the most viable avenues for escape from dire social circumstances, with a plethora of role models to choose from over the past five decades illustrating success. Orchestra's conjure up images of a large musical ensemble and are rarely associated with youth or urban communities, but youth of color and other underrepresented youth can be a part of this musical experience if it is made available to them as an option (Heath, 2015). The Youth Orchestra of Los Angeles (YOLA) is an example of one such ensemble that incorporates all of the elements associated with an orchestra (Flenaugh, 2012).

Review of Relevant Literature (Focus on Marginalized Youth)

Why is music so important in our lives, and why is its absence deeply felt, although unknowingly so? Music can help youth face particularly difficult transitions, facilitating self-reflection or helping to elicit positive memories that can serve as a basis for engagement in activities with both current and future benefits (Lippman & Greenwood, 2012). Music can be significant in altering a present-day situation and setting the stage for a more promising future, especially if it can be tied to the development of life skills and the closing of the political divide (Brinner, 2009).

Music goes far beyond a narrow focus of being entertaining or of being a way to fill idle time. Such a stance would seriously miss the importance of music as an art form, with its countless benefits to those playing music and those listening to it (Levy & Byrd, 2011):

> Listening to music is an emotional and educational experience that has the potential to shape an individual's values, actions, and worldview . . .. Although it can be applied to virtually any subject area, critical reflection and discussion of music can especially complement courses related to the concept of social justice.

Participating in music with others (collective experience) results in youth having the potential to assume multiple roles such as listening, singing, playing, composing, and improvising together (McFerran, 2011). If we bring the audience into this experience, it connects performers to them in a special way.

Benedict and colleagues (Benedict, Schmidt, Spruce, & Woodford, 2013) argue that there has been a historically tense relationship between music education and social justice; opening up music education to a wider and more diverse audience necessitates that the music be grounded within the cultural and social backgrounds of those studying it if it is to help us achieve a just and humane society.

The power of music is very often taken for granted, and nowhere is this power more prevalent than when it is closely tied to a social injustice or a politically significant historical event, as in the case of this nation's Civil Rights Movement. The concept of music as resistance is not new, and it is well understood that music is a method for creating collectivity and giving voice to social justice (Kauzlarich, 2012). Hip-hop has been conceptualized as youth resistance (Porfilio, Gardner, & Roychoudhury, 2013), and resistance, oppression, and marginalized youth are closely associated (Collins & Bilge, 2016).

Music has been conceptualized as having the potential to be a culturally indigenous method for spreading knowledge and historical accounts and engaging in much needed praxis among those who are marginalized (Biggs-El, 2012; Urban, 2012). All of these elements can speak to social justice concerns and issues without forcing. Music can be organic. Music can be about learning and teaching. The paucity of Latino and African-American/Black music teachers makes it arduous for youth of color to find role models within schools and makes it necessary to reach outside school boundaries to find (DeLorenzo & Silverman, 2016).

Music plays an important but often overlooked role in the lives of youth (Hickey, 2009; Kerchner & Abril, 2009). Its role within the history of social work with groups can be traced to the birth of the profession (Kelley & Doherty, 2016). Music can play a key role in helping youth during particularly difficult social and emotional periods in their lives because of how it encourages retrospective and contemplative outlooks that can be quite distressing (Dowdy, 2012).

Miranda (2013) analyzed the role of music in adolescent development and identified three significant themes: (1) music influences important aspects of adolescent development, (2) music can represent either a protective and a risk factor, and (3) music can serve as a component in prevention and intervention. Music, when conceived as a collective experience focused on a major social concern, introduces the power of the group in shaping transformative experiences.

Campbell (2015) argues that music is much ingrained in children's culture from very early in their lives, so it is not a subject that is new to them and it can help them achieve various instrumental and expressive goals. The same can be said for singing. Children's singing and playing go well together, bringing a dimension of fun so that each reinforces the other and serving as a foundation from which we can associate singing with a pleasurable moment as we mature (Countryman, Gabriel, & Thompson, 2015).

Wang (2010) describes how aboriginal youth became empowered through a hip-hop music youth development project, illustrating its potential to reach across conventional urban settings and hemispheric boundaries: "An irrepressibly popular musical phenomenon, hip-hop is close to spoken word and focuses on lyrics with a message, reviving local traditions of song that tell histories, counsel listeners, and challenge participants to outdo one another in clever exchanges."

Wang's cultural perspective reinforces Campbell's claim and illustrates the potential power of music and song to bring together youth from different backgrounds in pursuit of a common goal and activity. Origin-centric orientation builds upon cultural awareness, with Afrocentric being a popular example and a counterbalance to Eurocentric views of music. Hip-hop can be conceptualized as cultural capital (Adjapong & Emdin, 2015). It should not be a surprise that music and culture continue to exert influence across the life span. Music evolves and shapes youth identity as children mature, taking into account culture factors (Halverson, Lowenhaupt, Gibbons, & Bass, 2009; Hodkinson & Bennett, 2013) including the life span (Bennett, 2013, 2015).

Music, youth, and culture are inseparable and worldwide, highlighting their interconnectivity (De Kloet, 2010; Dimitriadis, 2008; Gazzah, 2008). Adult conceptions of what constitutes music and culture must be expansive and based upon youth voices. This may appear simple at first sight, but adult conceptions of what we think of as music and culture will be tested.

Tinsley, Wilson, and Spencer (2013, p. 83) eloquently outline the vast parameters of music and its potential as a vehicle for achieving a variety of goals, including giving voice to social justice for urban youth:

> Music is an essential component of life for many and represents a critical vehicle for meaning and self-representation. As a specific art form, it communicates thoughts, feelings, reactions, and perspectives about noteworthy issues. For many, it allows for the relief of stress; it encourages celebration among others; and for some, it serves as a soundtrack for social protest.

The proverb "music soothes the savage soul" captures the magic of music, which can be transformative when it successfully captures social injustices, as in protest music.

The role of protest music/songs goes far beyond entertainment, and its power rests in how it captures a social condition and brings together the power of the collective (Blake, 2012; Opara, 2012). Irish folk singer Frank Harte (quoted in Moloney, 2005) brings an added and often overlooked dimension to song: "Those in power write the history, while those who suffer write the songs." History is written by elites, with those suffering the consequences of historical events having few outlets for sharing since there is an emphasis on the written word as represented in historical accounts in history books. Songs are within the grasp of the non–formally educated, providing an outlet for expressing a collective history not shared by the elites.

Hip-hop music and culture is one of the most significant urban youth arts movements to emerge over the past three decades, and hip-hop captures the sociopolitical dimensions discussed above (Baszile, 2009; Love, 2015; Low, 2011; Veltre & Hadley, 2012). Hip-hop education and activities are not restricted to select organizational settings and can be found throughout a community, providing programming flexibility and broadening its reach (Hill & Petchauer, 2012). Hip-hop is international, and this attests to the power of music as a mechanism for social protest that crosses national borders (Ballivían & Herrera, 2012; Bischoff, 2012; Hammett, 2012; Maira & Shihade, 2012; Nzinga, 2012; Skinner, 2012; Thannoo, 2012).

Hip-hop does not enjoy universal appeal among urban youth—not to mention adults—and efforts to integrate it into programming and curriculum as a means of attracting and engaging youth have raised questions about the value of these efforts (Gosa & Fields, 2012). Deconstructing hip-hop messages helps urban youth develop critical analytical skills that can be the basis for praxis (Basham, 2015; Chung, 2007). Stereotyping youth must be guarded against; they are not monolithic, and the more we can individualize them, the higher the likelihood of tapping their strengths and meeting their needs.

Hip-hop culture is usually thought of consisting of four different elements (rapping, breakdancing, graffiti art, and deejaying), with each element having particular appeal to different youth segments (Brown & Kwakye, 2012). Hip-hop as music provides urban youth with an outlet for lyrics or narratives that resonate in their lives and those of their friends and loved ones (Tinsley et al., 2013).

Gitonga and Delport (2015) explored how hip-hop music helps shape identity by providing the space to encourage exploration of self, including initiation of transformation and agency, and using youth's own reality and language to do so. Engaging in this reflection also creates agency and corresponding empowerment and resistance.

Butler's (2010) book *Let's Get Free: A Hip-Hop Theory of Justice* provides a well-researched and scholarly connection between hip-hop's central oppression messages and key scholarly work on social justice, illustrating its particular appeal among youth of color. Pulido (2009, p. 67) argues that youth of color use hip-hop music in multiple and overlapping ways, increasing the significance of this art but also broadening its appeal:

> [E]ngaging hip hop music as both a pedagogy that centers the perspectives of people of color and a framework to examine daily life. Specifically, youth used hip hop discourse to make sense of the ways race operates in their daily lives; to more broadly understand their position in the US racial/ethnic hierarchy; and to critique traditional schooling for failing to critically incorporate their racialized ethnic/cultural identities within official school dialogues and curricula in empowering ways. Succinctly conveyed by one youth, the theme "Music fit for us minorities," explores the ways that students link hip hop music to the disempowering cultural identities they encounter about Latinas/os, the structures that marginalize them, and to broader systems of inequity.

Youth of color can use music as pedagogy and as a sociopolitical interpretive lens to socially navigate and challenge the racialization and criminalization in their lives (Bischoff, 2012). Music as a sociopolitical instrument (no pun intended) facilitates its use in social justice youth practice, providing youth with an alternative way of expressing their feelings and concerns.

Criticism has been leveled at hip-hop music, particularly from adults, focused especially on how some of the music portrays male–female relationships and violence. These critiques have been generalized and failed to take into account other mediating factors such as family, religious, and spiritual beliefs (Bryant, 2008). No music/song genre can be encapsulated into a simplistic analysis, and this also applies to hip-hop (Brooks, Daschuk, Poudrier, & Almond, 2015; Leland, 2016).

When the prefix "critical" is associated with hip-hop, it helps to ensure that this musical form embraces themes of liberation and social justice, and, at the same time, it resonates with the listeners of this music. Hip-hop can go beyond fulfilling an entertainment role, providing uplifting inspiration rather than reinforcing negative themes (Clemons & Clemons, 2013). The critical prefix is further reinforced when the artist looks like the listeners, bringing a high degree of realism to the artist–listener/audience interaction. Sharing common narratives related to social oppression and using language that captures these experiences reinforces the message.

Rap provides a context or window through which to understand youth, as well as being a vehicle for achieving social justice (Collins & Bilge, 2016). Travis, Jr. (2013, p. 139) sees tremendous value in capturing the power of rap music to act as a window to better understand urban youth and to develop a youth intervention strategy for engaging them by tapping into their interests:

> [R]ap music is a discourse in lifespan development. Rap music's developmental narratives may be used by practitioners, parents and researchers. The narratives exist within a framework and model that (a) provides a template for better understanding these narratives and (b) positions this understanding for use as a tool to promote and research positive change strategies for individuals and the communities that they value.

Travis points out a that adults can understand the power of narrative's role in appreciating youth of color if we take the time and make the effort to listen to the lyrics as a narrative or story. Such a step may prove challenging because of the words used and how they are strung together to make rhythm and convey a message or story.

Smith (2012) discusses the use of a pilot project that explored the use of popular music, songwriting, technology, music, and video production with urban "at-risk" youth and found that participation resulted in youth developing a positive group identity, having a sense of control over their creative process, and experiencing a "safe space and place" for them to channel their creative energy. Datoo and Chagani (2011, p. 22) note how the performing arts involve multiple types of intelligences: "Performance arts offer a powerful representational mode to express and address individual and collective self and identity. It involves variety of senses; kinesthetic and visual intelligences, that influence our emotional intelligence."

The performing arts capture many different media that can be used concomitantly, increasing the power of a performance and opening the door for contributions from youth with different talents. Music, song, and visual media, which often involve dance, can be integrated, as evidenced by the popularity of music videos to promote music and song among youth (Subrahmanyam & Smahel, 2010), which led to the creation of the MTV channel in the early 1980s.

One musical performance that may be new to many readers—it was to this author—is drum and bugle corps. It is worth commenting on a musical act that may have strong regional influences and features a strong teamwork component (Vance, 2014). This performance not only entails music, but also marching, which is not easy to accomplish. Drum and bugle competitions illustrate the popularity and level of organization of this music in certain circles (Odello, 2016), although lack of familiarity is probably very common overall (Odello, 2016, p. 241):

> The performances of youth drum corps in the United States reference both the history of the activity and the past practices of individual ensembles. These references create an insular form of performance where only cultural insiders who are familiar with both drum corps tradition and the performance histories of individual organizations are able to fully understand a performance. . . . Participants disagree on how large a role tradition should play in shaping these performances, so performance choices become both aesthetic and political statements.

Drum and bugle corps meet a niche and show the diversity and power of music and how it responds to local culture and local circumstances, even if they may not hold prominent positions within the music world in certain regions of the country (Ekstrom, 2015).

Marching bands are ubiquitous and are familiar across all regions of the country and among all demographic groups, and they, too, can be incorporated into youth practice (Adderley, 2009). It is hard to imagine a parade without marching bands of various types. Marching bands, which are always considered an afterschool activity, can be either a service or an entertainment. They, too, can bring a social justice message when these bands are incorporated into local social protests.

This power to create mood change and corresponding behavior strikes at the essence of music's transformative potential (Calvert, 2013). Moore (2009) notes that Western Africa and African-American music often integrates music with singing, playing instruments, and dancing.

Trevarthen and Malloch (2000, p. 3) discuss music's power to influence musicians and listeners at many conscious and unconscious levels, highlighting why it wields such sway in people's lives:

> Music making is a human activity that communicates motives—the underlying impulses for action, by which experience is gained, and which are accompanied by feelings. Music evokes narratives of experience, based on our innate

ability to share the passing of expressive "mind time," an ability that may be called "musicality," which is inseparable from the impulse to move with anticipation of rhythmic sensory consequences and varied emotional evaluations. Communicative musicality is the source of the music therapeutic experience and its effects.

Music is much more than using an instrument to make a sound. Music has the potential to uplift the spirits of a person as well as having the potential to put someone into a pensive, if not sad, state of mind. When done as a group, music's collective impact on performers and attendees only increases its power.

Music has the potential for social interventions to address a range of problems, and this should be acknowledged because of its effectiveness in accomplishing this goal (Robb, Burns, & Carpenter, 2011). The popularity of music therapy is a case in point (Allen, 2005; Bunt & Stige, 2014; DeCarlo & Hockman, 2004; Forrest, 2014; Thaut & Hoemberg, 2014). When viewed as an activity that is not "problem-focused," music is destigmatized, thus increasing the likelihood that it can be empowering and thereby lending this performing art to social justice youth practice.

Using music as a social intervention necessitates that we have a comprehensive understanding of its role across the life spans of the marginalized. Our understanding of the importance of music among very young children of color in their homes is very limited. This knowledge gap has implications for youth practice music if we do not have a historical context upon which to build. This gap is not limited to children of color and can exist among all children (Hari, 2009).

Advancements in our understanding of the cultural and social meaning of music are largely due to the work of ethnomusicologists, folklorists, sociologists, anthropologists, and educators, a relatively small but multidisciplinary list who consider the importance of music in people's lives (Campbell, 2010). Adding youth practitioners to this illustrious list brings a new and exciting dimension that emphasizes music as a social justice intervention.

Music is usually associated with an expert playing of instruments, although such an observation does a disservice to this performing art. The popularity of digital music production and performance has provided an emerging window for engaging youth and serving as a vehicle to teach a variety of academic-related subjects (Brader & Luke, 2013).

Music gives expression to both hopes and fears (Kiruthu, 2014). The role of an instrument, as in the case of Violins of Hope, as described in the following quote, brings to life the close associations among social justice narrative, instrument, and music in a manner that is inspirational (http://www.violinsofhopecle.org/):

> Each instrument has a capacity to create music that has the power to transport individuals to another place and space. Instruments go from being an object to an extension of oneself. "Violins of Hope," a Cleveland exhibition and concert, illustrates the power of a musical instrument, in this case violins: "For

Jews enduring utter despair and unimaginable evil during the Holocaust, music offered haven and humanity. The strains of a beloved song supplied solace, even if only for a few moments. The chords also provided a vital reminder that even the most brutal regime could not rob them of their faith. No matter what, their souls could be free. In some cases, the ability to play the violin spared Jewish musicians from more grueling labors or even death. Nearly 50 years ago, Amnon Weinstein heard such a story from a customer who brought in an instrument for restoration. The customer survived the Holocaust because his job was to play the violin while Nazi soldiers marched others to their deaths. When Weinstein opened the violin's case, he saw ashes. He thought of his own relatives who had perished, and was overwhelmed. He could not bring himself to begin the project. By 1996, Weinstein was ready. He put out a call for violins from the Holocaust that he would restore in hopes that the instruments would sound again.

Although Violins of Hope captures a narrative that has nothing to do with urban youth, it shows the power of music to encompass more than a performance and to share with the world a narrative that must not be forgotten. It also shows the potential for music to transcend time and space, as well as addressing a social justice theme(s).

Musical heritage and nostalgia have emerged in the literature to provide a window into how music can play a role in shaping generational identity, a different perspective on identity formation (Brandellero & Janssen, 2014; Van Der Hoeven, 2014). Musical heritage for newcomer groups has deep roots in their homelands, with youth straddling their homeland and a new land in ways that may separate them from the cultural heritage of their parents. Music targeting youth in this situation takes on added cultural and social significance.

Roberts and Cohen (2014) examined the role and significance of social memory and its manifestation in musical heritage through an appreciation of the cultural and social significance of popular music and of efforts to classify it. The authors developed a three-stage framework for classification: (1) officially authorized popular music heritage, (2) self-authorized popular music heritage, and (3) undocumented popular music heritage. Each brings forth a series of serious arguments and captures the sociopolitical considerations of different groups.

It is appropriate to end this section by discussing music in the African-American community. Moore (2009, p. 279) notes the totality of the oral tradition and musical experience involving African-Americans and examines how gospel music and jazz are instrumental in making performances both transformative and part of a deeply profound historical and cultural context:

In the African American culture, music permeates every facet of life, as it does in West Africa, its ethnic ancestor. It functions similar to Gioia's House of Music. Whenever there is a gathering, appropriate music and dance are performed. Consequently, when African Americans gather for worship, whether in church, concert hall, a home, or the street corner of a community, singing and movement (dance) are a part. When available and depending on the venue, instruments become a part of the performance . . .. Otherwise, the body provides the instrumental accomplishment through polyrhythmic hand-clapping and foot-stomping.

Creating a climate that induces participation at a primal as well as a collective level enhances the transformative power of the performance experience. When the performance transpires within a sacred space, it enhances the impact of these songs and musical performances.

Rewards and Benefits

Any comprehensive assessment of youth benefits derived from participation in music-focused youth practice programs will be difficult to arrive at simply because of the vastness of this arena. But this task is essential if we are to move forward in this field and set the stage for evaluation and research substantiating the benefits of engaging in music programming and the lasting nature of such benefits. Benefits cannot be time-limited, with those extending over a lengthy period of time—preferably a lifetime—holding greater significance than those that are temporary to the participation period and that disappear once youth stop performing.

Participation benefits can be extensive. Cain, Lakhani, and Istvandity (2016) found in their literature review on a participatory music program for marginalized youth that participants experienced increased school attendance, self-esteem, cultural empathy, confidence, feelings of empowerment, and healthy nutrition. Any one of these benefits can transfer to other realms in the life of youth. Clift (2012) notes that the arts and health ` face challenges in moving toward building a "progressive body of knowledge" that will set a foundation for future studies.

1. Cultural Grounding. Music has often been referred to as the universal language (math has also been referred to in a similar manner) for very good reason. We do not have to be deeply knowledgeable about a musical rendition to appreciate its aesthetic and moving qualities. Obtaining a historical understanding of its origins brings insight that cannot be obtained from a history book or listening to someone share their experiences in attending a performance. Understanding music's cultural grounding helps youth appreciate their cultural heritage.

Mexican music is easily recognizable in this country, and this recognition is not restricted to the Southwest. The increasing significance of Cinco de Mayo celebrations (Mexican's day of independence from France) is closely associated with its music and cultural symbols and very much ingrained in the national fabric. (Cinco de Mayo was originally appropriated by the alcohol industry to provide greater opportunities for alcohol consumption [Delgado, 2017; Hayes-Bautista, 2012].)

Mexican culture is transmitted through its music, and youth have been exposed to it throughout their lives, so integrating music into a cultural grounding and pride program provides another avenue through which to teach history and traditions while providing a counter-narrative to the assaults that Mexican-origin youth face in this society that integrates social justice in a highly engaging manner (Macías, 2008).

2. Connected Disruption and the Building of Bridges. Urban centers are growing in diversity, and youth community programs are in propitious positions to help build bridges between different segments seeking to find their places within these communities. "Connected disruption" is a concept that is gaining in saliency and captures the barriers that exist between groups occupying the same places within these communities (Harrell & Bond, 2006). In a discussion of music's benefits, it is only fitting to identify building bridges as a theme in breaking down interpersonal barriers.

Music can be a vehicle that reaches across groups within a community and in a manner that is nonthreatening and highly engaging. Hayes (2007) describes the use of a GLBT chorus as a mechanism for bridging community divides and educating audiences about their lives. Bradley (2006) also uses a youth choir (Mississauga Festival Youth Choir) to bridge racial and ethnic divides.

3. Bridging Intergenerational Divides. Music can bridge intergenerational divides that are only getting wider because we live in an age-segregated society where few institutions have the potential to embrace all age groups (Flora & Faulkner, 2007). We generally do not associate generational divides with urban communities, and that is a failing in any programming. Youth programming, too, can be faulted for furthering this divide. Music can bring together disparate groups, and age differences can be minimized.

Darrow et al. (Darrow, Johnson, Ollenberger, & Miller, 2001) describe the value of an intergenerational choir (bringing music and singing together) performance on adolescent and older adult audience attitudes. Price's (2011) edited book, *The Black Church and Hip Hop Culture: Toward Bridging the Generational Divide*, brings together the Black Church and popular hip-hop to provide an innovative view of how to break down generational differences in the African-American/ Black community. Haskett's (2013) analysis of the historical development of Phoenix's The Desert Winds Community Steel Orchestra, a form of music that has generally gone unstudied, illustrates how a youth–adult divide can be minimized through music.

Conclusion

Music appeals across the life cycle, and it is not unusual to have music genres associated with particular life stages and youth subgroups. Even within genres that is a range, making generalizations arduous and misleading. There is general agreement that music has the potential to meet a variety of needs and be socially transformative. When transformative, it causes controversy because it challenges the status quo.

This chapter highlighted a range of music from gospel, choir, social protest, and hip-hop. No practitioner can be expected to be an "expert" in all music types. Having musical abilities is as important as having athletic ability with sports and film and video expertise with those favoring this medium (Mitchell & de Lange, 2012). Enlisting those with requisite competencies to fill in the "gaps" in competencies within organizations is a skill set worth developing. Youth practitioners then become social brokers, matching youth interests with performing arts resources.

7

Song

Introduction

Separating music from song might be considered misguided and a fool's errand because many consider the two one and the same. In this book, however, I discuss them as two separate performing arts. The discussion of hip-hop in Chapter 6 illustrates how music and song can be inseparable from a social justice perspective.

It is possible to sing and dance without music and to simply have music as a performing art unto itself. It is also possible to sing (hum) without using words, bringing an even greater range of possibilities to this activity, including engaging those without vocal gifts to also participate, but a social justice message will require words to resonate and further enhance the singing experience.

If we can sing in the rain, where and when can we not sing? Singing can be done with or without accompanying music, bringing tremendous flexibility in cost, preparation, and site selection as to when and where it transpires. Those attending worship services where music and song are instrumental parts of the experience can attest to the attractiveness of a well-planned service.

Singing is not restricted to those who are truly talented or to any age group. That is one of the wonderful dimensions of song: it is welcoming of all regardless of their talent. One can sing by oneself or as part of a group or choir. When done as part of a group activity, song introduces a set of dynamics that makes the collective experience that much more memorable. Very young children can learn language through singing, too (Kultti, 2013).

With the exception of team sports, a collectivist view of the performing arts introduces an often overlooked aspect of youth practice: ensemble performances are a collective effort and offer opportunities for youth to engage in activities that necessitate constant feedback, aural and visual signals, body movements, anticipation and reaction, gestures, and eye contact to reinforce the group experience (Goodman, 2002). This experience parallels that found in team sports, which often emphasizes group over individual performance. Individual performance stands outs out when it occurs but not at the expense of the members of the group. This requires a very different level of thinking and behaving.

Singing can occur in a variety of settings and may even involve performing with strangers (Wei, 2013). Song does not require music, but there is no disputing that it is enhanced when singing accompanies music, with each giving greater meaning to the other. Singing is an activity that does not require an outlay of funds and lessons, and it is not restricted to any particular geographical or organizational locale.

Song, too, can be a vehicle for transmitting cultural values and customs in an inclusive manner, thus further adding to the importance of cultural traditions, many of which are usually accompanied by music (Kiruthu, 2014). Songs are definitely storytelling, and they are even more moving and memorable when telling a story about a people or group and social injustice (Pitzer, 2013). One can see the potential of song acting as a kind of "glue" for other performing arts.

Studies of singing and children have enjoyed considerable popularity in the scholarly literature. Those with scholarly interests in children/youth and singing will be able to find ample material to meet their needs. An extensive review of research on children's singing reveals the importance of matching the level of teaching to the abilities of learners, particularly as this relates to pitch and timbre (Hedden, 2012).

Definition

Various forms of singing exist, and the vastness of this field can seem overwhelming to practitioners and academics alike, making an encompassing definition difficult. This richness allows this performing art to accommodate youth interests that can range from conventional to unconventional styles. Youth may engage in various types of singing since youth programming does not have to focus on one type.

Several types of singing will be touched on to capture the breadth of song and its potential for use in urban youth practice because of how these song forms tap cultural traditions and bring together youth from different ethnic and racial backgrounds. Special attention will be paid to choir/collective efforts because of how they require the development of skill sets that reinforce a group experience.

There are numerous definitions of song and singing. I have purposefully selected a very succinct definition of song/singing that captures the ubiquitous nature of song and singing (Urban Dictionary, n.d.): "The act of using ones voice to produce musical sounds, often with the use of words." It is very easy to memorize this definition, but delving into its meaning and scope will not prove easy.

List (1963) notes that song, like speech, has several distinctive characteristics that highlight its universal qualities across cultures, making it a popular activity for reaching youth from varying backgrounds: it is (1) vocally produced, (2) linguistically meaningful, and (3) melodic. These qualities open the door for variability to take into account culture and local circumstances. Appert (2015) illustrates this relationship and discusses "hardcore" rap songs from the 1990s, noting that rap conflates "singing" as a melodic vocal practice with "singing" being performatively affirming, bridging interconnecting historical and present-day issues of power and oppression.

Review of Relevant Literature (Focus on Marginalized Youth)

Reviewing literature on singing and youth community programming encounters the same challenges as the other performing arts discussed in this book. When this review is specifically focused on marginalized youth, it is unmistakable that singing has an important role to play in helping these youth navigate difficult terrain and even thrive under the right conditions. There are certain forms of song and singing worth noting.

Folk songs are often rooted in the history of a people to capture an experience. They have been used to teach musical reading and writing skills at the elementary level and performance repertoire (choral and instrumental) at the advanced level, and used as a means of encouraging personal and cultural expression (Adams, 2013).

Of prime importance to social justice programming, songs in the African-American tradition of spirituals, gospel, and blues epitomize the role and power of song in giving voice to oppression and marginalization (Clemons & Clemons, 2013; King, Clardy, & Ramos, 2014; Radano, 2016). These songs have social meanings that transcend conventional boundaries of singing and illustrate the power of this activity for all age groups, and more so when singing is viewed as collective expression (Pascale, 2013).

Singing can involve a variety of singers. Choir singing brings personal and social benefits for singers and taps the power of the collective experience. Einarsdottir and Gudmundsdottir (2016), in a study of amateur choral singers, found that personal enjoyment of singing and a positive and conducive social atmosphere were the most significant factors in motivating choral singing. They consider choral singing the most popular art performance, particularly in Western countries, because ordinary people are able to create music without formal music education as a prerequisite.

Choral singing has appeal across the entire life cycle (Southcott & Joseph, 2013). Kivnick and Lymburner (2009) describe the success of CitySongs, an out-of-school program in an inner-city locale and premised on social justice principles addressed through a youth choir. The intergenerational potential is far greater with singing when compared to music or dance, although this is subject to debate.

Youth of all backgrounds can be attracted to choirs, although males may experience some hesitancy that requires specific outreach (Abrahams, 2012; Freer, 2009). This hesitancy is not restricted to singing: O'Neill, Pate, and Liese

(2011) note that girls are more likely than boys to engage in dance as an activity. Efforts to be inclusive often necessitate special endeavors to achieve this goal for all marginalized groups. Youth with various kinds of disabilities also can engage in singing, thus helping them achieve valuable social skills (Vaiouli, Grimmet, & Ruich, 2015).

Social protest songs carry a unique perspective and have the capacity to remain in one's memory because of how well they tie together a moment in time, an event, relationships, crowds, and the emotional climate of the time (DeJaeghere & McCleary, 2010; Peddie, 2006). Protest songs carry an explicit political message, making them particularly attractive when viewed from a social justice perspective (DePass, 2012). Bensimon (2012) discusses the sociology of collective singing during "intense moments" of social protest, concluding that it generates morale, vents negative emotions, strengthens group solidarity, provides spiritual transcendence experiences, and fosters hope and empowerment.

Rewards and Benefits

Tshabalala and Patel (2010, p. 73) identify the multiple benefits that youth derive from this performing art: "Music was experienced as uplifting and transforming. A 'sense of connection' was a common response emerging from their involvement in the group, in praise and worship, and the music." Spiritual singing also provides a forum for learning and exercising leadership skills within a supportive environment (Kleinerman, 2010) and in an institution that is well trusted and associated with social justice.

Hall (2014) found singing benefits to be of far-ranging social, cultural, and emotional significance. Flores-Gonzalez, Rodriguez, and Rodriguez-Muniz (2006) describe the importance of providing Chicago's Latino (predominantly Puerto Rican) youth with a community place and space (Batey Urbano) for exploring their culture and for undertaking community social action (fighting gentrification) through the use of hip-hop (hearing and collectively sharing their voices); this promotes self-awareness (developing an understanding and pride) that leads to social awareness and a search for social justice.

Youth, in addition to reclaiming their history and culture, also seek to enhance their strengths. The example of Batey Urbano could easily have found a home in the chapter on music but was placed here instead, thus serving as an example of how song and music are interrelated and the difficulty of separating the two. Three of the most important benefits of song are listed here.

1. **Providing a Collective Voice/Identity.** A key theme found throughout this book is the potential of the performing arts to generate a collective identity that builds on goals, processes, and an explicit embrace of a search for a just future (Datoo & Chagani, 2011, p. 22): "Performance arts offer a powerful representational mode to express and address individual and collective self and identity."

Bada (2014, p. 142) discusses the arts and Chicago's Mexican community and how singing and music often fall outside of conventional agency programming and thereby miss an opportunity of using a vehicle that can help create a collective identity: "Informal practice—such as singing with a mariachi band at a family gathering . . . often fall outside traditional nonprofit and commercial arts experiences, but occupy a significant place in the social infrastructure of Mexican migrant communities. These practices help to build individual and collective identity, bond Mexican nationals within Chicago and between Chicago and Mexico, and bridge Mexican immigrants with other US-born groups." Collective voice and identity become sources of strength among marginalized youth by providing an opportunity to learn about their cultural heritage.

Martin's (2013) study of a youth choir found that participation provided a constructive outlet for singing but also served as a vehicle for youth cultural identity construction and increased resiliency. Mutual engagement and support obtained through singing as a group also provides a shared and affirming experience (Whitaker, 2016).

2. Sharing a Story of Hope. Singing can inspirational in a manner unlike that of other performing art. Generating a story with conviction, symbols, and emotion is quite powerful for youth who have an abundance of energy and feelings that seek a positive outlet, particularly from a collective perspective. Singing can be an individual endeavor, but its collective aspects bring the power of the group to this art form.

When songs convey a social justice narrative, they take on significance because they connect youth from different ethnic and racial backgrounds and give meaning to a shared lived experience (Barz, 2014; Nasir, 2015). DeCarlo (2013) has proposed singing (in this instance rap) as a therapeutic group technique that taps the power of song and narrative to achieve therapeutic goals. Sharing a story through a collective process reinforces that story and its meaning in a way that individual singing or song would have a difficult time accomplishing.

3. Providing a Vehicle for Civic Engagement. Civic engagement has often been narrowly defined as volunteerism involving a particular cause. Singing can be thought of as civic engagement when it has this engagement as a central goal and seeks to entertain and inform a particular audience. Civic engagement has been found to be fostered by civic associations, and these settings can provide opportunities to gain valuable knowledge and skills that can translate into other forms of community engagement (Malin, 2015; Rizzini & Bush, 2013).

Community choirs, particularly those that are racially homogenous, provide a conducive climate for creating safe spaces and bonding social capital, which can be a stepping stone for civic engagement and social capital bridging (Baggetta, 2009). Activities that bring a community together have the capacity to generate goodwill and to develop relationships that strengthen a community. When these ties cross conventional geographical and ethnic/racial lines, they can be powerful in creating community spirit that can be tapped in other types of endeavors.

Challenges

Although most of us are capable of singing, some of us are only able to do this in the confines of our homes, and that includes me. The gift of possessing a voice that should be shared with the world is rare. By contrast, the other performing arts offer the potential for participation without having to be on stage through the carrying out of countless numbers of tasks associated with performances. Singing and song can easily be incorporated into other performing arts.

Singing can be integrated into youth practice; it does not have to be relegated to those programs that focus on the performing arts, and this makes it easier for practitioners to use song. One only has to remember singing in a bus while taking a school trip to capture how easy it is to tap singing as a no-cost and readily available activity. When music conveys a social injustice story, its significance is greatly increased as is its potential for personal transformation.

Telling these stories requires finding the right place to convene, practice, and eventually perform. This requires the guidance of those with expertise, time, and commitment. Youth programs often have this capacity, providing a setting and reaching out, finding, and engaging the requisite experts if that talent is not available within the organization. A performance often represents an "end point," and effort must be made to ensure that a group can sustain participation post performance. In addition to these more obvious challenges, the chemistry that is needed and enhanced through a group performance is unique and difficult to replicate with the addition of new members.

Conclusion

Engaging in singing and even song writing can be a passion or just a passing activity like any other in the lives of youth. Regardless, singing can hold a prominent place within any youth activity that takes place either within or outside of school, and it does not require an audience to hold this prominent place.

When singing is a major programming activity in the lives of youth, a social justice message ensures that its potential significance goes beyond the actual singing and performance. The learning of a song's history can help youth with a limited appreciation of their histories to learn about a subject that is usually associated with boring history lessons. Singing is much more than an actual event, and, when conceptualized as such, its potential impact on youth can be quite significant.

8

Dance

Introduction

Dance is a performing art with appeal across the entire life cycle, with no particular age-group owning claim to it. Nielsen and Burridge (2015a,b, p. x) see dance as transformative, especially when its power is understood and harnessed for the greater good: "Dance has the power to change the lives of young people. It is a force in shaping identity, affirming culture and exploring heritage in an increasingly borderless world." This power is increased when dance embraces principles that are associated with engagement in praxis and social justice. Critical pedagogy can be integrated into dance by creating space for youth resistance to unfold (Hickey-Moody, 2015).

Dance is not monolithic, and it can incorporate many different forms, particularly when taking culture and local context into account (Maira, 2012; Vaughan, 2012). Dance, unlike its performing arts counterparts, requires the use of extensive energy and sufficient physical space for it to have significant physical benefits that can result in weight loss and improved physical condition. Engaging in an activity that is fun definitely helps in achieving the right state of mind to endure the demands of physical activity.

Kerr-Berry (2012) shares the observation that the field of dance education is "not immune to conflicted discourses about race in the United States." Thinking of dance as being "pure" in motion and message misses the potential of this art form for creating dialogue and seeking social justice. Dance does not have to be apolitical and can address issues of social injustices in a manner that cannot be easily displayed in any other art form, making it a powerful social method with unlimited potential (Women-Centred, 2012). Its unique position brings with it immense responsibilities for community organizations staging dance performances and those participating in dance compositions. An opportunity not capitalized upon is an opportunity lost in seeking social justice for a particular group or community.

How can dance be separated from music without engaging in a futile semantic distinction? Swing dance is but one example (Doane, 2006). The same can be asked about music and song, and dance and theatre. Campbell addresses the artificial distinction between music and singing (2010, p. 250):

> How many times have we heard children distinguish between singing and "music" (meaning instrumental music)? Such a quip can irritate singers, who do not consider themselves outside the sphere of music! Yet the distinction could be taken as an innocent reference to vocal music as the most personal of all types of musical expressions as opposed to the somewhat more "distant" performance as extensions of the body.

Border crossing between dance and theatre is not an out of the ordinary goal, as witnessed by George-Grave's (2015) *The Oxford Handbook of Dance and Theater*. This book seeks to provide a multifaceted and in-depth perspective on this fascinating field and how these two art forms can inform and shape each other.

Ethnomusical, anthropological, and ethnochoreological perspectives address this distinction (Fogarty, 2015; Harrison, 2012). Dance offers practitioners a range of opportunities to use this art form in youth practice and collaboration (Langeveld, Belme, & Koppenberg, 2014). For those without performing arts backgrounds, it means that engaging in close collaboration with those who do, as applies to all other performing arts forms as well. Dance also lends itself to social justice themes (Woodley, 2013) and brings surprises concerning language and how values get conceptualized and operationalized.

Definition

Any definition of dance must capture its multiple dimensions and purposes to do justice to this performing art. Levesque (2014, p. 599) defines dance from an encompassing perspective to include music, props, and costumes, providing a solid grasp of the role of movement and separating it from other performing art forms: "Dance refers to sequences of body movements (and lack of them) that are purposeful, intentionally rhythmical, and culturally influenced expressions that typically are accompanied by music and sometimes by props and costumes."

We usually think of props as being associated with theatre, but props also can play important roles in dance (Chen, 2015):

> The prop is a kind of common phenomenon in dance creation and performance, and it is prevailing from ancient times to the present. With social development, the dance props are also changing. As an organic part of creating dance image, the dance props often play an important role in dance works. Actually, since the labor produces dance, the props are closely related to dance. In ancient times, people dance with wooden ware and stone tools beating. However, as the time goes on, the dance props of different nationality and different local feature are formed due to difference in geographical

environment, politics and history, religious faith, and folks. Different props can reinforce different theme and shape different figure.

Props enhance a dance performance and serve to communicate cultural symbols, providing opportunities for input and participation from non-dancers, as well as dancers themselves.

Prop design and construction opens the door for contributions from youth who are reluctant to perform on stage or have talents with few outlets within school settings. Props can have profound social messages regarding justice issues and can be created using participatory principles to enhance process and outcome (Howard, Carroll, Murphy, & Peck, 2002).

Defining dance is open to debate (Karoblis, 2010; Tholley, Meng, & Chung, 2012). In similar fashion to the other performing arts, youth should be involved in helping to define dance, and their interpretations should help to shape how this activity is used in programming targeting them for participation (Stark, 2009). How dance is defined is predicated upon a set of beliefs and values that often go unchallenged and are worth noting. McCarthy-Brown (2009, p. 120) raises provocative questions about the relevance and influence of Eurocentric conceptions of dance education:

> There is a need for culturally relevant teaching in dance education. Many dance teachers have heard the buzz words "culturally relevant teaching methods." Yet these dance educators acknowledge that the "dance culture" is not always synonymous with "culturally relevant." This paper examines the issue of culturally relevant teaching methods in dance education and makes suggestions for development in this area. . . . While many students of color adapt to and accept this system [traditional training and hierarchy] there are countless others who are turned-off by the exclusive approach of their dance instructors, therefore never fulfilling their potential as dancers. What impact, then, does the traditional dance training process have on students of color, their artwork, and consequently their teaching methods?

Cultural values cannot be separated from the social marginalization of these values for youth of color who come from low-income households. (I emphasize low-income because youth of color also come from middle, upper-middle, and higher socioeconomic class families living in urban communities.)

Culture must be addressed if the performing arts are to have a social impact on youth and their communities. Chacko and Menon (2013, p. 97) introduce the concept of "cultural competition" (*bhangra* and *raas-garba*) as a site and vehicle for the production of multiple identities by Indian American youths through dance:

> [T]hese competitions appear to resist hybridity and produce rhetoric that marginalizes diasporic culture in favour of the "pure" and "authentic" culture of the homeland. However, the goal of expressing uncontaminated

"authentic" culture is not realized as diasporic identities and cultures consistently interrupt and undermine homogenizing narratives of "tradition" and "authenticity."

The authors go on to note that these folk dance groups serve to reinforce ethnoregional distinctiveness rather than a hybrid or pan-Indian identity. Incorporating cultural traditions is never a simple process or one without tensions and even conflicts, and it will require extensive research on the part of youth. The skill sets learned while doing this research can be applied to other aspects of their lives, thus bringing an added dimension of benefit.

Teaching dance in urban centers provides teachers—and, one can add, community practitioners—with an opportunity to also learn and evolve in their philosophy and techniques related to this performing art by incorporating local culture (Gerdes & VanDenend Sorge, 2015). Dance can incorporate cultural and social justice themes so that it entertains and educates, raises consciousness, and informs social change (Franklin, 2013; Nielsen & Burridge, 2015*b*; Ward, 2013).

Dance can be socially transformative and therapeutic, and this aspect has received considerable attention in the scholarly literature of the field, in a similar fashion to music (Benson & Scales, 2012). Riggs et al. (Riggs, Bohnert, Guzman, & Davidson, 2010) discuss the importance and benefits of afterschool settings for Mexican-American youth and the use of traditional Mexican music and dance as culturally based activities to attract and maintain youth in the program. Cultural themes also are attractive to their families and communities.

Grounding dance as a vehicle for youth engagement in practice scholarship faces numerous challenges. Levesque (2014, p. 599) comments that the dance scholarly literature based on empirical research has not been comprehensive, with significant aspects being overemphasized and others generally ignored, thus limiting a comprehensive understanding that can inform youth programming:

> Somewhat surprisingly, for example, researchers essentially have ignored how the dance that may come to mind when thinking of dancing, a sort of play and spontaneous response to music, actually has not received much attention. Instead, research has focused on formal dance, dance as an after-school group activity, dance as a form of therapy, and dance as a social event that can bring hazards to youth.

Dance as an activity is not just about physical exercise: it has an intellectual or cognitive component as well, and never more so than when it has deep cultural roots and strong ritualistic symbols within a particular ethnic or racial group. Dance is an art form that requires that a trusting relationship exist at every stage through open communication and respectfulness (Stewart & Alrutz, 2012).

In turning to how dance can have an immediate effect on youth, one only has to look at the obesity crisis and see its impact on urban youth of color. Lack of exercise is the second part of the equation regarding excessive weight, with the other part being poor food choice and eating habits.

The social justice of fast-food establishments targeting urban groups and communities has received serious attention in policy and academic circles, and this has important implications for youth of color (Delgado, 2013). Introducing dance as a "fun" activity that can transpire both within organizations and during free-time brings with it the potential for increased health. Bringing together dance and social justice increases the significance of this activity.

Review of Relevant Literature (Focus on Marginalized Youth)

The dance field has benefitted from major literature reviews. Walker, Nordin-Bates, and Redding (2010), although not specifically focused on marginalized youth, in identifying and developing talent in dance, found conceptualization of what constitutes "talent" to be a major challenge in this field. Their review is important because not every youth wants to continue on a path to becoming a professional dancer, and programs must be adept at providing avenues for those who have the requisite talent to do so, but with the understanding that learning dance may be simply a stage in a participant's life, as with Atlanta's Moving in the Spirit (Chapter 12).

Chua (2014), building on the work of Walker, Nordin-Bates, and Redding, recommends viewing talent from four perspectives: (1) abilities and traits, (2) creativity, (3) motivation, and (4) support. Cultural and contextual factors must inform this "naming" process if marginalized youth are to be seriously considered to counter a Eurocentric perspective on who is "worthy" to be at the top of ladder in this field (Sanchez, Aujla, & Nordin-Bates, 2013).

Dance can be thought of as an umbrella with countless numbers of spokes. There are many different types of dances that can appeal to youth. The following are several (some of which may be surprising to the reader) of the more popular types: ballet, partnered dance, private jazz/hip-hop, Latin-flamenco, Latin-salsa/ballet folklorico, and tap (Lopez Castillo et al., 2015). Slam dancing, a form of dancing in which dancers collide into each other, will not appeal to all youth (Borgeson & Valeri, 2015).

Street dance, with hip-hop being the most popular type, can be considered a backlash against Eurocentric visions of dance (Bodén, 2013, p. 6): "Street dance started as an urban way of expression, in one way a rebellion against the classical dance forms, of the kids who could not afford to go to a dance school. The music scene was a great influence, hip hop music demanded its dance form companion, funk music likewise." Urban-centric positions on dance reveal deep divisions between what is acceptable as dance and who controls this conception, a prime example of internal versus external control.

Each of these types of dance brings forth its potential to incorporate social identity, culture, and social justice. One can no doubt see the appeal of Latin dancing to Latino youth and how it is deeply rooted within Afro-Caribbean history and traditions. The addition of hip-hop—and breakdancing if we go back several decades—opens up the appeal to a range of tastes and preferences among youth and brings together different youth groups to share in a common experience.

Dancing's sociocultural context helps us to understand and appreciate why and how particular dance styles were shaped, including the challenges associated with staging and performing particular dances with deep and important cultural roots that are non-Eurocentric. Dance, such as Latin salsa, can be used to break down misconceptions and educate participants in the sociocultural history and forces that shape this cultural expression (McMains, 2016).

Breakdancing has deep roots in urban communities (with its origins traced to the South Bronx), and issues of oppression, marginalization, and social justice add a social context that aids us in understanding its multifaceted message (Magaña, 2015, p. 5):

> Breaking developed partially due to the isolation of communities in the economic conditions in the late 60s and early 70s, where people of many ethnicities, but mostly Blacks and Latinos, had few options but to live very close together with minimal safe opportunities outside one's own neighborhood that would cause or allow one to travel outside their own borough.

Breakdancing and its music received considerable publicity nationwide, although movies and media coverage rarely grounded this performing art with the social marginalization that led to its creation and popularity across the country. Breakdancing, many a scholar would argue, can be considered the precursor to current-day hip-hop and shares a common etiology.

The identification and development of talented young dancers with disabilities can be an explicit or implicit objective of youth practice, particularly when it embraces an inclusive curriculum and programming (Aujla & Redding, 2014; Whatley, 2007). Gender issues—more specifically getting boys to dance—will be a challenge that will emerge when discussing youth practice and dancing.

Programming must openly challenge normative discourses on boys and masculinity (Holdsworth 2013). What it takes to be a "man" is a painful discourse because of the values that will be uncovered in the course of engaging in this dialogue. No urban youth program can be successful without such a conversation, either directly or indirectly. Any discussion of social justice will undoubtedly touch on this and lead to other types of discourse.

Dance can be combined with nontraditional art forms, expanding this performing art to incorporate innovative manifestations and the introduction of social justice messages. Lerman and Zollar (2015, p. 183) comment on the tension that dance has encountered regarding the introduction of narrative to this performing art, although this expands options for including messages of social importance that can be integrated throughout a performance:

> This concern has been the subject of an ongoing tension within the dance world. One fundamentalist camp says that if you have narrative, you are putting dance in the service of something else, which diminishes the art form. The other fundamentalist camp believes that any "art for art's sake" is irrelevant because it is not of service to a community, but neither extreme is very helpful.

Narrative and video can be introduced as a backdrop or enhancer, and can accompany dance, thus expanding the options that are available to share a message (Cormier & Gorman, 2014). This message can be delivered in various languages within a performance when using translation technology.

When the central message is social justice–focused, no medium is more or less important than another because the importance of this central message is the guiding achievement of this goal. Dance is a vehicle that is meant to transmit a message rather than having entertainment as its central purpose, but this does not mean that it cannot be entertaining and this should never be minimized.

Rewards and Benefits

The great Alvin Alley stated it well when he said "I believe that dance came from the people and that it should be delivered back to the people." Grounding dance within this context helps to ensure that its relevance is not lost and that it becomes a viable option for engaging those within the community who are so inclined. Dance can be therapeutic and socially significant, and it can address a multitude of social goals that can have individual and collective purposes, including highlighting how social injustices permeate the lives of particular groups and how to seek redress.

Dance can introduce an individual and group mechanism for transmission of culture, and this takes on added significance when youth have cultural backgrounds that are often overlooked by society or have been seriously devalued, thus impacting negatively on the identities of youth (Bennett, 2015). For example, obesity is a seriously under-recognized social justice (Delgado, 2013; Rasquinha & Cardinal, 2015).

Dance encompass a variety of benefits because of the different youth program goals that it can address. Dance has achieved a range of goals such as developing youth faith at an evangelical church (Larson, Pearce, Sullivan, & Jarrett, 2007); promoting healthy eating (Engels, Gretebeck, Gretebeck, & Jiménez, 2005; Lipman et al., 2011; Seo & Sa, 2010), physical activity (Strong et al., 2005; Wagener, Fedele, Mignogna, Hester, & Gillaspy, 2012), and cognitive and creative development (Giguere, 2011); physical healing (Shank & Schirch, 2008); cultural grounding (Melchior, 2011; Mmari, Blum, & Teufel-Shone, 2010; Shay, 2006); and well-being (Quiroga Murcia, Kreutz, Clift, & Bongard, 2010; Connolly, Quin, & Redding, 2011). Dance can be used with youth of all ages, starting with those in pre-school (Lobo & Winsler, 2006; Lorenzo-Laza, Ideishi, & Ideishi, 2007), and this makes it an attractive way to enlist and maintain youth throughout key developmental periods.

Four key benefit themes are highlighted here. These may appear disparate but they actually share much in common, showing how dance can be an attractive element of youth practice: dance (1) is affirming and inclusive; (2) provides cultural identity; (3) enhances physical activity and health; and (4) fosters nonverbal learning and creativity.

1. Affirming and Inclusive. Are all dances equally amenable to introducing a social justice perspective? The short answer is "no," particularly if stressing aesthetics, but this is open to debate, and rightly so. A Eurocentric perspective brings with it a bias that goes far beyond a focus on race and ethnicity and will implicitly encompass views on a host of social factors including age, gender, body type (including weight), and physical abilities/ideal body types.

People rarely think of someone who is struggling with excessive weight as a dancer; instead, most envision someone who is thin and muscular in build. A dancer will certainly not be envisioned as someone with an obvious physical disability (Burt, 2007). Gender stereotypes are also present and must be confronted (Morad, 2016), and Bodén (2013, p. 11) addresses this point: "In most dance forms, men and women participate but have different roles. Women are more often displayed and do tricks, while men carry, lift or lead them. As masculine as this might seem, male dancers are often faced with prejudices of homosexuality."

Atencio and Wright (2009) discuss ballet through an analysis of how it is held to a high status at the expense of socioeconomic class, race/ethnicity, and feminist values and principles. Stereotypes are reinforced pertaining to the ideal body type, conduct, and who can be prima/principal ballet dancers. Dance inclusiveness can be enhanced to include different body types and not be restricted to an idealized image.

Dance can be modified to incorporate participants with disabilities. There is no group that, regardless of abilities, cannot engage in dance. Youth with disabilities, too, can engage and benefit from dance. Zitomer and Reid (2011) found that their participation in an integrated dance program can have multiple positive impacts on children with disabilities' perceptions of dance ability and able-bodied participants' perceptions of disability. Able and non-able youth benefited from engaging in dance together.

Hackney and Earhart (2010) provide recommendations for introducing tango classes for people with disabilities. This is a purposeful dance form: it is highly scripted and associated with a serious view of dancing. Tango is a dance that has a historically grounded meaning that goes along with its disciplined approach.

Dance provides an alternative for youth with various intellectual and physical challenges to achieve positive student outcomes while incorporating diverse learner educational needs in a manner that can be fun and instructional (Munsell & Bryant Davis, 2015). Eales and Goodwin (2015) describe the success of a highly innovative use of dance as a vehicle in an integrated dance program (wide range of embodiments and capacities) that conceptualizes disabilities as social justice and thus opens the door for care-sharing ("life-sustaining, communal acts of radical interdependence; practices of consensus-building and the sharing of discomfort; and a commitment to negotiating complex power relations").

2. Cultural Identity. Dance helps marginalized youth of color reclaim their identities (Goldbard, 2006), and this is best understood when we use contextualized historical backgrounds to understand how dance shapes national and cultural identity (Lerman & Zollar, 2015; Lin & Man, 2011; Wengrower, 2015). The Tango (Argentina), the Samba (Brazil), Step Dancing (Ireland), and Salsa (Latino Caribbean) are much more than dances (Hutchinson, 2013).

Although dances can be taught through lessons at dance studios, these expenses are not necessary. The democratization of dance makes this performing art particularly appealing in low-income communities. Newcomer youth, too, can find dance an attractive mechanism for recapturing or learning their cultural heritage (Ngo, 2009).

The association between Native Americans and dance is ingrained in the American psyche. Tribal dances in the Native American community are a vehicle for grounding identity historically and providing an opportunity to engage in an intergenerational exchange between the past and the future (Schweigman, Soto, Wright, & Unger, 2011; Wexler, 2011). Intergenerational connections can be an unexpected benefit of efforts to enlist the support of community adults and older adults in sharing oral history that is simply not available to these youth in formal educational programs.

Coppens, Page, and Thou (2006) describe the challenges of evaluating a Cambodian youth dance program. Using non–culture-specific techniques, and balancing the demands of different funding sources while keeping the goal or mission focused on youth, is a perennial issue in discussing programming that is ethnic and racial centric and when placing culture as a central guiding component for recruiting and engaging youth from nondominant cultural backgrounds.

3. Physical Activity and Health. In discussing dance benefits, we must see its relationship to other performing arts, such as theatre. It is artificial to separate dance and theatre from physical exercise, and this is never more true than in a Boal-inspired production (Auslander, 1994, p. 124):

> Augusto Boal's theatre is immensely physical in nature, everything begins with the image, and the image is made up of human bodies. Boal's theatre takes the body of the spect-actor as its chief means of expression. The body

also becomes the primary focus of the ideological inscriptions and oppressions Boal wishes to address through theatre. The initial apprehension is of the body; discussion of the ideological implications of the images follows upon the apprehension.

Separating performing arts into discrete activities is artificial and unproductive. Theatre can easily be as demanding as dancing, necessitating a tremendous amount of physical exercise by the time a performance is completed.

Dance is closely associated with maintaining a healthy lifestyle, particularly when combined with a proper diet (Gao, Huang, Liu, & Xiong, 2012; Gao, Zhang, & Stodden, 2013). The case of urban youth who have difficulty maintaining a "healthy" weight because they do not have ready access to nutritional food and/ or exercise increases the importance of engaging in dance in a safe environment. Dance is a nonstigmatizing activity not associated with any one level of weight or physical fitness.

Dance provides physical activity that is enjoyable, inexpensive, and cannot be minimized in the lives of low-income youth. It is an activity in which they can engage in a large forum or in the privacy of their own homes. Dance routines can be learned in a program but with expectations that youth will go home and practice new routines, thus making it exercise associated with one setting and broadening it to include more familiar surroundings, bringing flexibility in programming. Practicing in the home has the potential to engage families in this activity.

4. Fostering Nonverbal Learning and Creativity. The performing arts can foster learning in many different academic subjects. And there are other aspects associated with learning that also can be addressed through dancing (Boydell, Jackson, & Strauss, 2012; Giguere, 2011; Nurmi & Kokkonen, 2015). Gilbert (2015) explores creative dancing (mastering movement and creative expression) through concepts that can assist youth in developing "deeper" learning and memory.

Hanna (2008), too, puts forth dance as a nonverbal language that lends itself to imagining and learning—critical elements in creativity—and reviews how dance has historically been viewed by theorists. Six of these views stand out: (1) aesthetics; (2) agency; (3) creativity; (4) lived experience and transcendence; (5) learning through the body; and (6) the power of the arts to shape alternative possibilities in culture, politics, and the environment.

Challenges

Hanna (2008), although acknowledging the contributions of various dance perspectives, still believes that they do not capture the full potential of dance, with recent research on nonverbal communication and cognition illustrating the potential of this art form to foster problem-solving and the acquisition, reinforcement, and assessment of non–dance-related knowledge. The merits of dance as an art form can be open to critique, and this is healthy for the advancement of this performing art.

Page (2012, p. 1) raises the provocative point of dance having a prominent place within the Black Arts Movement, drawing attention to the insidious nature of ranking of the arts according to their perceived prestige:

> The Black Arts Movement brought together a diverse range of African American artists who used their art to disseminate the African aesthetic nationally, yet dancers are rarely recognized or even mentioned in the historical literature of that social and political movement . . . .. In spite of overwhelming challenges African American dancers were able to use concert dance as a form of social protest and political commentary, not only during the Black Arts Movement but also during the development of the Civil Rights Movement. Black dance has historically been marginalized from two directions: Western ideologies about the function of dance and the Black Power Movement's devaluation of European aesthetics.

An arts "pecking order" must be avoided because the arts are not intended to signify order of prestige and importance, be it in the Black Arts Movement or any other movement. The arts provide a voice for expression, and not everyone shares the same voice, message, or method for expression. Youth engaging in one form of art are not more or less important than youth who perform in other forms of art.

The challenges and limitations related to dance as youth programming are closely associated with the goals dictating how it unfolds. Simpler goals correspond to simpler challenges and complex goals result in complex challenges. Practitioners have flexibility in how dance programming unfolds. The integration of social justice brings additional challenges but is worth addressing.

Musil (2010) identified three major challenges confronting the dance field with implication for youth practice: (1) the increased globalization and emergence of multiculturalism and its implications for how dance education should transpire, (2) the existence of long-standing divisions and tensions between performing artists and educators, and (3) philosophical and practice-based conflicts between what constitutes "educational" and "studio" dance. Two challenges will be highlighted here and were selected because of their significance when compared to the challenges identified in the other performing arts in this section.

1. Integration of Social Justice Themes. Dance by itself relies on movement to tell a story. A social justice theme can be introduced if innovation is welcomed and encouraged. Backgrounds (pictures and props) to dance performances can have scenes that are familiar to an audience, particularly when the dance is locally grounded. Building and street pictures can be strategically placed across the stage, including in and around an audience, thus allowing youth with artistic skills to participate.

Dance can also incorporate poetry as a message backdrop or enhancer during critical aspects of a performance, to enhance a key message or theme that would be difficult to express through dance alone. Adding this dimension also expands the possibility of including youth without an interest in dance as an activity. A multi-faceted perspective that sees dance as a foreground and other supporting arts as backgrounds necessitates a carefully orchestrated performance and a major commitment of time and effort in all facets, starting with recruitment.

2. Inclusive of Dancers with Various Physical Disabilities. Inclusivity is a topic that has only recently started to receive attention in the dancing professional literature because youth with disabilities, regardless of type, can participate and benefit from engaging in dance. Bodén (2013, p. 5) addresses the benefits of dance but also the challenges associated with this performing art:

> Dance is a universal language, a basic form of expression, whether it is for entertainment or communication. It is found in all corners of the world and as far back in history as can be seen. In the modern, western world though, it has become something embarrassing; most people (especially males) only dare enter the dance floor after a few drinks, if even then. Still, it is a built-in reflex, to move your body to the rhythm—just look at small children when they hear music! The health benefits of dancing are well researched and besides from being an excellent physical exercise form, they include many psychological aspects such as increased self-esteem and creative thinking.

Although an affirming and inclusive theme can be found throughout the other performing arts, this has been highlighted as a particular reward of dance and physical movement.

Youth slam poetry can be used to focus on particularly difficult periods during the telling of a story. This increases the number of potential contributors to a performance and can encourage youth with various disabilities to be integral to a dance performance. Integration into the actual dance will prove challenging but also equally rewarding when accomplished in an unforced or artificial manner, by embracing the concept that dance is open to all comers.

Conclusion

It is not unusual to hear someone say that they cannot sing or will not do so in public, but that this does not stop them from singing in private. Although some will say that they cannot dance in public, few will they say that they dance in private. Dance as a performing art takes a special kind of person who can go out in public and dance, either as a soloist or as part of a group. This chapter provided an encapsulated review of how dance can be included in youth practice highlighting social justice and cultural themes.

Dance as a youth practice can accomplish many different goals. Once a social justice focus is introduced, it opens up exciting new possibilities and challenges. Dancing provides youth and programs with an opportunity to engage in an activity that can be practiced at home and does not require expensive lessons and musical equipment. It is democratized art because it is within everyone's reach regardless of their station in life.

9

Theatre

Introduction

The term "great" is unique to theatre. Who is not in search of a great theatre experience as either a performer or as an attendee? Avid theatre-goers seem to be in a perpetual search for great theatre. Great theatre has a tremendous impact on an audience, touching on all of their senses and bringing them into the performance in a manner that few other performing arts can do. Theatre does not require a beautiful hall, great seating, elaborate sets, and accompanying music to make it great, as long as it has social meaning for audiences and casts.

Great theatre, too, prepares youth for life's many challenges (Richardson, 2015). We are not talking about big budgets or elaborate productions; instead, we are talking about a significant story to be told by youth to the broader community. Expanding our vision of theatre to include puppet shows, for instance, provides youth with a vehicle for sharing stories in a manner that may be less threatening to the performers and audiences (Tham-Agyekum & Loggoh, 2011).

Story is a central organizing force in how social justice–inspired theatre unfolds within a community context. When the story has relevance for an audience, residents see themselves and others they may know as represented in the plot and performance goals. Community ownership of performances is essential, and tapping local stories helps increase the chances that this occurs (Cocke, 2015). Theatre can transpire in places other than the typical venue, thus facilitating its integration into different types of community settings (Hughes, Jackson, & Kidd, 2007). Theatre can be an educational and social change tour de force, with its potential still in its infancy (Gallagher & Booth, 2015).

Understanding the medium of theatre is never easy, although the same can be said about music, song, and dance, and even more so when introducing a social justice message. Separating out theatre from music and song is often very difficult to do (Symonds & Taylor, 2014). Theatre presents unique challenges and rewards, particularly when incorporating other arts and taking on even greater complexity (Rizk, 2015).

Lobman (2015, p. 349) introduces the role and importance of play as an activity that can transpire in a multitude of ways for reaching youth:

> A review of the use of theater outside of the confines of traditional theater first needs to synthesize two historically different understandings of play: the theatrical one, as in creating or putting on a play, and pretend play, the activity traditionally associated with early childhood. One way to understand the relationship between these two types of play is through the lens of performance.

There are few practice activities that require a tremendous amount of time and energy and can still be thought of as a play in the conventional sense. Combining fun with learning and competency development is a tough formula to beat for any age group.

Many theatre variations have roots in Boal's pioneering work, Theatre of the Oppressed. *Applied theatre* is another example of a variation on Boal's work that has enjoyed tremendous popularity (Taylor, 2006), drawing upon the work of notables such as Giroux, Kincheloe, and McLaren (Landy & Montgomery, 2012). The term "applied theatre" can confound a comprehension of theatre as a field. Prentki and Preston (2009, p. 9) provide a definition that illustrates its attractiveness for social justice performing arts:

> "Applied theatre" has emerged in recent years as a term describing a broad set of theatrical and creative processes that take participants and audiences beyond the scope of conventional, mainstream theatre into the realm of a theatre that is responsive to ordinary people and their stories, local settings and priorities. The work often, but not always, happens in informal settings: schools, day centres, the street, prisons, village halls, an estate or any other location that might be specific or relevant to the interests of a community.

Applied theatre's broad research base provides another window through which to appreciate the vastness of this field and the terms that are used to describe it.

These terms share much in common because of a commitment to using theatre to make a difference throughout the life cycle. Street or community theatre, as addressed in the following section, brings an exciting dimension to this performing art by taking it out of the confines of a particular place and space—a large auditorium in a central location—and placing it within unconventional places and spaces, including museums (Alrutz, 2011).

Fox (2007) describes Playback Theatre, another example of Boal's Theatre of the Oppressed that uses trained performers to act out life stories shared by audience members to shine light on major social issues and problems and how best to achieve change. Playback Theatre, in the spirit of Boal, gives voice to groups that are ignored by a community and society. Playback Theatre is predicated upon performers grounding themselves in the local culture and language by living in the community, providing them with an opportunity to listen to stories (Meer, 2007).

There are outstanding books chronicling the transformative power of theatre applied to social justice (Woodson, 2015). In addition to Boal's classics, the following seven are illustrative:

Bowles & Nadon (2013), *Staging Social Justice: Collaborating to Create Activist Theatre*

Broyles-González (1994), *El Teatro Campesino: Theater in the Chicano Movement*

Elam (2001), *Taking It to the Streets: The Social Protest Theater of Luis Valdez and Amiri Baraka*

Gallagher (2014), *Why Theatre Matters: Urban Youth, Engagement, and a Pedagogy of the Real*

Kuftinec (2003), *Staging America: Cornerstone and Community-Based Theater*

Woodson (2015), *Theatre for Youth Third Space*

Van de Water (2012), *Theatre, Youth, and Culture: A Critical and Historical Exploration*

This list does not do justice to capturing the countless number of scholarly articles and research reports on the subject, indicating that theatre has a huge following and great potential to be a social intervention for the marginalized across all age groups.

Theatre debatably represents the most attractive mechanism for social justice youth community practice. Theatre provides a broader and more encompassing arena for including other performing arts, and this chapter is lengthier in comparison to the others to do justice to this topic.

Community Theatre

Community theatre is singled out for attention before moving on to other forms of theatre because it has a long tradition in this country. It seems as if every town and city has one or more community theatres with a long tradition of offering theatre at a community level, and most readers can tap into their own experience in reading this chapter.

Community theatre generally eschews focusing on a "star," instead being inclined to embrace an egalitarian stance in selecting a cast and thus increasing the likelihood of assembling a cast that is inclusive and reflective of the communities they reside within (Cohen-Cruz, 2006). This fits well with the collectivistic stance that has been a recurring theme throughout this book. Those youth with a collectivistic value stance will not find the traditionally individualistic and competitive approach of conventional theatre attractive and may eschew engaging in programs where this is stressed.

Kuftinec (2003, p.1), in describing community theatre, highlights the close relationships among its transformative potential, creativity, and its grounding within the local community: "The hope mainly emanates from experimental student and community-based productions, grounded in locality, place, or identity. These community-based productions . . . integrat[e] local history, concerns, stories, traditions, and/or performances." The "community" prefix in community theatre makes it imperative to have performances be reflective of where they transpire. There are limits and challenges regarding community-based theatre when models are developed that do not take into consideration local cultural values and traditions, as in the case of HIV/AIDS (Johansson, 2010).

Definition

Arriving at a consensus definition of theatre requires several different books specifically embracing this goal. Defining a performing art such as theatre without bringing in other art forms is not common. Performances that mix theatre, music, poetry, dance, and song allow a range of contributions to be made that offer new perspectives and interpretations (Jocson, 2008; Leonard & Kilkelly, 2006*b*).

Theatre is universal; it can be defined as a live performance that captures a narrative grounded in time and space. It encompasses actors, design, and movement, and it engages an audience on a journey that resonates in their lived experiences (Tillis, 2003). This definition is purposefully simple so that it captures various theatre forms.

Theatre unifies place and process (space) that encourages meaningful participation (Cohen-Cruz, 2006, p. 4): "I have identified the linked characteristics of these theatres as: primacy of place, deep interaction with constituents and commitment to goals including and exceeding the creation of great theatre. These characteristics are not just linked, they are inseparable from each other." Urban place and space can help elucidate a message of social justice (Glick Schiller & Schmidt, 2016).

Review of Relevant Literature (Focus on Marginalized Youth)

If life is drama, then theatre is how it is captured and shared with the world. There is no paucity of scholarship on drama and social justice (Freebody & Finneran, 2015). Theatre has great appeal for social justice youth practice because it provides flexibility for youth to engage in all facets of a production according to their competencies, goals, and personalities, yet it affords a collective experience. Introducing the prefix "social justice" opens up a world of theatre that is appealing for youth in highly marginalized situations.

What an audience experiences can be conceptualized as the tip of an iceberg, with most of what goes into a production being invisible to all but the most knowledgeable. A social justice message heightens the purpose of youth theatre (Shaw,

2014; Wernick, Woodford, & Kulick, 2014). Youth-focused theatre can address issues that are highly sensitive from a cultural point of view, as in the case of Latino youth and sexuality (Noone, Castillo, Allen, & Esqueda, 2015).

Flint, Graves, and Morong (2015; p. 207) provide a theatre model based on social justice values and principles to illustrate how civic engagement can transpire; although this theatre is based on a university-initiated effort, it still has the potential to be adopted within and outside of school settings:

> Creation of a play production examining ideas/principles of social justice. The Department of Theatre and Crossroads Charlotte at UNC Charlotte created a semester-long theatre collaboration course with the stated objective of (a) demonstrating an understanding of the demographic changes within the community and on campus; (b) defining and applying concepts of social capital and social justice including access, inclusion, equity, and trust; and (c) articulating and demonstrating the connection between theatre, community-building, and social change. Students were required to go out into the community and interview subjects relevant to the chosen issue and then create, write, design, and present an original work on that topic. Interview subjects and other members from the campus and local community were then invited to view the performance and have a talkback discussion about their thoughts on both the production and the larger community issue presented.

Theatre as civic engagement and service-learning brings tremendous potential for adaptation, particularly when crafted by youth with an explicit social justice purpose. This case example can be modified to cover different time periods and simplified accordingly.

Elam (2001, p. 139) notes that theatre, like protest music, played an instrumental role in social protest movements over the past few decades, setting the stage for theatre's current and future roles in such movements and bringing social justice issues into the center of theatre performances:

> Each historic moment and cultural constituency has its own specific demands and defines its own particular social protest theater. With each new cause of urgent social need, new social protest theaters have emerged, each believing in the singularity of its purpose and the individuality of its efforts. And yet the performances of these various groups bear striking similarities. Implicitly and explicitly, they reflect the transformative, generative, and regenerative power of ritual. The ritualistic social protest performance remains a potentially dynamic and powerful theatrical event.

Theatre, social protest, and ritual have great relevance for social justice youth performing arts, representing a continuation of a long tradition, one that is now directed at a new generation, and one that is of color and increasingly undocumented and urban-based.

Thinking that theatre as a youth social intervention is a phenomenon with short historical roots, as noted by Dutton (2001, p. 42), is an oversight that does a disservice to this art form:

> The arts are not a new concept to either youth organizations or social workers. Alongside other services offered by settlement houses, arts programs for youth began to emerge by the late 1890s. . . . During that time in our country's history, social workers were a vital part of many youth serving organizations . . . and consequently were often involved in building arts related programs. Although the use of the arts by social workers was common historically, today it is a rare occurrence.

Theatre's historical beginnings can be a powerful foundation upon which to base social work and other professions that have made contributions to the field of youth practice.

In 1909, Jane Addams (2010, p. 35), a Nobel Peace Prize winner and an early founder of the social work profession, addressed theatre as a mechanism with tremendous potential for reaching and engaging youth:

> The Children's Theater in New York is the most successful example, but every settlement in which dramatics have been systematically fostered can also testify to a surprisingly quick response to this form of art on the part of young people. The Hull-House is constantly besieged by children clamoring to "take part" . . . although it means weeks of rehearsal and the compete memorization of "stiff" lines. The audiences sit enthralled by the final rendition and other children whose tastes have supposedly been debased by constant vaudeville, are pathetically eager to come again and again.

Jane Addams is describing a youth practice activity involving a performing art (although not named as such) well over a century ago, and it still has saliency for a different set of urban and immigrant youth.

Hughes and Wilson (2004) report on research commissioned by the United Kingdom's National Association of Youth Theatres (NAYT), funded by the Arts Council England (ACE) and carried out by the Centre for Applied Theatre Research (CATR). The term "youth theatre" describes a variety of organizations that actively seek to engage young people in theatre-related activities in their own time.

Research findings suggest that youth theatre can fulfill important functions for young people, positively contributing to their personal and social development. Key findings emphasized the importance of youth theatre in helping youth transition to adulthood within a less than positive social-economic-political climate. Youth theatre provides a process that is participatory and meaningful to their life situations (Hunter & Milne, 2005).

Practitioners unfamiliar with the performing arts can find material to help them conceptualize how to initiate such an intervention. Rohd's book (1998), published almost 20 years ago and titled *Theatre for Community, Conflict &*

Dialogue: The Hope Is Vital Training Manual, outlines for practitioners numerous techniques and approaches that can be tapped for the engagement of youth in fostering dialogue on this art form. These youth-friendly activities are not restricted to the theatre and can be transferred over to other spheres of practice, often with minimal or no modifications.

Tapping academic subjects introduces a myriad of approaches for using theatre. Datoo and Chagani (2011) highlight one approach toward learning that introduces a critical pedagogy into teaching social studies through street theatre, which can trace its roots to the Theatre of the Oppressed. This form of street theatre increases their consciousness regarding oppression and empowers them in the process, illustrating how theatre can be social justice youth practice. Slater (2014) notes that cultural festivals, which can incorporate multiple forms of arts and performing arts, help ground youth within their cultural heritage, which helps them socially navigate difficult terrain.

Theatre is more than the staging of plays, rehearsing, and memorizing lines (Urban, 2012). This perspective is too mechanistic or formulaic and fails to capture the breadth and depth of an experience that can be transformative and is open to the introduction of innovation (Grewe et al., 2015). Theatre is about action, energy, fun, hard work, the telling of a compelling story, and experiences that are enhanced when viewed collectively from both participant and audience perspectives.

Fisher (2009, p. 3), inspired by Boal's Theater of the Oppressed and *Rainbow of Desire*, tackled obesity, a critical health issue in marginalized urban communities, and made it receptive to engage in and listen to:

> So why bring theatre into the issue of obesity? What can theatre do that doctors, nutritionists, fitness experts, and journalists cannot? Theatre is an interactive medium. It involves connecting with others, putting one's thoughts into actions, and delving into one's feelings. When people are directly involved in theatre, they are connecting their thoughts, feelings, and physicality. Obesity is also about connections or, more accurately, disconnections between the mind, feelings, and the body. As a theatre artist, I can think of no better way to tap into those areas of disconnection than to explore obesity through theater.

A stance that says that there are no social problems or issues that theatre cannot tackle when grounded within the views and needs of participants allows it to address obesity, violence, trauma, or virtually any another topic for that matter.

Elam (2001, p. 1) articulates the potential of theatre in addressing oppression and poses provocative questions in the process, bringing its relevance to social justice youth practice into focus in a natural way and increasing its relevance for this group:

> Repeatedly, in the modern as well as the postmodern United States oppressed peoples and new political movements have turned to the theater as a means to articulate social causes, to galvanize support, and to direct sympathizers

towards campaigns of political resistance. Consequently, the use of theater as a social weapon presents the dramatic scholar, critic, and practitioner
with questions of immediate and enduring support. Why use theater—an art
form—as a means to effect social change? How does the audience's commun-
ion, participation, and emotional empathy inside the theater dissipate or even
purge their energy, outrage, and desire to engage in protest activities outside
of the theater?

The potential transformative power of theatre is, again, only limited by our imagination and desire to use this art form as a vehicle to engage in praxis. Performing
theatre is not bound by a need for a particular architectural structure, scenery,
music, or any other element to exercise its power. It just has to be "authentic" and
based upon performers' and audiences' operative reality.

The teaching of theatre using youth development values and principles
necessitates that adult teachers, as well as youth teachers whenever possible,
bring competencies in this performing art as well as providing life lessons that
transcend the theatre (Jensen & Lazarus, 2014). Acting is an activity that can
enhance youth character strengths and bolster inherent psychological resources,
and this can translate into increased well-being when faced with adversity
(Stauber, 2012; Taylor, 2014).

Resiliency is a well-known construct that has a prominent role to play in
social justice youth practice (Lee, Cheung, & Kwong, 2012), with particular relevance to youth of color (Delgado, 2000; Neblett, Rivas-Drake, & Umaña-Taylor,
2012). It is heavily dependent on local circumstances dictating its language (how it
gets expressed) and how it is defined and operationalized (manifested).

Quality high school performing arts experiences, as in the case of speech and/
or theatre participation, can have a positive impact that extends beyond adolescence and well into adulthood (McCammon et al., 2012). Theatre encompasses
numerous elements and manifests itself in varied productions such as drama and
musical productions; it can also involve numerous roles that must be fulfilled to
bring a production to fruition (Rusk et al., 2013).

Theatre can occur in a variety of settings, including prisons (Buis & dA, 2013;
Shaw, 2014; Taylor et al., 2011). In the case of drama, it can be a therapeutic method
in assisting youth with various disabilities, such as autism (D'Amico, Lalonde, &
Snow, 2015).

A cry for social justice is not alien to the world of theatre, including a call
for social change efforts (Gallagher, 2015; Schroeder-Arce, 2016). Varied productions and roles provide ample opportunities to engage youth in areas of particular
interest to them based upon local circumstances and the justice issues that confront them on a daily basis. We can conceive of these productions as a collective
activity that can only successfully transpire when everyone carries out their roles,
although this should not be conceptualized in a highly scripted manner that dis-
courages spontaneity.

Grazer (2012, p. 1) addresses how the teaching and learning of drama can detach this method from a social justice reality and thereby miss the potential to engage marginalized youth:

> Drama attempts to interrogate spaces in all echelons of social and economic standing and seeks to bring together dichotomous perspectives in the spirit of irreverent collaboration. The narrowing of creative, synthesis, higher-order cognition in courses meant to be free-thinking and expressive signals a dangerous turn towards even more sterile subject matter in education.

Making drama sterile by depoliticizing it and simply making it entertainment effectively makes it meaningless for marginalized youth, and they are astute enough to know when this happens. Social justice youth practice involving the performing arts would not fulfill its mission if this were to transpire.

Dramas based on local youth concerns and events related to violence, infectious diseases, and police brutality provide outlets for narratives on their lives and the issues that most impact them (Hickling-Hudson, 2013). These dramas also represent efforts to capture history and preserve it for future generations, and performances can be digitally recorded and shared with future generations and across communities. Libraries can store these recordings, thus providing easy access to community residents. Librarians can facilitate this process by advertising the availability of these recordings.

Theatre that embraces a social justice foundation can go by many different names. *Popular theatre* is one of the most common terms found in the literature, and it provides a collective mechanism for youth eliciting, representing, and questioning their experiences through theatrical means (Conrad, 2008). Lee and Finney (2005) use popular theatre to engage racialized girls of color in exploring identity and belonging and describe how this performing art facilitated understanding intersectionality and local context in this process, including discourses of resistance.

Popular theatre also can be used as service-learning, opening up possibilities within educational settings (Feagan & Rossiter, 2011). The emergence of popular theatre introduced a different variation on participatory theatre (Conrad, 2004, 2008), community theatre (Singhal, 2004), and grassroots ensemble theatre (Leonard & Kilkelly, 2006*a*).

Theatre Collective Creation (TCC) and Human Rights Education (HRE) are other terms used in bringing social justice to theatre (Marin, 2014; Morris, 2012). Saldaña (2011) discusses the emergence of "ethnotheatre" and how it brings an ethnographic (culturally based), social justice, and social change lens to the arts and its potential to capture and present narratives of the voiceless who have an important stories to share.

The popularity of Theatre of the Oppressed stands out because of its universal appeal to address issues of oppression. Its success in achieving social change in the lives of those who are marginalized (Boal, 2000; Cohen-Cruz & Schutzman,

2006; Ferreira & Devine, 2012; Picher, 2007; Schaedler, 2010) nationally and internationally is due to the fact that its emphasis is solidly based upon social justice concerns and principles. Theatre of the Oppressed had its birth in responding to human rights repression, seeking to counter the manner in which cultural institutions fostered oppression rather than enacting alternative relationships (social and political) to resist oppression (Malloy, 2016).

It seems as if "all roads lead to Rome" when referring to theatre that seeks to achieve social justice, and that Rome is, with little argument, Boal. Boal (2009, p. 131) summed up his goals for theatre quite well in the following statement: "I believe that all truly revolutionary theatrical groups should transfer to the people the means of production in the theatre so that the people themselves may utilize them. Theatre is a weapon, and it is the people who should wield it." Theatre is the "people's weapon" and it can be tailored to youth, too.

Youth relationships with those in authority are complex and profound, and Theatre of the Oppressed is a viable mechanism or vehicle for uplifting these relationships and opening them up for analysis and action (Snyder, 2008; Struch, 2011). Tapping these voices, and having youth play prominent roles in how these voices are heard, brings to the fore all of the values addressed earlier and captures the spirit and meaning of social justice youth practice and the performing arts.

Boal's *forum theatre* is arguably his most influential manifestation of his work when discussing development within oppressed communities (Dwyer, 2004; Goldbard, 2006; Prior, 2010; Sullivan & Lloyd, 2006). Forum theatre has even been used with "talented" youth of color to address issues of marginalization (Sanders, 2004). Boal's work is not restricted to particular settings or groups. Rutten et al. (2010) describe an example of using forum theatre in organized youth soccer to influence youth behaviors.

Boal (1997, p. 6) identified techniques that give voice to the oppressed, bringing flexibility in how theatre can be implemented and making it very attractive in taking into account local conditions and goals:

> The personal, collective, and societal psyche. Exploring shared 'perceptions, the perceived situation. Means of empowering the oppressed. Provoking a dialogue that leaps beyond words: dialogue that is tangible through innuendo's and embodied communication. Zizek's Unknown Knowns.

These techniques can be used by any marginalized group, and youth of color can apply it in constructing their social justice stories or narratives.

It is impossible to read and understand Boal's *Theatre of the Oppressed* without also reading Freire's *Pedagogy of the Oppressed* because it represented a performing arts counterpart to this classic work (Christensen, 2012). The similarity in titles is no mistake, and both advocate for human liberation and the role of active social responses to lived experiences (Vine, 2013). Boal openly acknowledges the influence of Freire on shaping his thinking about theatre and social justice and the importance of creating a vehicle that depends on active and meaningful participation.

Freire (2009, p. 310) discusses the interrelationship of culture and action, setting the foundation for using the performing arts to achieve social change, and describes why his work is so closely associated with that of Boal:

> Cultural action is always a systematic and deliberate form of action which operates upon the social structure, either with the objective of preserving that structure or of transforming it . . . cultural action has its theory which determines its ends and thereby defines its methods. Cultural action either serves domination (consciously or unconsciously) or it serves the liberation of men and women. As these dialectically opposed types of cultural actions operate in and upon the social structure, they create dialectical relations of permanence and change.

Freire and Boal make a formidable team in advancing cultural action and its manifestation through multiple avenues, embracing and advocating for participatory and empowerment principles in the process.

Boal was clear about using theatre to achieve social change by creating a participatory process of engagement: "Theatre is a form of knowledge; it should and can also be a means of transforming society. Theatre can help us build our future, rather than just waiting for it" (1992, p. xxxi). Theatre of the Oppressed is both a philosophy and process method for participants to learn to be human and seek liberation from oppressive forces (Harlop & Aristizabal, 2013; Lacy, 2006). Its appeal is not restricted to adults, and it can find a receptive audience among youth expressing various forms of oppression (Bradley, Deighton, & Selby, 2004; Sullivan et al., 2008).

Theatre of the Oppressed transforms spectators from passive to active performers by stressing the importance of their voices in shaping the performance (Catherwood & Leonard, 2015). Listening and learning take on special significance: in this form of theatre, participants and audience develop scripts by having the actors stop action so that the audience can leave their seats and go on stage to recreate a scene; those remaining in their seats engage in dialogue/critique until there is a satisfactory ending to the play.

Boal's *Theatre of the Oppressed* has been translated into more than 25 languages since its original publication in 1974, and that statistic is dated (Schutzman & Cohen-Cruz, 1994). Theatre of the Oppressed is responsive in how it unfolds and involves audiences, increasing its appeal for incorporating local situations and circumstances. Beck and Purcell (2010, p. 110) address this appeal:

> The Theatre of the Oppressed offers a range of ways to help people explore their past, present and future. It provides an abbreviated experience of transformed social relationships; people can feel what it would be like to live in a world where they have a voice and power to act. The ability to transcend the

boundaries of language opens up creative spaces for transforming ways of both thinking and acting and can recharge the emotional reservoirs of people involved in social change. Finally, it is fun and challenging and acts as a real contrast to much of our committee-focused forms of practice.

This theatre has appeal among the marginalized regardless of their age. Importantly, fun must not be lost while addressing powerful social forces, and it can be a source of unexpected energy in this quest.

Theatre of the Oppressed can find manifestation in other forms (Boal, 1992, 1994, 1998, 2001) including *invisible theatre* (a group of actors perform a play without an audience realizing it is a play); *forum theatre* (a highly interactive process where actors and audience, who are referred to as "spect-actors," engage in exploration of how oppression comes to life in people's lives); and, often considered the signature element, *image theatre* (which uses of images, space, and physical evacuation of everyday concerns and issues rather than reliance on verbal expression). These were followed by *Rainbow of Desire* (therapeutic or psychodramatic acting to address anxiety) in 1995, and *legislative theatre* (an effort to change laws to create specific and concrete social-political impact) in 1998. Boal was once an elected member of Rio's City Council.

Beck and Purcell (2010) conceptualize Theatre of the Oppressed as an umbrella term that houses drama-based techniques that are social justice participatory-focused. Variations have emerged to capture the critical view of lived experiences. Each branch of participatory theatre has its share of participant/audience challenges and rewards and is sufficiently flexible that it can be modified to take into account local circumstances. Participatory theatre has found a receptive audience in international development (Abah, Okwori, & Alubo, 2009; Sloman, 2012; Winton, 2007).

Menke (2015, p. 3) notes how alternative views of theatre can transpire in unconventional public spaces and attract new types of performers: "It is played in spaces that are not traditionally defined as theatre buildings. The performances include participants who may or may not be skilled in theatre arts and audiences who have a vested interest in the issue taken up by the performance or are members of the community." Theatre can transpire in places and spaces not normally associated with this art form.

Rewards and Benefits

Bourke and Hunter (2011) point out the transformative power of youth as audience members in ushering in a new and more inclusive and responsive phase in theatre. This transformative power can have many different manifestations. The rewards of theatre can be quite significant in multiple ways for individual performers, audience members, and communities.

Theatre can accomplish a range of youth practice goals. Kelly (2015) provides a case example ("Voices") in using theatre as a vehicle for undertaking a youth rites of passage that helped prepare them to socially navigate entry into the broader community and be better prepared to encounter numerous challenges along the way.

Theatre can accomplish personal and social-political goals (whether by participating and/or attending), and these two are rarely separate from each other, as when building a sense of community within schools (Belliveau, 2015; Kisiel et al., 2006); gaining greater knowledge and tolerance of others (Greene, 2015); developing healthy social, cognitive, emotional, and physical competencies (Lobman, 2015; McCollum, 2015); and increasing social issues awareness (O'Connor & Colucci, 2016; Yoshihama & Tolman, 2015).

1. Affirming Exploration of Self-Identity. The arts and humanities provide youth with an opportunity for self-exploration in a manner that suits their interests and abilities, including cultural preferences. Theatre is a method that allows them to explore their own identities in a manner and at a pace that encourages and supports this exploratory process. Preston (2011) calls for new paradigms that resist tendencies to have youth conform to existing definitions of who they are and must be (macro forces on race and power), allowing for individuality to emerge from a positive or self-confidence stance, which translates into efficacy. Theatre provides the space and place for exploration and affirmation to transpire both individually and collectively.

2. Learning Educational Content. Theatre lends itself to creative approaches, making this performing art particularly attractive for use in school settings. Drama can be used to learn a range of academic subjects and to do so in a manner that is integrative and empowers youth in the learning process (Chan, 2009; María, 2015). Fleming, Merrell, and Tymms (2004) report on the success of using drama in teaching language and mathematics.

Drama has also been shown to hold promise in helping students connect with writing as a communication method (Cremin, Goouch, Blakemore, Goff, & Macdonald, 2006; Etherton & Prentki, 2006) and to learn social studies (Datoo & Chagani, 2011). Although in need of further research, it appears that when learning emphasizes a group approach it introduces many elements that can enhance the learning process, interpersonal skills, and ultimate ownership of the content being learned. Theatre can be a site for informal learning, too (James, 2005), an effective vehicle for bringing together other performing arts in teaching social justice (Hickling-Hudson, 2013).

3. Addressing Community and Interpersonal Conflicts. A major challenge that urban youth face when socially navigating their daily existence is the presence of conflict and violence within and outside of their communities. Understanding and addressing these issues is of paramount interest to these youth. Theatre must play an important role in helping them acquire knowledge and skill sets to de-escalate or prevent conflict and violence.

Crean (2013) illustrates the role and importance of creativity in describing the Once Upon a Time in the Bronx project, where a group of adolescent girls from the South Bronx created a storytelling card game that served as a mechanism through which to share their stories to an outside audience. These stories, through use of interactive theatre, proved highly successful in empowering them to facilitate community dialog and proposed alternative approaches to violence in their lives. Critical thinking and creative problem-solving were encouraged throughout the process.

Interpersonal conflicts can be found in all settings. Those related to living in urban communities are of great importance to urban youth and can be addressed through the performing arts in a manner that identifies and crystalizes these tensions for youth and provides them with a vocabulary and strategy/approach for minimizing them in their everyday lives (Enciso, Cushman, Edmiston, Post, & Berring, 2011).

Conflict-resolution is a critical skill set in neighborhoods with high rates of violence, and it stands to reason that these competencies must be taught in schools or in out-of-school settings. The performing arts, and particularly theatre when it integrates other arts, are excellent media through which to present these conflicts and engage the audience in proposing solutions that are contextually grounded because they are based on real-life situations. All parties benefit from these types of sessions.

4. Creation of Interpersonal Bonds and a Sense of Community. Youth-focused theatre can create a supportive community with important outcomes related to peer and friendship relationships, and, when social justice–inspired, praxis (Nelson, 2011). Capturing youth disaster stories is often overlooked in any recordings of the impacts these events have on communities, and theatre provides a forum and method for youth to share their experiences (Gibbs, Mutch, O'Connor, & MacDougall, 2013).

Daykin et al. (2008) reviewed the literature on the impact of participation in performing arts on adolescent health and behavior and concluded that the field was still in its infancy from a research point of view. Drama was the most beneficial performing art covered in the research, and this speaks to the need for an expanded vision for research and evaluation in this field to more fully achieve a comprehensive understanding of its significance.

Theatre provides a mechanism through which difficult stories can be shared (Gallagher, 2014, p. 16): "Storytelling, or as we often experienced storytelling through theatre that draws on symbol and metaphor, realism and abstraction, can act as a 'methodological release point' to invite the unsaid, the masked, the contested, the contradictory." These stories invariably deal with social justice and inequality, including the failing of youth-focused institutions such as schools and out-of-school settings, which are key institutions outside of their families.

Snyder-Young (2012) introduces the concept of "every single day" and theatre as a cultural artifact and site for critical inquiry, a means of providing a time period and space to unify a case study theme through which youth in a high school setting can represent social antagonism or micro-aggression. Students are able to deconstruct their peer and adult interrelationships, in this case focused on bullying.

Heathcote (2009, p. 290), in describing the role and power of drama, describes how a prominent and highly emotional theatre experience uplifts the transformative potential of this performing art and why it has tremendous potential for achieving change at both individual and community levels in a manner that resonates with participants and audiences alike:

> Let us look at what is special about drama itself. The most important manifestation about this thing called drama is that it must show change. It does not freeze a moment in time, it freezes a problem in time, and you examine the problem as the people go through a process of change. If you want to use drama as education, you have to train people to understand how to negotiate in that the people go through a process of change.

Drama is an excellent mechanism to showcase a problem frozen in time for urban youth, and it can create critical interpersonal bonds and a sense of community that enhances its potential for a transformative experience.

Challenges

The potential of theatre to encompass multiple social justice youth community practice goals, particularly when envisioned as incorporating ambitious goals, also represents one of its greatest challenges facing practitioners. Of a number of challenges that can be discussed, one stands out and is worthy of focus in this section. Translating awareness into action post performance is a challenge that increases when the social injustice is of tremendous magnitude and difficult to address within a short timeframe. This challenge includes numerous logistical considerations such as finding appropriate staff funding and dealing with the emotional upheavals for youth (Alrutz, 2013; Blake, 2016; Grewe et al., 2015; Hickling-Hudson, 2013; Lima, 2016; Snyder-Young, 2013; Tarasoff, Epstein, Green, Anderson, & Ross, 2014). When theatre also seeks to create and tap creativity, it challenges how the process and evaluation unfolds (Toivanen, Halkilahti, & Ruismäki, 2013).

Evaluation must be central to organized efforts at using theatre as a vehicle for achieving change in participants. The evaluation of theatre and its impact on participants is very challenging because the gains youth make can be multifaceted and lie beyond obvious goals (Halse et al., 2013; McCammon, Saldaña, Hines, & Omasta, 2012; Mohler, 2012a, 2012b). These gains can be immediate, but the true test of an intervention is its long-lasting benefits and this necessitates longitudinal evaluation.

Translating theatre experience into a social change campaign, particularly one that is youth-led with adult allies, can be quite threatening to adult stakeholders and more so when it threatens stereotypes (Edell, 2013; Wernick, Woodford, &

Kulick, 2014). These efforts make youth programs sponsoring these efforts particularly vulnerable to political backlash. These change efforts, even when they fail to achieve the outcomes they wish to accomplish, are still valuable lessons.

The journey is as important, if not more so, than the destination (Halse et al., 2013). Helping youth realize how much they have gained and why a long view of change is often needed is critical because failure is part of life. Failure is not restricted to youth, and adults have a long track record of failing, too. What we can learn from failure has significant meaning. One can learn more about a person by how he or she handles failure than by how he or she handles success. The ability to "bounce back" (resiliency) should never be underestimated in the lives of youth.

Conclusion

It is quite natural to associate theatre with luminaries such as Shakespeare and Beck, for example, and to think of this performing art as social class-based, primarily appealing to those from privileged backgrounds. But theater's potential reach goes far beyond socioeconomic class and can encompass so much more that is social in nature, including justice and language that resonate with a nontraditional audience.

The following Section III provides four different case examples that bring the performing arts and theory to life in a manner that provides insights into how social justice, marginalized youth, and urban settings come together within the field. These cases show how organizations conceptualized practice, with each case sharing similarities with the others and also showcasing significant differences that take into account local circumstances.

SECTION III

Case Studies and Illustrations

Case studies have a prominent place in helping us understand better the potential role that the humanities can play in the lives of marginalized youth (Wishart & D'Elia, 2013). Case studies and the performing arts seem very natural together because this research method facilitates storytelling and the integration of visual images and sound to be documented, with the nuances associated with the performing arts.

Four cities are represented in this section (Boston, Chicago, Atlanta, and Los Angeles). Each case consists of six sections involving a degree of overlap: (1) Brief Literature Grounding; (2) Organizational Setting (school, youth organization, non–youth-focused community organization); (3) Brief Organizational History; (4) Program Components and Major Activities; (5) Evaluation; and (6) Key Lessons Learned and General Observations. Not all cases feature an equal amount of detail, based on available information. These cases relied heavily on publicly available information, but this limitation does not detract from the value of the lessons learned.

10

Music

ZUMIX, BOSTON

Introduction

"Popular music" goes beyond a narrow definition or range of types and can play a critical role in shaping memory (Bennett & Janssen, 2016). The popularity of music is fostered by a range of music programs in the nation's schools, although these offerings are often limited in type and shy away from social justice themes. Music is an integral part of all cultures, regardless of ethnic and racial background. Out-of-school settings are positioned to tap these two streams in a community-focused and youth-informed manner.

Boston's ZUMIX case study brings an exciting and highly ambitious dimension to youth practice because of its location in a section of Boston (East Boston) that has undergone a rapid change in composition and has a history of attracting newcomers to the United States, but is now undergoing gentrification. Youth organizational ability to "evolve" as its participant base changes will prove to be a hallmark of a responsive organization, and one that is destined to expand beyond its original mission.

In my history of writing about youth organizations, I have generally avoided writing about Boston organizations in an effort to showcase a more national representation. I did a case study of the New England Aquarium (Delgado, 2002), and, until this case study on ZUMIX, it has been the only one undertaken in Boston. My relationship with ZUMIX has been through student internships, alumni on the board, and classroom lectures. It is an exceptional organization and worthy of inclusion in this book, and my familiarity with this organization facilitated the decision-making process to include it, although there are countless other youth organizations in Boston and throughout the country that could have been selected for inclusion in this book.

Brief Literature Grounding

Music brings a rich cultural tradition and a multitude of approaches and instruments. It is not a far stretch to see how mastery of an instrument, score, and/or equipment can have great appeal for youth. Musical learning can transpire in formal, nonformal, and informal contexts and spaces, thus broadening the potential for learning this performing art (Lonie & Dickens, 2016). Music can be very empowering (Warrington, Hart, Daniels, & Block, 2016). The knowledge, skill set, and relationship skills garnered while engaging in music can easily transfer to many other aspects of the lives of youth, including the academic sphere (Crowther, McFadden, Fleming, & Davis, 2016).

Music is well grounded within a social and cultural contextual meaning, especially if an audience takes the time to listen to the words (when singing accompanies music) and the emotions surrounding them (Marsh & Dieckmann, 2016; Soley & Spelke, 2016). One has only to turn to movies to see the role of music and song in capturing and enhancing key scenes (Dyer, 2013). Music, through its regulation of emotions and social connections, also shapes youths' sense of well-being and interpersonal relationships (Cohen, Silber, Sangiorgio, & Iadeluca, 2012; Papinczak, Dingle, Stoyanov, Hides, & Zelenko, 2015).

Music does not require expensive instruments, expensive lessons, or elaborate scores, and it can attract youth with varying language abilities since music is a language of its own (Urban, 2016). Fostering inclusiveness, particularly in newcomer communities where music becomes a language for bridging divides (Edge, Newbold, & McKeary, 2014), can be a central goal of music programs. These programs take an asset approach toward newcomer communities, seeing them as possessing qualities that have the potential to increase our understandings of people from different backgrounds, but also helping us connect in a manner that does not require verbal or written competencies in another language (although that helps).

Organizational Setting

Urban youth organizations have a prominent role to play in communities by aiding in a variety of spheres, and music can be a force of attraction and the glue that keeps youth engaged over an extended period of time and thereby increases the likelihood of achieving much needed benefits:

> ZUMIX is an East Boston-based nonprofit organization dedicated to building our community through music and the arts. A core belief is that music is the most powerful means of developing adolescent self-identity . . .. Through community events, ZUMIX provides access to top-quality arts experiences for a low-income, under-served neighborhood.

ZUMIX provides venues for youth to showcase their newly acquired or refined musical abilities. Providing support and an extensive network that can be mobilized in service to youth is an attractive element that ZUMIX possesses and makes it the envy of many organizations. Its long history is an asset that only comes with age.

Brief Organizational History

ZUMIX's has existed more than 25 years (the name ZUMIX was created by one of the early youth participants), and this longevity can be traced to the passion and commitment of two individuals who wanted to do something about what East Boston youth faced in their daily life. They began the program in their livingroom, with a drive to provide positive alternatives for those youth who wished to engage in positive pursuits against a backdrop of urban tensions and conflict:

> Like a lot of good ideas, ZUMIX started in someone's livingroom . . . in 1991 as a response to Boston's worst wave of youth violence. ZUMIX began as a summer songwriting program with 24 youth, $200, and the simple idea that giving youth something to be passionate about could transform lives and elevate communities. Our programming quickly expanded. In 1993 we created a free outdoor Summer Concert Series in order to serve the broader community.

No one at the birth of this organization could have foreseen the growth of ZUMIX, its encompassing such a broad view of music, or its impact on the lives of countless youth and their community.

Programmatic Components and Major Activities

ZUMIX has purposefully taken an encompassing view of music because of an understanding that youth, too, take a broad view of this performing art field. It has sought to reach youth along an age continuum, with an appreciation that not all youth will be interested in a career in music and that participation may be episodic and that, for others, it is a career path.

ZUMIX consists of five programmatic components that share similar philosophies and values: (1) Instrumental Music, (2) Song Writing and Performance, (3) Z-Tech, (4) Sprouts, and (5) ZUMIX Radio. Each component addresses specific goals but also serves to reinforce each other in the quest to keep youth engaged over an extended period of time.

1. Instrumental Music. Music can take many forms and represents both an attractive element and an organizational challenge as well, necessitating an extensive array of musical options. It is necessary to find the right talent to staff such a program (people with both musical and youth relationships skills): "If you want to shred on an instrument, jam with a rad band, or sing yourself silly, we got what you need."

> **African Drumming:** "Take part in a high-energy drumming ensemble where you'll learn team work, communication skills, and rhythm. To end the semester, students will participate in a recital-style performance with members of the audience being invited to make music too."
>
> **Drumline:** "Rhythm is a movement and this is the group to move with. The ZUMIX Drumline will let you develop skills on the snare, tenor and bass drums with a team of other percussionists. Build your technique, confidence, and concentration as you march to the team's cadence in parades and events."
>
> **Las Mariposas:** "Discover the rich and diverse music of Latino America, from folk to pop to rock en Español! Learn, listen, make music, and explore your roots. Do you play an instrument and/or like to sing? Then this program is for youth. Open to youth ages 10–18."
>
> **Music Theory:** "How does music work? Take an in-depth look at rhythm, melody, harmony, structure, and form while getting a chance to compose works of your own. Whether you are a guitarist, singer, pianist, songwriter, or rapper, your understanding of music and skill level will increase through this class."
>
> **Performance Ensembles:** "(For our more advanced musicians). These groups represent ZUMIX at public concerts and events and offer a taste of being a professional musician. Membership is by invitation only . . . so hone your skills if you are interested! There are four groups representing different music traditions: (1) DiverCity Band—rock/pop; (2) Latin Ensemble— Latin Soul Ensemble; (3) ZUMIX Jazz Allstars—jazz standards with a modern flavor; and (4) Miyagi & The Kids—rock ensemble."

2. Songwriting and Performance: Songwriting is a skill that plays an instrumental role, no pun intended, in music and song. Teaching this skill or art rarely gets highlighted in the literature, but ZUMIX has elevated it to a major activity.

Songwriting, critical to singing, has not been folded into other activities but has been considered of sufficient importance for attention from a programmatic perspective. Not all youth want to take a spotlight approach to their participation. The activity of songwriting provides youth with little or no interest in performing the chance to participate in a meaningful way. They can write and perform the songs, but that is not a requirement to engage in this activity.

Songwriting is a creativity outlet, and there are few formal settings where youth can learn or enhance this talent: "ZUMIX's songwriters use their voices, rhythm, and energy to express what's on their minds. They take their messages to the street, performing locally and touring throughout the Northeast. From Hip Hop to Rock, students express themselves through a range of popular music. Our studio allows more advanced students to record their original music to CD."

Eight songwriting outlets are provided to ZUMIX participants, with each offering a distinctive avenue for cultural expression, including the use of theatre, which enhances music as a performing art and takes into account demographic factors. ZUMIX reaches out to all age levels, as evidenced through it Sprouts Program: "Younger participants (7–12) interested in getting involved with us have an opportunity to find out what we have to offer. This is an introduction to music, theater, and dance with an emphasis on stage and performance techniques."

Con la Corriente: The high percentage of Latino youth in East Boston and ZUMIX made offering a Latino music program natural: "Keep with the current and the styles of Latin dance. You will learn how to tighten your moves in salsa, merengue, and bachata on your own and with a partner. The class will finish with a choreographed performance. Open to all levels of dance experience." The integration of dance brings an added dimension.

Droppin': "Hip Hop at ZUMIX is back. This is a drop-in class that offers you the chance to work on your performance skills and to create, build and produce with others. Make time for your inner-artist. This group will incorporate all elements of Hip Hop (rapping, breakdancing, and graffiti) and participants will be encouraged to produce work and direct events to showcase their talents and build community."

Hi-Def: "Craft your thoughts, feelings and ideas into a music video. You will not only write your own music, but learn to conceive, direct, and edit your own music video. It doesn't matter if you are a poet, lyricist, emcee, musician, break-dancer, aspiring filmmaker, or are just curious to learn about how music and video come together. Become part of the movement of empowered young people using arts and technology to create change."

Rock Ed: "A unique opportunity to play in a live band! Come together with people who have different tastes in music to play rock and roll, hip hop, or Latin covers, and your own originals. Each band rehearses weekly and will be given opportunities to play in live gig(s)! This is a chance to discover what it takes to be in a band."

Street Program: "As the weather heats up, kids hit the street. Those who are musical and creative are invited to join the Street Program. This songwriting & performance series gives developing young artists opportunities to write songs, produce music, showcase their other artistic talents, and perform for other teens in an action-packed tour that includes performances in . . . around New England!"

Streetwise: "Have you ever dreamed of recording your own music? In StreetWise you learn how to write, produce, and record original music. Your songs will express what you want to say. Together, the class will produce an original album available to the public."

The Write Rhythm: "They say truth is stranger than fiction . . . and its often more interesting. Especially if you can translate that truth into fascinating art pieces by learning the craft that goes into creative nonfiction. Unleash your creativity as a writer, while learning the tricks of the trade and creating an original production. See with a writer's eyes, spark ideas to life, gain confidence, and experiment with music and nonfiction writing. When you know how to express yourself with words, you've got a special power."

Theater Troupe: "Theater is an art where music, dancing, and acting all come together. If you are an actor, artist, or musician, this is a great chance to learn the basics of scene study, improvisation and stage design. This class will finish with a rehearsed production for a live audience."

3. Z-Tech (Music Technology): Music takes many different shapes, and technology is a major force in this field: "If you are you interested in how music is made? Producing, recording, and engineering isn't easy, but these classes will put you on track . . . literally."

Music is a team effort even in the case of solo artists. Much needs to happen to bring about a performance, and this often requires numerous individuals carrying out technical jobs, including setting the stage for a performance: "Z-Tech programs give you access to state-of-the-art equipment in our recording studio, multimedia lab, and live sound audio equipment. Some Z-Tech graduates join the ZUMIX Tech-Crew as audio engineers in our recording studio and paid technicians at live gigs."

Beatmakers: "Learn how to produce music on the computer. Create your own original instrumental tracks or beats for vocalists to sing/rap over. Using computers you'll learn about music theory, music production software, sampling, sequencing, and synthesizers."

Fix-It: "Are you the type of person who likes to take things apart and put them back together again? Come learn basic audio technology repair, maintenance, and troubleshooting. Learn how to use specialized tools and equipment to build or fix cables and basic circuits."

Recording Lab: (Restricted to graduates of Z-Tech Studio.) "You need: to keep your skills sharpened by getting professional hands-on experience in audio recording, editing, and mixing."

Z-Tech Live!: "What goes on behind the scenes to make concerts work? Are you interested in controlling the equipment that gets the music to the audience? Join Z-TECH Live and learn how to set up the sound system for concerts, events, and festivals."

4. Z-Tech Studio – Creative Technology: ZUMIX youth interested in the behind-the-scenes work receive didactic as well as hands-on training to prepare them to carry out a multiplicity of tasks associated with this activity:

Z-Tech is a technical training program that introduces young people to audio and computer technologies using an experiential and interactive approach . . . training is divided into four sections: 1) Live Audio Engineering,

2) Beatmaking & Music Production, 3) Studio Recording, and 4) Audio Troubleshooting & Repair. Z-Tech empowers young people to apply their newfound skills in an entrepreneurial way, as it includes hands-on training and year-round paid contract work for all graduates.

Youth interested in a career in this area are provided with experience in helping them decide early on whether this is something they want to devote their lives to. There is an understanding that it is OK not to pursue music as a career:

Z-Tech Studio trains participants in the basics of Audio Engineering. Learn about the equipment, techniques, and people skills needed to become a great recording engineer. The artist can create the 'magic' but it takes someone with great ears and skills to capture it.

ZUMIX's (2014) annual report provides additional information:

ZUMIX Programming SONGWRITING & PERFORMANCE – These programs are designed to help youth address life's challenges in a positive way. Participants develop critical thinking and literacy skills as they analyze, write, and discuss issues that affect their lives. Projects include the creation of original musical, dance, and theater shows, monthly open mic events, and the production of a compilation CD and music videos. INSTRUMENTAL MUSIC – ZUMIX offers private and group music instruction in piano, guitar, bass, drums, voice, brass, woodwinds, and African drumming. As participants continue their studies, young instrumentalists improve their artistry through Music Theory classes and learn group-building skills in ensembles which allow youth to perform at a variety of events throughout the city.

For youth interested in combining music and visual technology, Zoom In is a great activity. It is natural to combine music with video, but it requires access to technology and specialized training, and it should not be surprising that ZUMIX entered into this medium:

Craft your thoughts, feeling and ideas into video. You will learn filmmaking techniques like directing, cinematography, lighting, sound, and editing -basically all the skills you need to be a filmmaker! As a team, you will get to create several different projects including music videos, promotional videos, video journalism, and artistic videos. Video can be a powerful tool for social justice. Become part of a movement using arts & technology to create change.

Visual arts and technology open up an influential window for youth to exercise creativity and provide new avenues for crafting meaningful narratives.

5. ZUMIX Radio: Radios can be found in the homes of virtually all people regardless of their background and socio-economic means:

ZUMIX Radio promotes youth and community voices in East Boston, while supporting teens to learn valuable 21st century skills in technology, radio production, communication, and journalism. Radio classes train participants to host their own live radio broadcasts, produce their own radio stories, and develop meaningful relationships with adult mentors. ZUMIX Radio, our online radio station, also serves to connect us to our community and invites participation by community members.

Radio Active: Assuming a "background" role in radio is an option for youth not interested in assuming a performing role: "If you love listening to, talking about, and sharing your love for music, then this is the class for you! You will learn how to run equipment, structure a music program, and how to use your voice effectively over the airwaves. Join the growing roster of ZUMIX Radio DJs and develop a following for your own weekly radio show!" Youth can still assume a team role and benefit from peer interactions in carrying out radio programming.

Reality Radio: "News" is rarely associated with youth, but the importance of narrative creation is critical in urban communities. Those youth interested in assuming reporter roles and other supporting roles have an opportunity to do so: "Are you an aspiring journalist, artist, poet, scientist, or activist? Do you want to know more about your community? Everyone has a story to share . . . what's yours? In this class you will connect with community members of East Boston, conduct interviews, record and edit audio, and use a state-of-the-art radio studio to produce the stories you uncover on ZUMIX Radio. All you need is a curiosity about the world around you! (Graduates of this class are eligible for paid positions as ZUMIX Youth Radio Journalists)."

Reality Radio II: For those youth interested in a more "serious" involvement in reporting, they can enroll in an advanced course: "(Restricted to graduates of Reality Radio.) Deepen your skills in audio journalism/storytelling, while getting PAID to contribute stories to ZUMIX Radio! Students will visit local radio stations and distribute their stories. They will also prepare a portfolio of stories to be used in college applications, while honing their skills in technology, communication, journalism, and media literacy."

ZUMIX Radio Youth Advisory Council: Participatory democracy is a key value in ZUMIX, and this can be exercised through involvement in an advisory committee: "In June of 2016, ZUMIX will begin broadcasting on 94.9 FM! As a recipient of a license to a Low-Power FM frequency in Boston, we have an opportunity to share youth and community voices with listeners throughout East Boston and beyond. How can our station tell an authentic story of East Boston? What will our station sound like? What does it mean to define a 'community?' How can we promote volunteerism to include as many neighbors as possible? Youth interested in answering these questions to develop their leadership skills, become more civically engaged, and to be an ambassador for our station, please join us!"

5. ZUMIX Sprouts: Children can develop and sharpen their interests in music at an early age if provided with a warm and affirming environment: "These classes offer introductions to music, theater, and dance with an emphasis on stage and performance techniques. Sprouts participants share their performances on the ZUMIX stage and often tour their community to bring music and joy to others."

> **Sprouts Chorus:** Singing is not restricted to any one age group, and opportunities to engage children early in their lives provide a window for participation: "Calling all kids who like to sing! Spend your afternoons singing *with* others and *for* others! Improve your singing skills, sing songs from around the world, learn basic music theory concepts, and be part of a team that enjoys making music together! No previous experience needed, just your singing voice."

> **Sprouts Musical Theater:** Theatre, too, can engage youth of all ages: "Once upon a time there was a group of students who liked to act, sing, and dance. They met to act out different fables and fairytales, and presented them at the end of the semester to happy audiences. They had so much fun and lived happily ever after!"

> **Sprouts Orchestra:** The attractiveness of instruments can serve as a mechanism for engaging very young children and possibly casting them into a lifelong pursuit of music: "Have you ever wanted to play an instrument? Explore the world of music in the Sprouts Orchestra! Have fun playing and performing songs with your friends. Learn about all different types of music and instruments through hands on activities as well as demonstrations from special guest musicians."

> **Warmth Program:** Venturing into the community and engaging in civic pursuits provides youth with an opportunity to give to the community and for the community to see them in a different light as valuable members of the community: "Deep in the winter months it gets wicked cold outside . . . that many people stay home as much as possible. This is a chance to bring the warmth of music to them. You will create and rehearse an original show of popular music and take it on a tour of local nursing homes."

Evaluation

Evaluation brings inherent tensions and challenges. If organizations using the performing arts are to continue to evolve, evaluation will take on great significance, including disseminating results. Getting the impact message out can be accomplished in a variety of ways, including annual reports. ZUMIX reported on outcomes in their 2014 Annual Report, and these measures cover a variety of perspectives:

> On average, we offer 220 hours of youth programming at the ZUMIX Firehouse each week. In the past 4 years, 99% of our seniors graduated from high school (compared to 58% of East Boston High School seniors, and

66% of BPS seniors city-wide). In the past 4 years, 90% of our seniors were accepted to college (compared to 65% of East Boston High School graduating seniors, and 70% of BPS graduating seniors city-wide). During the past year, we served 1,170 youth—506 through on-site programming in the Firehouse and 664 through partnerships. . . . This year, our high school seniors have been accepted into colleges. . . . In the summer of 2014, we celebrated our 20th anniversary of our partnership with the Vermont Arts Exchange with a special tour featuring performances from both our Street Program and DiverCity Band. In January 2014, the ZUMIX Jazz Allstars taught and performed at the Panama Jazz Festival, our second international tour. Over the past year, a total of 50 youth collectively earned over $30,000 through skills they learned at ZUMIX—30 as performing musicians, seven as live sound technicians, and six as teaching assistants, four as youth staff, and three as radio journalists.

This description of how ZUMIX changed the lives of countless youth, including the funds generated by participants, illustrates the career paths that have been shaped because of this program and its potential reach in shaping youth futures.

An international perspective is essential in immigrant/refugee communities if culture is to play an instrumental role in shaping participation experience, and it is represented in ZUMIX's Ethiopian-American pop band (ZUMIX 2014 Annual Report):

> This year, ZUMIX is proud to partner with Boston-based Ethiopian pop band, Debo Band, as our second annual Artist Ambassador. Debo Band is an 11-member group led by Ethiopian-American saxophonist, Danny Mekonnen, and fronted by charismatic vocalist, Bruck Tesfaye. Since their inception in 2006, the band has won raves for their groundbreaking take on Ethiopian pop music, which incorporates traditional scales and vocal styles, alongside American soul and funk rhythms, and instrumentation reminiscent of Eastern European brass bands. To learn more and listen to their music, visit www.deboband.com. Debo Band will provide unique performance and learning opportunities for ZUMIX participants and we look forward to this exciting partnership! 'As long-time fans of the inspiring youth programs and mission of ZUMIX, Debo Band is thrilled about the opportunity to serve as their Artist Ambassador.'"

It is safe to say that ZUMIX's Debo Band is rare and reflects well on how ethnic and cultural identity influences music and its power to bridge cultural divides and enhance youth self-identity.

Julianna Quiroz (age 19) and Mario Jarjour (age 14) illustrate the transformational process of music and the extensiveness of this impact across a variety of social spheres (ZUMIX 2014 Annual Report):

Julianna Quiroz: Julianna first came to ZUMIX as a quiet, introverted 11-year-old. She loved theater and was searching for creative outlets. "ZUMIX answered my prayers. I knew I had a lot of creative abilities, but I was so shy. ZUMIX really pushed me out of my shell." Julianna first participated in Theater programs and piano lessons, and quickly branched out into Songwriting & Performance programs, ensembles such as Voices and African Drumming, and Z-Tech programs. In fact, Julianna is a member of a very elite group of ZUMIX youth and alumni—she is a Z-Tech Wizard, meaning she has graduated from every single Z-Tech program we offer. Now 19 years old, she spent this past summer working at ZUMIX as our Z-Tech Fix-It Scholar through the John Hancock MLK Summer Scholars Program. . . . Julianna is a sophomore at Skidmore College. . . . She plans to build a career combining her love of education and helping people with her love of creative arts.

Mario Jarjour: Mario started playing the trumpet in fifth grade in his elementary school band and quickly realized how much he loved making music. His middle school didn't offer any music programs so his guidance counselor recommended that he look into ZUMIX. Mario didn't waste any time getting involved. Over the past three years, Mario has participated in nearly every ZUMIX program area, including Z-Tech Studio, Fix-It, Recording Lab, Rock Ed, Streetwise, Street Program, Con la Corriente, Reality Radio, and Theater. He has also taken private trumpet and drum lessons, and is a member of the ZUMIX Jazz Allstars and Miyagi and the Kids, ZUMIX's Rock Ensemble. Mario is now a freshman at Revere High School. In addition to being an incredibly active ZUMIX participant, he has also found a passion in photography and graphic design, and often volunteers his skills at ZUMIX events . . . he's most drawn to the intricacies of Z-Tech's creative technology programs. "It's cool being on the back end of a finished product. I get to use all of the tools that look really complicated but aren't, work with artists, and be an important part of really fun and unique projects." Mario has a few different options in mind for his future, but his number one dream is to earn a scholarship to Berklee College of Music to study Electrical Engineering. He's grateful for the opportunities available to him through ZUMIX. "ZUMIX has opened up so many doors for me. It's made me more responsible and a better communicator, and I've made so many great friends here. I'm 14 and I get to work in a recording studio, gaining knowledge and skills in the field I want to work—it's pretty awesome."

Juliana and Mario concretize the outcomes of ZUMIX's success, put a face on data, and show how the varied interests of youth can be met through a music program that is broad in scope and mission.

Key Lessons Learned and General Observations

Empowerment is a key value in ZUMIX, as it is in the other case illustrations used in this book, and this value is closely tied to participation and decision-making.

This is evident in how this organization systematically integrates youth in its planning activities (2014 Annual Report):

> Looking Forward Over the past two years, ZUMIX has been implementing a strategic plan focusing on increasing the depth and breadth of our service to young people while diversifying our revenue streams.
>
> In June 2014, we held a youth-led retreat. With the assistance of an adult facilitator, a group of dedicated ZUMIX youth participants formed a committee, planned, and ran a retreat for ZUMIX youth, staff, and board members, ranging from 8–60 years old. . . . In the summer of 2014, we hired five youth and recent alumni to work at ZUMIX through the John Hancock MLK Summer Scholars Program. They worked with program and administrative staff, leading classes, and planning events. We currently have seven ZUMIX alumni on staff, connecting us to our past and helping lead us toward our future.

There are numerous ways that participants can be integrated into a youth practice organization. Summers provide ample opportunities for engagement because of weather and the freeing-up of time schedules, thus serving as a platform for activities throughout the forthcoming year.

Discussion of using music to keep urban youth engaged in programming must cast a wide net, as evidenced by the extensive range of programming involving music. ZUMIX understands the importance of offering a varied menu of options because one size does not fit all. This embrace of music's diversity speaks well to how accepting the organization is about is flexibility. Providing youth with a radio experience broadens the program's reach beyond the geographical boundaries of East Boston.

A review of the music options reveals a richness of cultural heritage as well as conventional music options. This embrace allows the organization to respond to changing community demographics occurring with the influx of newcomers. The need for an organization to have the ability to respond quickly to changing demographics, a factor in many urban communities, is a constant threat.

Not every youth wishes to perform before an audience, and the option of being behind the scene can be attractive for some youth. Again, a key theme that can be found in the cases selected for inclusion in this section is a willingness to broaden the age range of youth and an understanding that not every participant wishes to make a career in the performing arts. There is an understanding that participants can acquire important academic and social skills in the process of engaging in music making.

Conclusion

ZUMIX's success is the result of its mission and the flexibility, time, and energy devoted to recruiting, training, and supporting its staff. Its birth in response to social injustices carried over into its evolution in reaching urban youth. Its ability to reach youth across the life cycle is a key factor in its success, and its ability to provide a range of approaches has managed to tap varied musical interests. Through flexible music programming, youth-serving organizations can make a difference in the lives of all youth, including those who are newcomers to this country. Many of the same themes that reflect ZUMIX's evolution will also be found in the following chapter on song in Chicago's Good Life Organization.

11

Song

THE GOOD LIFE ORGANIZATION, CHICAGO

Introduction

Singing can transpire in a multitude of ways and a variety of settings, making this method particularly attractive for social justice youth practice and the performing arts. Although singing does not have to involve words, the integration of story-telling is greatly enhanced when words capture critical themes and issues in the lives of youth and their communities. When singing is supported by music, you have a formula that can be powerful in addressing social justice, one that carries increased appeal for urban youth.

Out-of-school settings sponsoring youth singing must be attuned to their interests and challenges if they are to effectively reach youth who have few positive outlets for their interests and talents. The introduction of a group experience harnesses the power and potential of collective forces and memory that can be transformative at both individual and group levels. It is the kind of experience that everyone can relate to, even those of us without the gift of song or talent in this performing art.

Chicago's Good Life Organization was selected because of the social tension found in that city resulting from neighborhood violence specifically perpetrated on youth of color by the city's police force. The organization shows how hip-hop has been a key mechanism for reaching youth and addressing social justice. The convergence of these various factors led to the development of an engaging and transformative performing arts organization.

Brief Literature Grounding

It is appropriate to start this literature review with a reference to the Civil Rights songs of the 1960s. Becker (2016), in an interview of Professor Cheryl Boots, reminds us of the presence of song in racial justice campaigns: "From 'We Shall Overcome' to 'Blowin' in the Wind,' the 'freedom songs' of the civil rights movement helped motivate people of all ages and races, from Student Nonviolent Coordinating Committee (SNCC) activists and Freedom Riders to the thousands who marched on Washington, Selma, and Montgomery."

Songs together with social justice are a powerful mechanism for conveying narratives that are compelling and move crowds to action. The Jamaican song titled "Get Up, Stand Up, Stand Up for Your Rights!" captures how social justice and song can be interrelated (Ferguson, Boer, Clobert, Prade, & Saroglou, 2016). Basham (2015) provides an evolutionary perspective on how hip-hop has incorporated themes of race, crime, and violence in its lyrics and why these themes are salient for urban youth of color. It is no mistake that the Good Life Organization has tapped hip-hop to get youth involved.

Brief Organizational History

The Good Life Organization's history follows a path that should not be surprising, with its origins starting in a school and expanding beyond this confine to one involving multiple states. Its base of operation has remained in Chicago:

> The Fulfill the Dream program began at Social Justice High School almost three years ago. It started when Roberto and Mr. Crye (math teacher) began dreaming about giving youth space to think about their lives, share stories, learn about Hiphop, and how to use it as a tool to create change. The program started out small as it meet about twice to three times a month for about 2 and a half hours. Meeting during the colloquium time of school, or life skills time, the youth watched video's, met local artists, discussed issues going on in life and created art.
>
> The group started out by doing small performances for the school and eventually expanded to include other schools on Chicago's West Side. CCA joined the Fulfill the Dream family as Phenom partnered with Crystal Williams, the guidance counselor at CCA high school. The group met every week, and also discussed life and what could be changed for the better.
>
> The second year, the movement expanded to Manley High School. All three schools continued to develop their critical analysis of their realities while using their creative genius through Hip-hop to challenge and make change. The three schools started to collaborate and organize monthly open mic sessions.
>
> The three schools went off and organized the Hiphop Revival II-leaving a legacy. The event brought in legendary artist Kurtis Blow, and also help breaking battles, MC battles, graffiti battles, and had local performances. . . . Youth still meet and are now working on mentoring younger youth, and doing a

creative research project where they use data as a tool to allow their voices to not only be heard by officials but also respected. Click here to meet a few of the leaders from each of the three schools.

Year three allowed us to expand. . . . This was the first time that the Fulfill the Dream curriculum was taught as an entire course. Connecting with the aspects of performing arts, this class allowed youth to have a critical foundation to look at social issues while addressing them creatively through the arts. These youth were instrumental in the development of an open cipher at Batey Urban which allowed youth an opportunity to come together to share their stories through the elements of hiphop. This gathering was a major catalyst in the development of *Youth Voice Nation*, a book that was developed by youth themselves.

This chapter is unique in that it started with two groups: one being youth and the other being parents. The groups met for ten weeks and discussed the issues facing their communities, the assets available to them, and began working collaboratively in developing a plan of action to address these issues more creatively. The result was the Hip-hop Revival 2008.

This very detailed account of the origins and evolution of this organization is presented in its entirety because it is rare to have the history of an organization's clearly stated purpose written out and preserved to be shared with the outside world. There are many familiar themes in this history and how the organization expanded over time. The inclusion of multiple performing arts served to enhance singing. Youth mentoring youth is a theme raised earlier, as opposed to the more conventional model of adults serving as mentors. The two are not mutually exclusive of each other.

Organizational Setting

The following overview of the Good Life Organization grounds the concept of community capacity enhancement through the use of song in a multifaceted and highly responsive manner:

The Good Life Organization is starting a national movement to positively transform communities through unified strategic planning efforts. This strategic planning is unique in that it spans educational, after-school/nonprofit, family, faith communities, and locally cultivated youth leaders. To achieve this The Good Life Organization is developing educational curricula (The Fulfill the Dream Program) and accompanying products that can be utilized in school, after-school, in faith communities, between family members, and between peers.

This movement of "Hip-hope" which focuses on prevention is aimed at reducing the youth violence rate, high school dropout rate, murder rate, and incarceration rate focusing on youth between 8 and 18 years old.

Chicago's youth and community regarding violence is well understood nationally because of the intense publicity that has been generated nationally, and it should not be surprising why the role of violence is focused on in this program. Mass incarceration cannot be separated from violence, including that perpetrated by law enforcement officers.

Program Components and Major Activities

Song cannot be separated from its cultural context. Understanding this cultural context helps youth express themselves in a manner that resonates and unites them in a common understanding and pursuit. For the Good Life Organization, this is accomplished through Hip-Hop(e) Education, which consists of five components:

> Hiphop culture is a phenomenon that affects youth from every background. In this talk Roberto distinguishes between Hiphop Industry and Hiphop culture. He also explores how Hiphop culture organically integrates best practices in engaging youth found in principles of youth development and culturally relevant pedagogy. This talk further examines how youth culture can inform educators in their pedagogical style and curriculum design in order to engage students in a way that is authentic, fun, and effective. Roberto shares his own research regarding the challenges and best practices of using this cutting edge 21st century approach and how it can and has helped youth raise G.P.A.'s, have fewer behavior issues, and increase attendance.

Helping educators and others develop an understanding of urban youth's operative reality is an important step forward in developing a social justice agenda based on a common understanding, with youth playing an active and significant role in shaping this narrative. Acquisition of "tools" that can help create an affirming climate is an important consequence and one that must be purposeful.

The Good Life Organization has five programmatic components of varying intensity and reach: (1) GLO Radio, (2) Fulfill the Dream, (3) Fulfill the Dream CD, (4) Youth Voice Nation, and (5) Fulfill the Dream Facilitator's Guide. Each of these components exists as a separate entity but still remain closely tied to the others.

1. GLO Radio: The Good Life Organization, in similar fashion to ZUMIX in the prior case, offers radio as an activity, thus adding a communication dimension that appeals to a subgroup of youth:

> "GLO Radio provides you access with a worldwide network of artists and organizations that are working to using Hip Hop, Spoken Word, and the elements of Hip Hop Culture towards social justice, youth empowerment, and the building of consciousness.

Nahume Diaz is a young man that transformed his life after going through the Fulfill The Dream program. He is now a community leader who works to create change by helping other youth find their voice and use them to offer solutions to community issues. We made a music video with a filmmakers from Disney to capture the change this young man is having in the world. Enjoy this song entitled "The Light"!

2. Fulfill the Dream: The journey toward engaging and preparing youth uses a curriculum that views this journey through an evolutionary perspective and has those playing active roles:

Fulfill the Dream is a social and emotional learning curriculum that engages youth in culturally relevant ways using media, movement, and music. The program is aimed at helping youth thrive by helping them to discover their unique gifts or "sparks," by aiding them in the development of healthy relationships with adults and peers, and supporting them in the discovery and cultivating their unique voices.

Youth empowerment and meaningful participation are essential ingredients in this journey of self-discovery through the deconstruction and reliance on self and community assets:

The Fulfill the Dream Program is a student-centered curriculum focused on . . . empirically proven principles of empowerment. It is directed toward developing leadership, relationship, and citizenship skills in adolescents. . . . Culturally relevant pedagogy uses "the cultural knowledge, prior experiences, frames of reference, and performance styles of ethnically diverse students to make learning more relevant and effective." . . . This program builds cumulatively as it gives students tools to critically examine and deconstruct their realities for the purpose of discovering and cultivating assets to direct themselves and their communities toward positive change.

The training journey is closely tied to tap youth culture and fun activities that serve multiple purposes, including life skills enhancement and the development of a clear purpose in life:

Students are encouraged to develop personal leadership skills as they prepare for "making dreams a reality" as they discover their resources, develop a plan, identify action steps, and reflect on their ideas of what "the good life" is. The ten workshops in this curriculum are strategically tied to youth culture because they use media, movement, and music to teach many lessons and communicate main points. . . . "Hip Hop is a very powerful educational tool; teaching has to change.". . . Since there are a variety of elements and activities included with this program, it can fulfill a variety of standards from social studies and English to health, life skills, art and design, theatre, and even science.

The expectation of a product at the completion provides a concrete accomplishment that encapsulates the insights and personal growth achieved in this journey:

> Youth are required to have a culminating project at the end of the program that represents what they learned and how they will apply it. Youth are encouraged to take the resources they have identified and communicate the lessons they have learned, creatively, with their class or their community. Youth can create a poem, a rap, a song, or a collage to represent what they have learned from the program. The second part of the culminating project will include a plan regarding how they can take what they have learned and serve a person or group of people in need.

The following curriculum excerpts illustrate content with a heavy social justice emphasis, including engagement in critical thinking, which is essential for empowerment and social justice:

> **Chapter 1 (Reality Check):** Reality Check – Mainstream media's marketing strategy to youth, and many Americans for that matter, is to create the belief that living the American Dream and being a consumer is the path to lasting fulfillment. In reality what ends up happening is people live a fantasy definition of success, that both empirical research and personal experience inform us does NOT bring lasting fulfillment. Sometimes to understand this, we need a reality check, which serves as a wake-up call, letting us know that we need to reevaluate our life's direction. Then we begin to realize that hustling to get money, or stealing to get that thing, or putting material things before people will not bring the lasting fulfillment that we are seeking. Hip-hop Culture, and the teens who created it, remind us that we have the potential power to redefine societal definitions of success, replacing them with ones that are truly fulfilling.

This chapter addresses values that resonate with youth by having them engage in critical reflection on what is important in their lives. These conversations can prove troubling because it is rare for this subject to be addressed in their lives, particularly in an affirming group context involving peers.

> **Chapter 4 (Your Crew):** Your Crew – Hip-hop is one of the first cultures that brings people together from different race, class, sex, religious, and ethnic backgrounds. This unity of diversity is transformative as it demonstrates that community is most powerful when each individual's unique voice is heard and celebrated rather than homogenized and assimilated. Inherited from Jazz, the activity of ciphering allows one to share his or her unique voice and energy with the community through call and response expression.

> **Chapter 10 (The Great Life Legacy):** In this chapter, youth are encouraged to examine the lifelong consequences of actions taken without thought and the

importance of understanding and embracing the meaning of a life that is reaction-
ary and reckless:

> The Great Life Legacy – You have heard the saying "you reap what you
> sow," but have you ever thought about what that really means? Of course,
> in terms of science it means that if you plant a green bean seed, you will
> grow a green bean plant. A person who plants corn in the ground will never
> reap a harvest of rice, lentils, or some other plant. If you plant corn, you
> will consistently reap corn during harvest time. How does this apply to life?
> What we plant will eventually grow up and become full-grown not only in
> dirt, but also in our hearts and life. We can at times be disillusioned about
> what it is we are planting and end up planting weeds thinking that they are
> something else.

3. Fulfill the Dream CD: Creation of a CD provides participants with an
opportunity to broaden the reach of their influence using a medium that resonates
with youth across the country. The CD production process seeks sought to have
youth use critical thinking skills.

4. Youth Voice Nation: Hip-hop curriculum is essential in maximizing its
potential to engage and increase the awareness of urban youth concerning social
forces operative in the lives:

> Youth Voice Nation: Taking the Voices of Youth Off Mute, inspired by the
> Good Life Organization's Fulfill the Dream Curriculum, is a powerful counter
> narrative that uses Hiphop to creatively and critically challenge those that
> say: "youth should have no input regarding the current crisis in America."
> Creating a movement of youth equipped with the artillery of spoken word,
> essays, raps, sketches, and murals.
>
> The best part of this book is that it is a living document that welcomes
> the contributions of other youth and youth workers. Centered on the tenants
> of the old school mentoring the next generation of youth to find their spark of
> genius and use that to create change. . . . You will also find the words and mes-
> sages found here challenge you to respond in your own way and share your
> responses with the collective community of change agents.

5. Fulfill the Dream Facilitator's Guide: The Good Life Organization produced a highly detailed and user-friendly facilitator's guide:

> This guide contains in depth explanations of the ten principles of the Fulfill
> The Dream curriculum along with step by step instruction on how to facilitate
> each workshop and meet each learning objective. This program is in align-
> ment with current SEL standards for secondary aged students and connects
> with all 40 Assets outlined by the SEARCH Institute. This program also meets
> culturally relevant pedagogical standards at it is embedded in youth culture
> with the usage of media, movement, and music to use this tool correctly,

facilitators must attend a 16 hour certification training. All trainings are available to university credit and can also go towards being certified as a professional youth development practitioner.

Youth organizations can use one of three ways of conducting evaluation: (1) internally focused, (2) external expertise, or (3) capacity enhancement (external working with internal). The Good Life Organization has tapped external resources in evaluation.

Key Lessons Learned and General Observations

Music's transformative (therapeutic and social) power is increased when confronting social justice and encouraging youth to share their message with peers and the world. The popularity of hip-hop and the fight to decommercialize it represents a dimension of social justice that resonates among many urban youth. Youth, to achieve their goal, participate in an ongoing dialogue that brings individual voices into a collective voice. This enhances agency, a critical element in seeking change in their lives and seeking social change.

Hip-hop's popularity, as well as its controversy, highlights music's potential to spark conversations and even heated debates that can further the cause of social justice. When urban youth themselves take this message on the road, they only enhance the message because we cannot separate out the message from the messenger. The Good Life Organization's effort to develop products enhances its reach beyond narrow geographical boundaries onto a national level.

Youth organizations that are highly successful have broadened the age groups that they serve. Developing a continuum of participation allows organizations to reach youth at a very young age without neglecting older and—quite frankly—less attractive youth for many youth-serving organizations because the issues these older youth are dealing with are highly contentious and have possible life-and-death consequences. This attempt to reach across the life span can be quite challenging because it requires staff with different interests and competencies, thus challenging recruitment, training, and staff retention.

Hip-hop's importance across the country and the world has been addressed. To see its influence in the development of a youth organization and to witness the role of social justice in shaping the message and the vehicle is essential in helping urban youth articulate their concerns and share their dreams for a more just future. The Good Life Organization is not satisfied with focusing their message on Chicago and has expanded beyond this city to include the West Coast.

Songs' collective benefits, when tied to music, can redress injustices and represent an attractive focus for youth organizations stressing the performing arts. Song can easily be added to programs that emphasize other activities of interest to urban youth because singing is a natural occurrence.

Conclusion

The power of song and singing has been demonstrated over the past 60 years by African-Americans in their search for justice and shows how protest and spiritual singing has furthered their cause for social justice. Urban youth are closely associated with music as culture and as a vehicle for conveying important messages in their lives, as evidenced by hip-hop's origins and evolution. Singing and songs provide an avenue for youth to express their hopes and fears and to do so in a manner that is natural, can tap symbols and language that is relevant in their lives, and can be done inexpensively.

12

Dance

MOVING IN THE SPIRIT, ATLANTA

Introduction

Dance challenges the social justice youth community practice field to integrate social justice themes that resonate with participants. These challenges can be often met in a highly innovative and engaging fashion, as demonstrated in this chapter. It is important to attract youth across the entire age span, and this goal provides youth organizations with an opportunity to be there during key developmental stages, as is the case with Atlanta's Moving in the Spirit program.

The selection was easy to make because this is not my first exposure to this organization. I included Moving in the Spirit in a collection of case studies undertaken in the late 1990s for a book titled *New Dimensions for Youth Community Practice: Use of the Arts, Humanities and Sports* (Delgado, 2000). At that time, the organization had been operational approximately 15 years and it left a lasting impression because of the staff's openness, cooperation, and propensity to document their efforts. I made a commitment to myself that I would visit this program again in the future.

Brief Literature Grounding

Youth engagement and disengagement in dance must not be thought of as a dichotomy but rather as a continuum (Bond & Stinson, 2016). Failure to engage in dance may be due to a multiplicity of reasons, such as fear of failure, lack of interest, or belief that skill sets do not match the demands of dance, for instance. Those who are attracted to dance may have an interest and emotional connection to this performing art, are excited by the challenge, and embrace the role of autonomy in setting their own measures of success.

Dance is closely associated with youth, regardless of dance abilities. Dance does not require music although the integration of music with dance reinforces the attractiveness of both. The benefits and range of dancing options attest to its appeal and potential for transforming the lives of urban youth. Dancing as an activity is associated with fun and is not restricted to any particular youth age group. The worldwide phenomenon of flash mob dancing has tapped the joy, fun, and camaraderie associated with dancing and youth culture, but is not limited to youth and thus opens up intergenerational possibilities (Molnár, 2014). Organizations wishing to maximize their impact on youth will need to offer varying dance forms across a range of ages.

Dance's cultural roots provide a mechanism through which youth can explore heritage and traditions in a way that is highly physical and fun, too (Buck & Rowe, 2015; Fürst, 2015). Dancing can be either sacred or secular in nature, thus bringing a different cultural perspective on this performing art (Kuwor, 2015). When dance introduces music and possibly song, too, it provides a broad canvas on which to introduce social justice and other themes and issues of relevance to urban youth of color, including those youth who are newcomers (Linton, Choi, & Mendoza, 2016). However, the performing arts are not universally embraced by all religious groups and this could be a potential barrier in outreach to youth who belong to these religions (McDonnell, 2015).

Dance presents a particular challenge in attracting and maintaining young males of color when they reach adolescence, so that special attention must be paid to recruiting and supporting them when they enter a youth dance organization (Aponte, 2013; Delgado, 2000). Youth dance organizations must actively work against stereotypical and homophobic forces undermining the development of an inclusive and affirming organization (Peterson & Anderson, 2012; Rogers & Sanders III, 2012).

Organizational Setting

Moving in the Spirit's philosophy fills an important void in the lives of Atlanta's youth of color, who are predominantly African-American/Black, and the program is welcoming of all regardless of their dancing abilities: "At Moving in the Spirit, we believe *every child* deserves to grow within a community that is rich in cultural assets, caring role models and safe places to learn. We exist to create opportunities for youth who might otherwise lack access to after-school enrichment programs, especially those focused on the arts." Moving in the Spirits is a viable afterschool alternative, filling a niche in Atlanta's afterschool field.

Its mission is transformative:

Moving in the Spirit is a nationally-recognized youth development program that uses the art of dance to positively transform the lives of children and teens in Atlanta, Georgia. Through programs that integrate high-quality dance instruction with performance, leadership and mentor opportunities, Moving in the Spirit impacts over 200 children and teens annually, encouraging them to overcome the obstacles they face each day and realize their highest potential . . .. Ultimately, Moving in the Spirit EDUCATES, INSPIRES and UNITES young people through dance, propelling them to become successful and compassionate leaders.

Brief Organizational History

Moving in the Spirit's organizational history dates back an impressive 30 years and taps into the power, vision, and commitment of two individuals wishing to make a difference in an America still reeling from the devastations of major riots: "Moving in the Spirit began in 1986 as the hopeful vision of Dana Lupton and Leah Mann, who believed they could unite their love for dance with their commitment to social justice."

The expansion during this period of time attests to its meeting the needs of Atlanta's youth interested in dance as vehicle for self-expression, but also introduces a range of challenges that are inherent in any organization wishing to expand its reach and services.

Program Components and Major Activities

Moving in the Spirits represents a sanctuary that is physical and symbolic, and this place and space is welcoming of all youth regardless of their abilities to pay and inclusive of all:

Moving in the Spirit provides a safe, nurturing environment in which young people can study the art of dance, make friends and develop leadership skills. Our curriculum focuses primarily on modern dance and incorporates ballet technique, creative movement and the creation of original choreography. We accept students ages 3–18, beginner to advanced. Need-based scholarships are available. . . . Moving in the Spirit's unique mission is to create compassionate leaders through the art of dance. We realize this mission by linking our class structure and goals directly with the Positive Youth Development Model, designed to transition children successfully into adulthood. Students are given a voice in class activities and choreography, set personal goals, problem-solve with their peers and practice leadership skills. . . . On average, they remain with Moving in the Spirit for 6 to 8 years.

Moving in the Spirit views dancing along an age developmental continuum and from a corresponding curriculum standpoint, with participants engaging at a relatively early age and staying with the program over an extended age period:

> **Stepping Stones:** Moving in the Spirit's open-level offering, Stepping Stones provides students ages 3–18 one hour of age-appropriate dance classes each week. Stepping Stones dance classes provide participants with creative movement experiences that encourage positive behavior and leadership skills. Students learn fundamental modern dance techniques while addressing core values of discipline, commitment and responsibility.

The following age and gender breakdown provides a glimpse into how each group is addressed using age-specific approaches across a developmental cycle that allows youth an extended period of time to remain engaged in this performing art:

> **Ages 3–4, Boys & Girls: Baby Steps:** Creative movement, improvisation and basic modern dance technique are used to introduce students to the primary elements of dance, build foundational locomotor and non-locomotor skills, and explore imagination and creativity.
>
> **Ages 5–7, Boys & Girls: Mini Steps:** Students continue building fundamental modern dance technique while learning dance terminology, refining body alignment, and exploring spatial relationships, timing/tempo and different movement qualities. They also create choreographic phrases with their peers, practice observational skills and experience opportunities to teach and lead their peers.
>
> **Ages 8–12, Girls: Girls in Motion:** Girls in Motion students expand their training in modern dance technique and learn basic elements of partnering. They study the fundamentals of choreographic structures, improvising and experimenting with new ways to combine movements and vary their use of the key dance elements. Girls in Motion students also explore ways to express meaning through dance, collaborating and problem-solving with their peers to create choreography for their class.
>
> **Ages 8–12, Boys: Boys in Motion:** Boys in Motion students study modern dance, hip hop and the basic elements of partnering. Led by alumnus Chris McCord, they study the fundamentals of choreographic structures, improvising and experimenting with new ways to combine movements and vary their use of the key dance elements: space, time, and energy. Boys in Motion students also explore ways to express meaning through dance, collaborating and problem-solving with their peers to create choreography for their class.
>
> **Ages 13–18, Boys & Girls: Collective Motion:** Collective Motion students study modern dance, improvisation and partnering. They gain a nuanced understanding of dance terminology and body awareness and deepen their facility with the key elements of dance: space, time and energy. Collective Motion students collaborate with one another to generate artistically

expressive dances that are interesting and varied in form and structure. Focus is also given to practicing critical and analytical thinking skills; students learn how to discuss their movement choices, provide constructive feedback to their peers and discover solutions together.

The Men in Motion program may go by many different names in other programs. This program's focus is on latency and early teen years. Calling it "Men in Motion" elevates the status of participants.

> **Men in Motion:** A place in which young men ages 10–13 can learn values, build confidence and practice leadership skills. Activities and choreography for the Men in Motion program are specially crafted to engage the unique energies and interests of young men.

The program structure emphasizes didactic and dance activities and performances:

> Meet for 90 minutes weekly to study modern dance, hip hop and choreography. Create energetic choreography with their peers. Deepen their understanding of dance terminology, anatomy, and the key elements of dance performance. Train with male guest artists from Atlanta's professional dance community who conduct workshops, set choreography and serve as role models. Participate in group mentoring activities through our Mentor Program. Take part in recreational, cultural and educational field trips. Present works they rehearse and create in their very own Men in Motion show, and in our year-end show at the Rialto Center for the Arts at Georgia State University.

Participation is formalized through a contract: "Men in Motion members must complete a placement assessment at the beginning of the year and sign a 'commitment contract' outlining their goals and responsibilities serving to highlight the seriousness of this commitment." This contract goes far beyond rules and regulations and necessitates that potential participants undertake self-reflection.

Director McCord, an alumnus of Moving in the Spirit, takes special care to provide counseling and encouragement. (It is important to highlight that many organizations feature a career ladder, and more so because it opens up career opportunities for alums, as in the case of Chris McCord.) "Men in Motion members also take part in monthly educational workshops covering topics such as puberty and health, violence prevention, self-esteem and peer pressure, and conflict resolution training." Education is a lifelong pursuit, and how this value is emphasized takes on great importance and has carryover to life outside.

SUMMER CAMP

Summer Camp provides Moving in the Spirit with an opportunity to continue to reach youth for a concentrated period of time and introduce activities that are not dance centered during a time period when many Atlanta youth may be without a structured environment:

> Moving in the Spirit's Summer Dance Camp, for young people ages 8–14, combines dance instruction with creative youth development workshops and adventurous field trips. The two-week program provides campers with a safe environment where they can have fun while learning dance technique, developing life skills and increasing confidence . . .. At the end of camp, students perform a special show for family and friends. The camp will consists of dance technique classes in Hip-Hop, African, Jazz and Modern; Game Time & Craft Projects; Health and Life Skills classes; Recreational field trip.

STUDENT TOURING COMPANY

Using a touring company reflects the importance of this organization's reaching out to new audiences and providing an opportunity to venture outside of their more familiar confines:

> ¤ Comprised of our most advanced students, Moving in the Spirit's Touring Company offers uplifting performances of modern dance that celebrate diversity and make a difference in the world.
> ¤ Our Touring Company has traveled across the United States and performed overseas in France, the Czech Republic, Panama and Hungary. To create their powerful pieces, our gifted teen artists collaborate with innovative local and national choreographers.

Evaluation

Testimonials by Dana Marie Lupton, Executive and Artistic Director, provide a face and narrative that numbers simply cannot capture:

> Over my past 29 years at Moving in the Spirit, I have watched thousands of young people transform before my eyes—students who walked through our doors timid, angry or aloof have emerged as confident, compassionate leaders. Often I'm asked how Moving in the Spirit accomplishes this powerful and lasting change in our students' lives. How does a dance program produce successful and courageous young leaders like Tenesia? I met Tenesia when she was 12 years old. Like so many students we serve, she had many wonderful talents but was unable to see the greatness in herself. She was afraid to express her opinion, avoided forming close relationships, and shied away from opportunities that put her in the spotlight. . . . Through weekly "check-ins" and monthly "family time" sessions, Tenesia found a healthy outlet for coping with stress and a nurturing place to express herself and assert

personal agency. Through the rigor of dance she learned self-control and discipline. Through opportunities to collaborate with her peers, she developed close friendships.

Tenesia came to Moving in the Spirit expecting dance lessons, but what she gained was so much more—critical life skills that would serve her beyond the dance floor.

My fondest memory of Tenesia occurred during a rehearsal for Iron Jawed Angels, a dance about the women's suffrage movement. I had asked Tenesia to create choreography that would embody the struggles faced by these pioneering women from our history. . . . When she taught the choreography to her peers, Tenesia communicated effectively and demonstrated intention. . . . Tenesia graduated this past spring from University of Georgia and is now a fierce leader and active member of Moving in the Spirit's alumni committee. . . . We are proud that, while the graduation rate for Atlanta Public Schools was 51% in 2012, 100% of Moving in the Spirit seniors over the past ten years have graduated high school and gone on to college, vocational school or military careers.

Key outcomes are measured throughout the program. In our most recently completed program year, students stated that Moving in the Spirit helped them improve in the following:

- ◻ Thinking about job/career opportunities (100%)
- ◻ Setting personal goals (98%)
- ◻ Showing concern for others (99%)
- ◻ Expressing anger without violence (99%)
- ◻ Avoiding drug and gang activity (97%)
- ◻ Working hard in school (93%)

Additionally, evaluations revealed significant improvement in Positive Youth Development goals including conflict management, behavioral and intellectual competency and self-esteem . . .. Moving in the Spirit's impact is best exemplified by our alumni, who have found success in their own live are returning to our organization to give back to the next generation of young people at Moving in the Spirit as teachers, mentors and donors.

Evaluation requires a multifaceted approach, and Moving the Spirit utilizes the following evaluation tools: Pro-Social Checklist, Piers Harris 2 Self Concept Test, Developmental Assets Profile, and a Modern Dance Technique Assessment. It is appropriate to end this evaluation with a short testimonial about what participation in this program meant for one youth member:

Moving in the Spirit molded me into a mature young person. They gave me that inner strength to communicate not only with respect, but with seriousness and assertiveness. Moving in the Spirit raised me, and I would not be the leader I am today without them. (Tenesia Benson, alumna, '11)

Key Lessons Learned and General Observations

Moving in the Spirit is multifunctional, with a long developmental history illustrating its success in securing stable and long-term funding, as well as an increased programming demand from youth. Dance is a performing art that can encompass many different forms and must do so if it is to be responsive to the community. There is an understanding that, for many youth, dance will not be a lifetime pursuit, yet there are youth who wish to make it a career and they, too, have an opportunity to pursue this dream.

Moving in the Spirit has evolved since its inception in 1986 and encompasses a variety of dance forms and age-groups. Providing opportunities for alums to come back as staff is a key element in maintaining the commitment it made when initially founded. Alums become effective ambassadors. When a program is youth-centered, its graduates have a long life span in this capacity.

The relationship between social media and youth is close, and it has provided Moving in the Spirit with a series of platforms from which to share its amazing mission and results with the world. It has also helped with recruitment. Word of mouth is still a powerful mechanism in reaching out to potential recruits. Their webpage, in similar fashion to the other programs highlighted in this case study section, is outstanding and reflective of the importance of communication within and across groups.

Conclusion

The reader must be impressed by the role that Atlanta's Moving in the Spirit has played in using dance as an activity to reach and engage male and female participants. Although social justice issues led to the creation of this organization and have manifested a role throughout its history, it is not as pronounced as in the other performing arts covered in this book. Providing dance opportunities across the life span allows youth to engage at an early age and stay engaged through their youth-hood. Practitioners and academics alike have much to draw upon in this case, and this is a credit to its propensity to document.

The case of the Unusual Suspects Theatre Company in Chapter 13 builds on Moving in the Spirit and pays particular attention to the presence and influence of trauma and how it has shaped the lives of urban youth individually and collectively. The reader will see how complementary these two organizations are, in a way that goes beyond an embrace of the performing arts.

13

Theatre

THE UNUSUAL SUSPECTS THEATER COMPANY, LA

Introduction

I was not at a loss in selecting the Unusual Suspects Theater Company of Los Angeles, California, for inclusion in this chapter, and this is a testament to this organization's efforts to outreach and engage urban youth. Youth in criminal justice systems and those under intense scrutiny are a growing percentage across the nation, particularly when discussing urban youth of color. Social justice practice has much to accomplish here, and there is general agreement that "conventional" approaches that have proved successful with other groups have not proved so with these youth (Bradshaw, Brown, & Hamilton, 2006; Fader, 2013).

Selecting the Unusual Suspects Company was very easy because of its mission, access to public information, and multifaceted approach. Some years ago I did a case study of Home Boys/Home Girls, a social enterprise focused on former gang members (Delgado, 2012), came across the Unusual Suspects Company, made a mental note of its unique approach towards youth, and wanted to revisit this organization.

Brief Literature Grounding

Use of theatre with youth offenders or those at great likelihood of offending falls within the category of "theatre practice with offenders." "Applied theatre" is often the label used to designate this theatre because of its broad reach within the field, although this label cover a great deal of territory (Hughes & Ruding, 2009). Giving youth an opportunity to describe, share, and dramatize their narratives before an audience is a rare chance in their lives (Armstrong, 2006).

Youth who are court-involved or have criminal justice experiences are often thought of as "hard core" and the most difficult to reach. Quite frankly, they not an "attractive" group to integrate into existing and more conventional out-of-school settings. If we follow this logic, then they also have the most to gain when given the opportunity to engage in youth practice. This may require greater resources than their non–court involved counterparts, but this group also has the greatest needs and potential for growth.

Turner (2007) draws on restorative justice as a major theme in using theatre with youthful offenders to provide them with a mechanism through which they can give back to their communities but also reconnect with their community on a positive note. Bintliff (2011) reports on success in reaching youth who have been labeled "at-risk" through the use of restorative justice and tapping into their eagerness to learn. Palidofsky and Stolbach (2012) address the therapeutic help that musical theatre can provide girls who are incarcerated in helping them deal with trauma in their lives.

The subject's popularity has resulted in a number of outstanding books that readers can turn to for greater depth of details. The following books are but several that stand out:

- ¤ Baim and Brookes (2002) *Geese Theater Handbook: Drama with Offenders and People at Risk* provides examples and tools that help youth express themselves in a manner that captures their reality and hopes.
- ¤ Balfour's (2004) *Theater in Prison: Theory and Practice* provides a theoretical foundation and practical application of theatre across a variety of prison groups and applications.
- ¤ McAvinehey's (2011) *Theater Prison* is a short but very informative book that grounds theatre within the broader society's propensity to incarcerate.
- ¤ Shailor's (2011a) edited book, *Performing New Lives: Prison Theater,* provides a range of examples to draw upon on how prisons shape inmate behaviors and how theatre can be an effective vehicle to allow them to express themselves within the confines of a total institution.
- ¤ Taylor and colleagues' book (2010a) *Performing New Lives: Prison Theater* illustrates the role that theatre plays in helping the re-entry process.
- ¤ Trounstine's (2001) *Shakespeare Behind Bars: The Power of Drama in a Women's Prison* does a wonder job of describing how women inmates found their experiences therapeutic and socially significant in their lives. The use of theatre in the setting of youth in detention has not benefited from the same level of attention as their adult counterparts.
- ¤ Thompson's (1998) *Prison Theater: Practices and Perspectives,* although dated remains highly relevant today; it brings a strong international perspective and uses the voices of prisoners.
- ¤ Tocci's (2007) *The Proscenium Cage: Critical Case Studies in US Prison Theater Programs* provides case studies for helping readers understand how theatre companies can undertake theatre within prisons.
- ¤ Landy and Montgomery (2012) discuss The Unusual Suspects Theater Company in *Theater for Change: Education, Social Action and Therapy,*

bringing attention to the importance of urban youth sharing their personal struggles. They emphasize that making the personal public is therapeutic but also essential to address social injustices.

Theater with the incarcerated or those with a high probability of being so represents a significant cohort of urban youth who are deserving of a first or second chance, as the case may be. The example of the Unusual Suspects Theater Company illustrates the power of theatre to address social justice and empower youth.

The concept of sanctuary has appeared in the correctional literature and has applicability to youth practice. Readers may be familiar with this concept as popularized by McLaughlin, Irby, and Langman's (1994) classic book *Urban Sanctuaries: Neighborhood Organizations in the Lives and Futures of Inner-City Youth*, with its applicability to programs focused on court-involved youth (Shailor, 2011b, pp. 22–23):

> Prison theater programs create sanctuaries where the distractions and degradations of the normal prison context are temporarily set aside. A safe container is established where focus and discipline can be exercised in the service of artistic goals. A sense of ensemble or community can develop, offering both challenge and support to each of the participants. An environment very unlike the prison cell, the prison yard, and most prison classrooms develops, where creativity and compassion, self-exploration and experimentation, playfulness and risk-taking can flourish and bear fruit.

Sanctuary as a concept can also be applied to theatre with court-involved youth. Theatre captures a space and place where youth can be accepted and can share and be provided with an opportunity to grow socially and emotionally.

Organizational Setting

The Unusual Suspects Theater Company was founded in 1993, by Laura Leigh, and it is located in Los Angeles. The association of Los Angeles with the performing arts is well known and represents an asset that few cities in the country can claim. The longevity of this organization is a testament to its embrace of innovation, caring, and willingness to reach out to youth whom other organizations would simply rather ignore. It is an ideal case illustration of an organization that has been able to not only survive but thrive to reach a milestone in existence. Mohler (2012a, 2012b) shows how a Los Angeles theatre company can play an influential role within the community.

Brief Organizational History

The Unusual Suspects Theater Company, sharing a similar history to many youth organizations across the United States, was born in responsive to the urban strife of the early 1990s, seeking to reach urban youth and young adults in a manner that was culture-specific and affirming (Fairman, 2014):

> Born out of the ashes of the 1992 L.A. Uprising, Unusual Suspects was founded on the belief that youth are our cultural barometer and that listening to their stories can help bridge divides and heal communities. In the 20 years since its founding, Unusual Suspects has helped bring people together by implementing theatre projects with both youth and adults all over L.A. County, including at youth prisons, treatment centers and L.A.'s most underserved schools and communities. And so, Unusual Suspects gathered together the school's principal, counselor, and parent representative to listen.

Few cities in the United States are as associated with gangs as Los Angeles. Youth organizations would be hard pressed to select an underserved group as great and as challenging as current or former gang members. The Unusual Suspects Theater Company focused on the needs experienced by these youth:

> Los Angeles is known to some as the "Gang Capital" of America. While many reports are expressing record lows in juvenile crime, the dips aren't consistent neighborhood to neighborhood, and incarceration rates are still spiking. Committed to meeting the needs of Los Angeles' most vulnerable youth, we identify and work with communities, schools, and detention centers with the most incidents of violence and crime, and the highest poverty, incarceration, and dropout rates.

Youth programming organizations in urban centers cannot ignore the presence and influence of gangs if they hope to succeed. An embrace of all youth, regardless of their involvement in the court systems, means that "business as usual" will be unsuccessful and that bold initiatives are necessary.

Outreach to settings with high rates of violence and crime means that issues related to social justice will be prominent in the lives of youth and will emerge in the narratives they share through their plays and the audiences they wish to reach. The theme of violence was raised earlier in this book, and this case highlights the concerns practitioners may have that violence will become endemic in the lives of youth as they age into adulthood:

> We are devoted to Los Angeles' youth, and believe that there is hope for *each* one if given the right opportunity and support, and that's exactly what we do. A majority of the youth involved in our programming (over 600 annually) live in poverty, have visions of futures shaped by violence and loss, struggle with reading and writing skills, and as a result, have low self esteem and broken relationships. Our team uses the stage as a vehicle for confidence, hope, reconciliation and belonging.

The theatre stage represents a wonderful and vibrant arena to showcase youth issues, dreams, and talents, and it lends itself to collective and interactive expression. The Unusual Theater Company has a place and role for all youth in tapping their interests and abilities and in creating a narrative that binds youth together and reflects their lives and those of their families and friends in the community:

> In theatre as in life, everyone has a role to play, and neither can be done well in solitude. By creating and performing as an ensemble, participants develop valuable social and emotional life skills. With a common goal, working in tandem with community and family members of all ages, participants learn choice and consequences, and develop tools of empathy and self-confidence that help to heal their homes and communities, and serving them long after they leave the stage.

The Unusual Suspects Theater Company's vision shaped its mission, and it is important to see how the following two statements are informative in providing insight into the forces shaping its unique stance:

> Our vision is to be a source of compassion, strength and support for youth in underserved and at-risk environments; to give them a voice that is heard, valued and respected; and to be a bridge that helps them make positive life choices.

The Unusual Suspects Theatre Company's mission draws upon many of the values identified in Chapter 4 and illustrates how they can be operational-ized in a manner that seeks to achieve positive social change in the lives of participating youth:

> The Unusual Suspects Theater Company's mission is to empower youth in underserved and at-risk environments with the means and methods neces-sary to explore personal and social conflicts and develop self-esteem, commu-nication and coping skills to make positive life choices and become productive members of the community.

The Unusual Suspects Theater Company has a keen understanding of the importance of occupying a unique niche within the Los Angeles theatre scene, in what is arguably one of the nation's most competitive performing arts fields, but one with room and encouragement for innovation, particularly when reaching out to new audiences and participants:

> Given the breadth of talent and access to industry, Los Angeles is home to many wonderful theatre arts, after-school, and mentoring programs; we are proud to call many of them partners and friends. Los Angeles is also home to a variety of nuanced communities and neighborhoods, and the tools used to address each one's particular needs must be as multifaceted as its people.

Success translates into organizational longevity, and a reputation for being able to deliver on promises through a variety of programs, and outreach to all youth.

Program Components and Major Activities

The Unusual Suspects Theater Company delivered on its ambitious vision and mission statement through an acceptance of youth as they are, and it developed a programmatic approach that does not make youth feel bad about themselves and their competencies:

> It's not easy to teach a child to write, it's even harder to teach them how to get in front of an audience to direct and perform their words, vulnerably, before their peers, families, and communities. Both in our school programs and juvenile detention centers—in conjunction with a county and state approved curriculum developed in-house—the youth write, direct, and perform their stories, uncensored, and in their own voices.

The Unusual Suspects Theater Company is heavily dependent upon group process and youth being accepted for who they are, and their life experiences are viewed as critical ingredients to successful youth programs (Fairman, 2014):

> Guided by half a dozen caring adults, our students work in groups of 25–30, in which every member is accountable to the rest, to complete the high-stakes project of writing and/or performing an original play in ensemble. Many students say that being in our program is the first time they have ever felt truly supported, that it is the only place they feel accepted for who they are, and that they feel that Unusual Suspects is a family.

Creation of a welcoming and affirming climate translates into a safe and trusting environment, which is essential for youth to be open to sharing and learning from each other and adults:

> Within this safe environment of the ensemble, our kids express their truth, and then learn to hone it into a story with a beginning, middle and end. They learn to create the inciting incident, how to create a dramatic arc, and that conflict and how the characters manage it is what makes things interesting. Within this process, they learn to think about life in new ways. For example, with our camp kids (those incarcerated in L.A. County probation lock ups), they're so used to violence that the term dramatic arsenal is sometimes taken literally. Imagine you're improvising a scene in which you have to convince someone to give you $20. How many of us would take out a gun and threaten to shoot the person?

Most youth have a range of responses to this assignment of getting $20. Exploring various actions and their potential consequences becomes an important process and learning experience for participants. The lessons learned through this group or collective process can have life-long consequences.

Youth engage in a two consecutive 10-week (60–80 hours each) workshop series. Engagement in the development of a play follows distinctive phases according to Program Director Denton (Fairman, 2014):

> Once the play is written, we have our first table read. The kids are always nervous and excited at this point, and the nerves are particularly apparent at the camps, where the average age is 16 but the average reading level is 5th grade. . . . A lot of the young people we're working with, especially those in the juvenile justice system, have missed out on the nurturing and education that most kids get growing up. Consequently, many of our teens are reading below grade level. . . . They do a lot of the writing on their feet through improvisation, so all the kids can participate in creating a sophisticated story regardless of their literacy level. It's always a great day when the kids get the formatted copy of the script that they wrote. They want to be able to read it so desperately. It's extremely motivating!

Reading and writing are closely associated with most forms of this performing art. Bringing a feeling of openness to how youth can contribute to this sharing and learning process and improvisation can be high energy, fun, and cathartic, too. Accommodating different levels of language mastery (verbal, reading, and writing) and being flexible in allowing youth to express their sentiments in their preferred manner makes the process inclusive, nonstigmatizing, and paced according to abilities, as noted by Senior Program Manager Joyce Lee (Fairman, 2014):

> At the table read, each young person gets assigned a part (not necessarily the part they'll play on stage) and the reading begins. Here's where having so many mentors really helps. The teens that can't read well are embarrassed, of course, and the process can be painful. To alleviate the tension, our mentors quietly sit next to any child that's having trouble and help. And, it turns out the ensemble is surprisingly supportive—there's none of the teasing that one might expect from adolescents. They're all pulling for each other at this point. . . . That's what makes our program so effective. In a play, and in our process, every voice is critical, and the kids know it. We raise the bar for our young people, and it works. The kids know they are important and that makes all the difference.

Group support taps into collectivistic and cooperative values in a society where education stresses individualistic and competitive values. Theater, at least as conceptualized by The Unusual Suspects, seeks to build bridges between youth rather than separate them according to academic abilities. This takes on even greater significance for participants with histories of being separated within educational systems.

Theater requires that youth develop or enhance their abilities to focus, which can be quite demanding; to be punctual; and to work hard, all qualities that serve them well both in the theatre and in the real world, and they still have fun in the process (Fairman, 2014):

> Unusual Suspects provides workshops that focus on rhythm, eye-to-eye contact, and on having fun when working hard. When the youth participants improvise with others in the ensemble they have to be present, focused and deeply connected to move the work forward. "Attunement requires committed adults capable of being emotionally present and developing trusting relationships and nurturing experiences," explains Sela-Amit. "That's what the exercises and the development of trust between the visiting artists and the participants do."

Activities also serve to increase participation and commitment when well conceptualized by youth; this provides important information for staff to gauge the degree of engagement and provides trust as the "the glue" to successful youth programming. Caring adults are essential for youth engagement and growth (emotionally, socially, and cognitively) in youth programs (Fairman, 2014):

> And, as it turns out, the part about being a kid and having a caring adult role model is key. When a person experiences trauma, as many of our young people growing up in high-crime areas do, the impact of it is lodged in the brain. Improvisation, through attunementα—a concentrated activity that is happening between two or more people who are being fully present—assists in processing trauma. It's a means of deeply focusing on one's state of mind, one's needs, and providing valuable feedback to those needs in a way that the other person feels deeply heard, valued, respected and cared for. This nurturing is something that many Unusual Suspects participants didn't get growing up.

Trauma is not a subject that is foreign to urban youth. Developing a willingness and ability to explore trauma, which is not a straightforward process, requires a safe and supportive environment, and having trusting and competent adults involved in this process is essential. The group can be a supportive mechanism, providing other members with an opportunity to share and support where appropriate.

This context of sharing and support sets the stage for a discussion of programs. Any successful youth performing arts program is not unidimensional, and the Unusual Suspects Theater Company features a multifaceted set of components in its efforts to be systematic and comprehensive in reaching and successfully engage urban youth. Unusual Suspects relies on six components that include active alumni services: (1) Youth Theater Residency Program, (2) Neighborhood Voices Program, (3) Voices for Arts and Social Theater Program, (4) Theater and Culture Access Program, (5) Teaching Assistant Training, and (6) Volunteer Program.

YOUTH THEATER RESIDENCY PROGRAM

Youth are not adverse to making a commitment or participating in a structured and lengthy training program if their engagement is viewed as meaningful and taps into their hopes for a better future:

> Hundreds of youth in middle schools, high schools, and juvenile detention camps take part in our cornerstone playwriting and performance workshops each year. These 20-week, two-part intensive after-school and in-camp trainings, instructed by industry and education professionals and mentors, reveal new insight and opportunity for each participant. Youth explore the personal and social conflicts that impact their communities via the creative process of writing and/or performing their own original plays. Workshop curricula are certified under California state education standards for English Language Writing and Visual and Performing Arts (VAPA), and utilize theatrical story development, script writing, improvisation techniques, and onstage performance to help youth develop self-esteem, respect, and tolerance of others, as well as the communication, coping, and behavioral skills necessary to make positive life choices.

This training is multifaceted, highly interactive, and uses youth narratives as the primary and sole source of motivation and material to create their own play, one that reflects their views of life and their priorities and, undoubtedly, those of their audiences, too. Relevance to their operative reality is effected in these trainings and eventual community performance.

NEIGHBORHOOD VOICES PROGRAM

Although community experiences and dreams are represented in youth-centered productions, the Neighborhood Voices Program specifically sets out to united these voices in an inclusive manner with those of their families and loved ones, thus serving to bridge intergenerational divides in a highly participatory and culturally affirming manner:

> These 12-week intensive workshops bring youth, parents and grandparents together to create and perform their own theatrical works. This participant-driven program offers writing workshops and culminates in performances designed to decrease social isolation and the destructive behaviors that negatively impact children's development, such as substance abuse and domestic strife. The workshops successfully improve self-confidence, social connections, and knowledge of community resources. Neighborhood Voices workshops end with interactive productions that engage the audience around the play's themes.

We can see Boal's influence in shaping Neighborhood Voices in how it brings performances and audiences together in a nonscripted and highly participatory manner. Breaking down barriers between theatre and audience in marginalized communities is a viable and worthy goal when values and methods seek to accomplish this outcome.

VOICES FOR ARTS AND SOCIAL THEATER PROGRAM

The performing arts are not restricted to out-of-school settings; schools also have the potential to benefit when goals and methods can be adjusted to take into account the challenges of time periods, narratives, and support by adults in authority:

> In multiple classrooms each year, hundreds of students participate in our in-class theatre workshops. These residency, in-class theatre workshops uniquely pair teachers, teacher's assistants, and The Unusual Suspects staff in training and mentoring students. Each workshop follows proven, standards-based curriculum, which enhances language and communication skills and helps strengthen students' ability to work effectively and respectfully with diverse teams. Trained teaching artists guide students through master theatre exercises that support communication skills, public speaking, and role playing, thereby enhancing essential 21st century skills such as critical thinking, creativity, and innovation in the classroom.

Breaking down barriers between schools and out-of-school settings is a worthy goal, meeting academic and social topics. Introducing or enhancing critical thinking benefits youth within and outside of school and can be accomplished through theatre's emphasis on collective participation.

THEATER AND CULTURE ACCESS PROGRAM

Youth recruitment can be accomplished through conventional referrals and unconventional approaches such as the Theater and Culture Access Program, which introduces innovative thinking and provides exposure to the world of theatre, which for many can be a new experience:

> Multiple times a year, we make it possible for low-income, underserved youth and adults to experience professional theatre together. Recently piloted, and in conjunction with Neighborhood Voices, TCAP brings together former and current program participants in intergenerational, professional theatre settings. Each TCAP outing is led by two of our highly trained TAs and/or staff, and is coupled with a pre- and a post-show workshop in order to foster active participation. Understanding the value of exposure to the arts, this new program connects those who might not otherwise have access to professional, live theatre, to some of the most impacting and enriching performances and training Los Angeles has to offer.

> Alumni are often a program's best spokespersons, and actively involving them in doing outreach is an effective recruitment mechanism. Peer-to-peer models

hold great potential in the performing arts. Broadening youth understanding of various theatre forms and ventures into areas of a city that they normally would not visit is an additional value to attending a performance.

TEACHING ASSISTANT TRAINING

The importance of preparing staff for the unique rewards and challenges of a performing arts program with youth who have had or are likely to have experiences with law enforcement and the criminal justice system cannot be understated. These youth have often had limited experiences of being valued and trusted by the broader community and rightly bring high levels of distrust to any effort to engage them in programmatic activities. This organization undertakes a bi-annual activity to teach novice and experienced artists:

> This content adheres to nationally recognized methodology and curricula which has benefited from input by professional artists, mentors and arts educators over 30 years. Teaching artists are helped in developing the strategies and skill-sets in creating a safe and affirming environment where youth are equipped to engage in exploration (personal and social conflicts), as well as helped in development of self-esteem, communication and collaborative theatre art making skills.

These training sessions feature speakers from child psychology and social and emotional development and involve setting up mock classroom situations to assist teaching artists to develop or enhance team teaching strategies and use of assessment tools, as well as to expand their theatre-making and improvisational skills.

Safety concerns often associated with engaging urban youth are addressed in a manner that helps ensure that staff are not encumbered with this onerous task:

> In addition, teaching artists learn to structure lesson plans by incorporating scaffold learning outcomes, which have been found to have a high probability of aiding youth transformation and self-discovery. Teaching artists . . . are not expected to enforce discipline. Rather, they are able to participate in what is referred to as "Arts Ensemble" feedback sessions to facilitate establishment of group norms and goals, which, in turn, seek to enhance youth listening skills, critical thinking, cooperative learning, and social skills.

Interpersonal skill acquisition is essential for youth. Reinforcing positive ways to communicate serves youth well within and outside of programs.

VOLUNTEER PROGRAM

Tapping human capital and providing mechanisms for engaging volunteers is an important youth program dimension. Youth organizations sponsoring performing arts must actively reach out to bring in resources from a variety of sources.

Civic engagement takes on even greater prominence when these organizations want to remain relevant to community issues and capital.

A volunteer program is one mechanism that increases the connectedness of these organizations to communities, with resources being devoted to reaching and supporting volunteers:

> US Volunteer Mentors commit to serving at one site, once-a-week, over a period of 10 weeks, and play a vital role in helping to build a creative, supportive team for playwriting and theatre performance workshops. US Volunteer Mentors serve as true role models, exemplifying discipline, enthusiasm, and willingness to take risks in ensemble workshop activities. US Volunteer Mentors check in with participants during workshops and actively listen to their needs, supporting creative problem-solving and social-emotional development. US Volunteer Mentors participate in reflection meetings; join in fun, engaging theatre exercises; and have opportunities to lead warm-ups and reflective group discussions.

Civic engagement can be attractive for enhancing program resources and increasing social-political ties between programs and communities. Programs must devote resources to this goal because "good" volunteer programs just do not happen by themselves. Recruitment, screening, training, and ongoing support are essential in making these programs a valuable resource.

FUNDING AND OPERATIONAL CHALLENGES

The Unusual Suspects hosts an annual spring gala. The 2014 event drew well with Hollywood celebrities such as Ed Asner, Viola Davis, and Mariska Hargitay attending the function. Universal Pictures Director of Development Sara Scott, who has been helping the organization for nearly a decade, first got involved when a college friend and she began researching organizations that could sponsor a nonprofit they were trying to start up.

Evaluation

The Unusual Suspects has received numerous awards, including The National Juvenile Justice Award (2000), The National Youth Arts and Humanities Award (2007), and the Otto Rene Castillo Award for Political Theater (2013).

Theater participation outcomes are multifold. Youth having a place to go where they feel validated is one that is difficult to measure but critical to the success of any intervention (Fairman, 2014):

> Asked about the specific benefits of the afterschool workshops, Denton says that the kids tell her that sometimes the only reason they come to school is

so that they can attend Unusual Suspects. Miguel, a student at San Fernando High School, is a perfect example. A bright young man, he was nonetheless failing his classes and assigned to afterschool tutoring. After joining US, he started doing better in school. "If I don't do well in my classes, I'm going to miss Unusual Suspects," he says. What's so special about theatre as an art form in reaching youth in under-resourced areas is two-fold. First, theater and the ensemble work is about reaching each youth on a very deep level and showing them they can be somebody; and second, it's about the fact that theater, by its nature, brings community together to witness our collective truth.

Incentives that encourage participants to do well if they are to continue in a program are well understood by staff. Eventually, doing well becomes its own incentive. Having a sanctuary to turn to where these youth can be safe (socially, emotionally, and physically) while participating in fun and rewarding activities only sweetens the experience. An exceptional youth program must make youth a part of the organization, audience, and staff, too (Fairman, 2014):

> And this is exactly what we saw at Vaughn Middle School. 'The Difficulty of Love' ends with the mother character becoming emboldened and standing up to her alcoholic, abusive husband and finally kicking him out of the house. As the curtain fell, the audience erupted with applause, and the parent leader, who had earlier complained, stood and presented flowers to the youth saying publicly how much she appreciated what The Unusual Suspects had brought to bear. As the excitement settled in and the audience explored the themes of the play during the Q & A, a woman in the back raised her hand, "Was it hard to write a story that doesn't have a happy ending?"

The following participant response does a wonderful job of showing how theatre provides an experience through involving various perspectives (Fairman, 2014):

> "This story *does* have a happy ending," one of the 12-year-old playwrights explained. "The children now know that they're accepted for who they are." Such wisdom from our youth. And all we have to do is listen. . . . For most, it will be the first time they've spoken their words aloud in front of a public audience much less heard the laughter, tears and excitement their play inspires. If you can come out and see them, you'll surely be glad you did. You might just go away feeling really good.

Speaking before an audience is a powerful experience and never more so than when a particularly painful (traumatic) experience is shared for the world to see and comment upon. Casting youth as experts is empowering and places them at the center of a conversation as opposed to being the object of the conversation.

ALUMNI

Any youth practice program worth its salt places tremendous emphasis on understanding and supporting graduates who have succeeded. This group represents the best that a program has to offer, with graduates becoming ambassadors to society and showing what is possible if attention and resources are devoted to youth well-being. Participants who have finished their programs have opportunities to continue their affiliation with this organization.

The Unusual Suspects, probably more so than any other program I am familiar with, has paid considerable attention to supporting its alumni. Several approaches have been identified to accomplish this goal of support: (1) Building Relationships, (2) Reaching Goals, (3) Achieving Greatness, (4) Alumni Reunion, (5) Internship Opportunities, (6) Lunch on Us, (7) Work and Community Resources, (8) Summer Alumni Program, (9) Master Classes, (10) Special events, and (11) Letters of Recommendation. These efforts tap human and cultural capital in service to the organization and community.

1. **Building Relationships:** The importance of initiating and maintaining relationships should not be surprising: "The Unusual Suspects strives to take our services to the next level by offering a free program for youth who have participated and completed a youth theatre residency program with us. The goal of the Alumni Services Program is to build on the relationships formed during the workshops and offer support services to alumni members by linking them to resources within their community." These relationships bring an intergenerational perspective that is critical in communities with changing and highly dynamic demographics and also introduce a historical perspective on a community's history.

2. **Reaching Goals:** Providing opportunities for further involvement for youth who wish to continue becomes an important goal: "After participating in this program, our youth will have access to opportunities including internships, reunions, Summer Alumni Programs and special events. We are here to help our youth reach their goals, whatever they may better."

3. **Achieving Greatness:** Successfully completing a program is a major accomplishment that must be celebrated, capitalized upon, and cast as a community asset: "When participants complete a program, they become official US Alumni receiving a Certificate of Completion outlining community service hours they accumulated by participating. They will also receive an alumni packet containing a letter from the Executive Director, a DVD of their staged reading/performance to share with friends and family, a copy of the script they wrote/performed, an Unusual Suspects t-shirt, and a personalized letter from their teaching artists."

4. **Alumni Reunion:** "Shortly after we say goodbye, we invite our alumni to spend an afternoon with their Teaching Artists and Volunteer Mentors,

where we play their favorite theater games, watch the DVD from their show, and enjoy some popcorn and snacks."

5. **Internship Opportunities:** "Alumni have the opportunity to become an intern with The Unusual Suspects, where they can build their resume by working at our central office or volunteering at the workshops. Some of our alums have even become paid teaching artists with our organization."

6. **Lunch on US:** "When youth participants who were formerly incarcerated contact us upon release, The Unusual Suspects will coordinate a time to take them out to lunch, along with their Teaching Artists and Volunteer Mentors, providing an opportunity for us to check in and provide our alums with guidance and support during their time of transition."

7. **Work/Community Resources**: "Youth in need of a job or someone to talk to can find resources on our quick reference list, included in the alumni packet they receive at the conclusion of their program. Specialized services, along with referrals to specific contacts at each organization, are provided for each community we serve."

8. **Summer Alumni Program**: "The Unusual Suspects offers intensive performance programs every summer at various locations in the greater L.A. area, open to all Unusual Suspects alumni. Participants produce a script written by youth in a previous US program, and are given an opportunity to act, sing, dance, design, crew, and stage manage a full play."

9. **Master Classes:** "Alumni interested in learning more about theatre have the opportunity to take advanced-level classes at local L.A. venues, where professionals in acting, directing, technical design, and theatre management teach our alums more of what they'll need to know if they are looking to pursue a career in the arts."

10. **Special Events:** "We invite our alumni to take field trips with US to professional theatre productions, music concerts, and other artistic outings, such as The Odyssey Theater and The L.A. Chamber Orchestra."

11. **Recommendation Letters:** "We do everything we can to help our alums get into college. If they need a recommendation letter for scholarships or applications, we'll be happy to write one."

Alums are a treasure trove, and this organization understands this. Alum civic engagement requires careful planning and a strategic understanding of their importance in the legacy of an organization and the role they can play in recruiting and helping future generations benefit from participation, as they have in the past.

Key Lessons Learned and General Observations

Youth need to be approached with dignity and respect; success and progress are not possible without these two ingredients. The youth whom Unusual Suspects seeks to reach represent a group that rarely have organizations attempting to actively engage them, and when they do, in a manner that starts the building of trust, an essential ingredient in any successful program. Youth voices must find an outlet throughout all performance facets, but it can result in tension and upheaval in the lives of youth, as evidenced in the following case illustration (Fairman, 2014):

> Unusual Suspects never tells our kids what to write. A key to their creative journey is that we honor the voice of our participants in every way. And so, as always, these young playwrights wrote from their hearts and from their experience. In "The Difficulty of Love," an autistic girl tries to fit in at school while dealing with her alcoholic, abusive father, a physician and pillar of the community, who's in denial about his daughter's struggle and the fact that his son is gay. When their mother starts to stand up for herself and her family, we watch as the family dynamics unravel. During the playwriting process, it turned out that the father character in the play wasn't the only person that wanted to keep these domestic issues under wraps. About mid-way through the 10-week workshop, Unusual Suspects staff got a call from the school's parent representative reporting that parents were upset about the play's content and that they thought the kids should not write about a gay character or an alcoholic father. They threatened to pull the plug."

Social justice, emotional turmoil, exercise of creativity, and clarity of purpose and awareness of situation, although therapeutically and socially beneficial, do not come without consequence, as evidenced by this example.

Youth who are court-involved or those with a high potential to be so are not an "attractive" group to target in out-of-school settings. Their designation as "hard-to-reach" is relative and based on local circumstances. Urban communities without high gang participation rates would not consider this group particularly threatening, and other groups may occupy this spot. Programs may unintentionally screen out those youth who have the most to gain from participation.

Unusual Suspects is not your "typical" performing arts organizations, and it occupies a place in a particularly exclusive grouping of youth service organizations nationally, with much in common with Homeboys/Homegirls Industries in Los Angeles (Delgado, 2012). In similar fashion to its exemplary counterpart, I do not expect The Unusual Suspects be adopted as a model for replication elsewhere because of the convergence of multiple factors unique to Los Angeles and the organization. Much can be learned and "borrowed," however, and then applied locally. The Unusual Suspects webpage is easily accessible and up-to-date, and is no doubt a key feature of their program's effort to connect with the outside world. Instagram Photos uploaded nearby the Unusual Suspects Theater Company.

The location of the Unusual Suspects in Los Angeles, which is a highly diverse city with a major gang-related challenge, represents two major factors coming together and into contact with adults with the vision and commitment to tackle a major social problem in this country. The ability of theatre to confront and give voice to trauma in the lives of urban youth is commendable because there are few outlets for this to transpire in this country. Undertaking this collective task, with youth playing supporting roles, increases the significance of the experience and its long-term benefits for participants, their families, friends, and, ultimately, their communities.

Conclusion

A case study is only as good as the availability of material to base a study upon. An organization that is responsive to youth and community needs has much to share with the world of practice and academia. The Unusual Suspects has been in existence as long as it has because of how well it has been able to reach out and engage urban youth and because of its openness to involve countless others with similar missions. This case study has hopefully done justice to the potential of social justice finding a welcoming home in theatre and will inspire other organizations across the country to incorporate the principles, program components, and activities that have proved highly relevant for urban youth. The following chapters will revisit the field and scholarly literature, but also include my perceptions and predictions about how social justice youth community performing arts will evolve in the future.

SECTION IV

Future Directions and Conclusions

14

Theory to Action

Introduction

The synthesis involving theory and action is essential to any social intervention if it is to be practical and attractive to practitioners and theorists. Social justice youth practice and the performing arts is not an exception. Some academics would argue that it is our role or mission to bring these two worlds together to facilitate advancements in the field. The field has a prominent role to play in shaping how theory evolves and is relevant to the world of practice.

This chapter provides a framework that emphasizes capacity enhancement and social justice youth practice. The performing arts will be addressed to provide concrete examples of how the paradigm and framework come to life. Other youth practice, such as mural painting, sculpture, and film/video, can easily be substituted because of the universal quality of the performing arts.

Framework

Bringing values and theories to life necessitates a "tool" that can aid practitioners and academics. A framework is one such tool, and there are many different types to select from. My experience in tapping assets using a community capacity enhancement framework has been effective in carrying out community celebrations; establishing collaborations with nontraditional community settings; and developing murals, gardens, playgrounds, and community-built sculptures (Delgado, 1999, 2000, 2016b).

Frameworks are dynamic and systematically guide practitioners and academics in gathering information to make informed decisions on how best to proceed and concentrate efforts to accomplish various essential tasks and activities and achieve results. The performing arts can be tapped to achieve transformative youth outcomes. Providing tools or a framework for assessment of social justice issues and capacity enhancement helps marginalized youth analyze the oppressive forces that shape their existence and destiny (Newell & Coffee, 2012). Integrating these elements into assessment leads to an intervention that is synergistic, enhancing all program aspects being proposed in this book.

Analytical and Interactional Dimensions

Any intervention that is community-focused and seeks to achieve significant social changes is bound to encounter numerous political (interactional) challenges or barriers along the way (Googins, Capoccia, & Kaufman, 1983). If an intervention is of any great significance, one hopes that it *does* encounter sociopolitical resistance. Each intervention stage can be conceptualized as integrating theoretical and political content. One without the other will not maximize resources in reaching urban youth.

Five Stages

An effective framework breaks down major activities into clear developmental stages that allow a focus on specific tasks and goals. Capacity-enhancement involves five stages that integrate key theoretical concepts while taking into consideration critical sociopolitical forces. Each stage is distinct and connected to the other yet brings distinctive goals that must incorporate key theoretical concepts and sociopolitical considerations: (1) Assessment, (2) Building Support, (3) Planning, (4) Implementation, and (5) Evaluation. The following is a brief overview of each stage:

> **Stage 1: Assessment:** It is most appropriate to start with an assessment phase because it represents the foundation of any programmatic efforts at using the performing arts. This phase seeks to balance needs with assets. What are the needs that youth are articulating about social justice and their desire to use particular performing arts? Any effort at identifying needs must take into account why they exist. For example, are youth expressing a need for a music program, and none exists within the community; or they simply are unaware of a program existing? The answer to this question has profound outcomes. In the former, it means developing a program. In the latter, it means playing a broker role in connecting youth with existing programs.

This phase also provides community practitioners with an opportunity for establishing important interpersonal relationships and agreements with youth and existing formal and informal organizations that either are performing arts–focused or have the potential for sponsoring these types of projects. The building of sociopolitical support is integral to this phase because a program must be owned by the youth and the community.

This assessment will prove labor intensive, but the time and effort devoted to this phase will pay dividends later in the process of establishing a performing arts program or helping to expand and strengthen existing programs. It also provides an opportunity to determine how much support or pushback the organization can expect later in the process, the best language to use, and even the best name for a program.

Practitioners can tap a variety of definitions of needs/assets to conceptually ground this phase, such as felt needs, expressed needs, normative needs, and comparative needs. Obtaining "hard" data will be much easier from a needs perspective because these are typically gathered by most organizations and governmental sources. "Soft" data provide a greater likelihood of ownership by youth and communities. Gathering data on assets can also be viewed as primary data gathering because practitioners will have to generate this information. It will be more expensive and time-intensive, but the results will be far superior and play an instrumental role in shaping how a youth performing arts program unfolds.

Doing an inventory and assessment of past and current efforts at using the performing arts is one way to identify and mobilize community assets in the enhancement of the performing arts. Identifying youth in the community who have been recognized for having talent and connecting them to organizations is a simple but highly effective in furthering youth performing arts.

Figure 14.1 shows how assets can be conceptualized as falling into seven types, and each can be operationalized with a goal of using them in support of community performing arts. Each of these assets can vary in availability and intensity depending on local circumstances and goals.

Identifying community assets does not have to be labor-intensive, and ambitious efforts can be expensive. Being cognizant of the countless "little ways" of identifying assets is constructive and can lead to more systematic and comprehensive efforts (Delgado & Humm-Delgado, 2013).

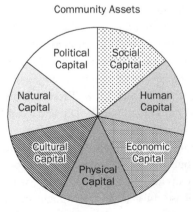

FIGURE 14.1 Community assets

Stage 2: Building Support: One can rightly ask why there should be a stage specifically focused on a goal of building support when this goal should permeate the entire framework. The response is quite simple—building relationships is of sufficient importance to be worthy of having an entire stage devoted to it as a means of consolidating relationships, but with an understanding that relationships are key throughout any intervention.

Development of an advisory committee is one mechanism that can be built into a performing arts program. The composition of this committee can consist of multiple members, with the majority of the seats being occupied by youth and the remaining seats being devoted to key community leaders and organizations who are selected based on what they bring to the table (instrumental, expressive, and informational benefits) and political considerations.

An advisory committee, in similar fashion to an orchestra, is composed with attention to different sources of legitimacy (expertise, institutional, ethical, and consumer) (Rein, 1969) and can incorporate current participants and alums—the latter because of their unique insights, but also as a way of bridging program participation and life after completing or aging out a program.

Stage 3: Planning: The planning of a youth performing arts intervention is probably what most people think of when the concept of "program development" is mentioned. This process has sometimes been referred to as the "meat and potatoes" phase of program development. This phase is only as good as the two previous phases because it rests on their foundation.

Planning consists of goals, objectives (process, output, and impact), strategies, tasks, and activities. Each of these elements provides practitioners using the performing arts for youth with an opportunity to apply key theoretical concepts covered throughout this book, with due attention to sociopolitical considerations. The values outlined earlier help guide practitioners through this and the other phases of this framework.

Stage 4: Implementation: As the saying goes, "to plan is human, but to implement is divine." Interventions are dynamic and can be expected to change. If practitioners have been systematic in their planning, including having built the necessary community and advisory committee support and enlistment of key stakeholders, changes to plans will be a natural occurrence rather than a fatal blow. These changes can be conceptualized as "adjustments" rather than roadblocks, and a careful assessment and plan can help minimize setbacks.

Stage 5: Evaluation: The evaluation phase must not be conceptualized as the final phase but rather as the step before the beginning phase. Program development is cyclical rather than linear, with one phase leading to another. This phase must never be thought of as the end. Evaluation is process- and outcome-driven, and it must be documented if it is to have meaning locally and in theory development.

These evaluation efforts must actively enlist the participation of current and former program members as a means of developing human capital but also as a means of ensuring that the results reflect the operative reality of participants. The recommendations that are forthcoming are relevant and have a high probability of being implemented.

Conclusion

It is hoped that the reader has developed a general grasp and appreciation of how to implement a youth performing arts social intervention. The preceding framework has proved to be effective, and it is not unique to the performing arts. No practitioner is expected to grasp each of the stages with equal fervor and competency, but this does not mean that we simply skip a stage. The five stages discussed in this chapter are highly interrelated, and none is more or less important than another. An intervention framework like the one presented in this chapter is not unique to youth community practice and the performing arts, but a focus on the performing arts brings an extra set of challenges and rewards for youth and practitioners.

15

Future Directions

Introduction

Any discussion about the future of social justice youth practice performing arts will raise questions about how this nation will ultimately view youth and if it will correct its current course to be affirming and empowering. Urban youth of color will continue to increase in numbers as the nation ages, in the process diversifying it according to race and ethnicity. Intersectionality challenges us, and unsuccessfully addressing this challenge means that significant progress cannot occur. Seven cross-cutting themes were identified that cut across all four performing arts in this book, with some themes being obvious and others being surprising.

It is important to note that this book did not deliberately set out to favor one performing art over another. Dance, music, theater, and song each bring unique strengths and challenges, with some (theater, for instance) lending themselves to providing youth with more opportunities to engage when compared others (song, for instance). But theater requires considerably more preparation and coordination, larger budgets, and bigger teams. Youth programming goals and local circumstances will dictate which one or combination of performing arts will be tapped.

Performing Arts Competencies of Community Youth Practitioners

What competencies are essential in the youth performing arts? I certainly have no natural abilities in this arena; so what do practitioners interested in using the performing arts in youth practice do when they, too, have limited or no artistic abilities?

This lack should not dissuade organizations from engaging the performing arts. There are a number of creative ways that organizations without histories of performing arts programming can obtain staff with these abilities. Sponsoring artist residency programs is one vehicle for bringing talented performers to an organization without a tradition of performing arts programming. Universities can initiate internships or field units in collaboration with these types of organizations.

Apprenticeships or internships can be developed when youth practice programs do not actively offer performing arts activities but may have participants with particular interests in the performing arts (Downey, Dalidowicz, & Mason, 2015).

Rohd (1998, p. 128) introduces peer education and a youth traveling ensemble model that goes into communities to help other youth and institutions wishing to conduct theater performances:

> Peer education means youths working with youths to raise awareness, instill activism, and problem solve around community issues through education . . . education is dialogue, therefore, the training of youths to go out and conduct theatre-as-dialogue workshops that can act as a resource in your community.

An ensemble model broadens youth theater's reach where there is a paucity of performing arts programs. It places youth in positions of authority, a rare opportunity in the lives of the marginalized.

Although there has been an increase in collaboration between performing artists and academics, epistemological and methodological differences have resulted in significant challenges in creating these partnerships (Rossiter et al., 2008, p. 284):

> Theatre provides both new and exciting forms of knowledge generation and knowledge translation, which in turn advances greater opportunities for doing interdisciplinary research. Transcending the boundaries between the arts and sciences holds great potential for broadening horizons, not only with regards to new areas and types of research, but also regarding how we come to know, interpret and make sense of phenomena under examination.

The importance of interdisciplinary collaboration is always raised and extolled in the scholarly literature. Tremendous barriers and challenges are endemic to these partnerships, going beyond language and encompassing thorny epistemological and methodological differences.

Anderson and Risner's (2012) surveyed teaching artists in dance and theater and highlighted the vast range of approaches to teaching dance and theater within a variety of settings. Many dance and theater companies have developed their own educational programs, and community organizations can contract out with these organizations or make youth referrals to them. McLean (2014) notes that artists can envision their role to be more encompassing, even to the point of arts-led regeneration strategies that can lead to social justice in marginalized communities.

Reach of Social Justice Youth Community Practice

The performing arts have been conceptualized rather narrowly in this book to do justice to several different forms. The arts, in the broadest sense, are but the latest wave of programming with the potential to transform youth lives. Youth also may be interested in composing poetry, producing films, and writing novels.

An arts "menu" is sufficiently broad to be able to accommodate virtually any youth needs, and making it a prominent part of an even broader youth practice menu bodes well for the field in general. Bringing in social justice as a guiding goal, with its corresponding principles, increases both its transformative potential and corresponding challenges.

Why Can't the Performing Arts Embrace Social Justice and Become Even More Politicized?

Why can't we just get along? This question strikes at the roots of why to engage in youth programming with marginalized youth. Staff have a deep moral commitment to making society more respectful and responsive to marginalized youth, and this does not encompass having them conform to society's expectations. Rather, it is to prepare youth to confront and achieve positive change in their lives, including acquiring the necessary "tools" to confront the sources of oppression.

The process of transformation from victim to victor requires a shift in thinking and having the competencies to translate knowledge (self and otherwise) into action (Banales, 2012). Finding the right outlet to accomplish this transition requires communities to offer a menu of programs that are attractive to youth. Not all youth will be interested in the performing arts; some will be interested in the sciences, working at local media outlets, and in sports. How does a community bring these disparate groups together? Sharing a social justice agenda becomes a unifying mechanism that benefits youth and their communities, regardless of their interests in activities or programs.

Is There One Performing Art that Stands Out in Social Justice Youth Community Practice?

The answer to this question is a resounding "no." If social justice is to hold center stage—no pun intended—then the performing arts are there to support the central message. The same can be said for any other activity that finds its way into youth practice with urban marginalized youth. The performing arts do not have to assume a full-scale production either.

A clear theme that emerged in the course of doing the case studies was how humbly these organizations started. It was not unusual to have them start with one or two individuals in the living room of their homes. One can no doubt be impressed by how these organizations evolved in a field where the life spans of organizations can be very limited.

A study of the founders of performing arts organizations that started with humble beginnings will find individuals deeply moved by social justice goals and the importance of investing in youth. Their vision, competencies, and commitment fueled these organizations in such a manner that they still exist today, many after several decades. An in-depth study will also find these individuals embracing the value of empowerment of youth and having them play decision-making roles in shaping how an organization evolves and is even named (as in the case of Boston's ZUMIX).

Urban Youth Abilities to Resist Oppression and Thrive

One must marvel at how urban youth still strive for a better future against the incredible odds against them. This does not mean that they have not suffered or will not suffer from marginalization. I am always uplifted when visiting youth programs and seeing the level of engagement and commitment to fighting for a better society for the participating youth and those in their communities. These youth are not selfish or self-centered, and they serve as role models for adults. They are not seeking justice for themselves; they are seeking justice for others, too.

The Black Lives Matter Movement, although born in response to social oppression, has managed to capture the imagination and engage countless youth across the country. It has encouraged them to participate in the most democratic of actions (peaceful protests) that led to the creation of this country and the embrace of democracy as a government. Black lives matter, and youth are there to make sure that we as adults to not forget this. (Youth, too, were at the Occupy Movement that addressed income inequality.)

Programs that can effectively tap the voices and experiences of adults who have had to contend with oppression take on great significant in the lives of youth. These adults, particularly when they are alumni of these programs, bring insights and legitimacies that have profound consequences for youth. Hiring of adult staff must take into consideration social justice experiences and not merely concentrate on competencies obtained through higher education.

Youth Performing Arts: All Things to All People?

The reader has no doubt raised questions about the inclusive abilities of social justice youth practice programs and their ability to have a reach broad enough so that all youth, regardless of their challenges, can participate in the same program. No one organization can successfully meet the needs of all youth in their program. Having youth who experiment with alcohol and drugs in a program with others who are young parents or pregnant necessitates allocating resources differently and having staff with different competencies.

We must eschew stigmatizing youth by having them be part of "special" initiatives that single them out in an obvious manner and marginalize them, regardless of our noble intentions. This dilemma is very real, regardless of the scale. It can often be found within programs that have actively sought to create a mix of youth from different backgrounds.

Adults: Cannot Live With Them, Cannot Live Without Them

Zeldin et al. (2015), in a cross-national study (United States, Portugal, and Malaysia), found that the likelihood of youth achieving positive results through programming is greatly increased when they exercise power (agency) over decisions while concomitantly experiencing trust and power-sharing from adults. Youth–adult partnerships are at the core of youth practices, whether occurring within or outside of schools (Antrop-González & De Jesús, 2006; Roach, Wureta, & Ross, 2013; Schiepers, 2012).

Relationships, for instance, are at the crux of youth–adult mentoring/working experiences, and this should not be surprising (Chhuon & Wallace, 2014; Kupersmidt & Rhodes, 2014; Sue & Craig, 2014). These relationships are considered one of the most critical elements of positive youth development (PYD) because they permeate the entire participation experience (Jones & Perkins, 2005; Khan, 2014; Rothman & Haydon, 2006; Scales, 2006; Snyder, 2006). Effective youth practice is only possible through an affirming and sustaining relationship between youth and adults (Bowers, Johnson, Warren, Tirrell, & Lerner, 2015; Kearney, 2014; Zeldin, Petrokubi, & MacNeil, 2008).

The role of adults and how they envision Positive Youth Development cuts across all theory, case examples, and experiences reported in using the performing arts. Flexibility, openness, a willingness to listening, and joining with youth in their struggle to achieve social justice are cross-cutting themes. The importance of trust stands out.

The process of youth and adults establishing trusting relationships is as important, if not more important, than the actual outcomes of those interactions. Success in outcomes is always welcomed, but, even when success is not achieved, the lessons learned and the trust established should not be minimized in any evaluation efforts. Process is never insignificant.

Youth decision-making always represents an important dimension or element in youth–adult relationships within youth programs, but particularly those programs that embrace social justice goals and principles (Serido, Borden, & Perkins, 2011). Trust is integral to the decision-making process by facilitating the sharing of power and providing youth with an experience that they can draw upon as they age into adulthood.

Zeldin and Leidheiser (2014, p. 6) make an important observation about society and how difficult it is for intergenerational relationships to develop based on mutual respect: "Our culture tends to separate persons of different ages thus minimizing the opportunity for youth voice and intergenerational collaboration." Opportunities for youth–adult relationships based on mutual trust and respect must be maximized (Schilling, Martinek, & Carson, 2007), and this can be seen in all four case studies.

A critical aspect of youth–adult relationships is the presence of caring, which is the "glue" that keeps youth engaged and filled with hope for a future that maximizes their potential (Ross, Capra, Carpenter, Hubbell, & Walker, 2015; Te Riele, 2010). Caring and trust are interrelated.

The paucity of marginalized youth having positive and caring experiences with adults in positions of authority makes these caring adults that much more significant when encountered (Gastic & Johnson, 2009). The absence of positive relational experiences only increases the importance and challenges of youth community practitioners successfully engaging them and creating opportunities for affirming relationship-building. If performing arts programs provide youth who age out with an opportunity to continue involvement in these programs, it helps ensure that adult graduates can serve as mentors and role models. Peer relationships in the performing arts also can be enhanced with peer mentoring, bringing a greatly underdeveloped approach to this activity (McCammon, 2007).

Youth–adult relationships can be fostered through a conscious effort at intergenerational teamwork (Cater & Jones, 2014). The performing arts have ample opportunities for intergenerational projects that can be modified to take into account youth interests and abilities, thus providing valuable experiences for youth as well as adults to partner in productions and including youth in leadership roles as directors and producers.

Conclusion

What is in store for the future as we discuss the performing arts and social justice youth practice? I cannot help but think that the best is around the corner. This chapter has touched on a few areas that will undoubtedly evolve in the next decade. An expanding universe metaphor symbolizes both the excitement and the challenges in developing an understanding of how social justice youth practice will evolve in the immediate future.

The performing arts are only the tip of the iceberg when discussing social justice youth practice. Other aspects of the arts were simply touched on in passing in this book, but I sincerely hope that this book has spurred the interest of other academics to undertake a book on youth practice that introduces exciting and highly innovative approaches to this field, particularly when those approaches are deeply grounded within the field.

16

Epilogue

Introduction

Writing a book is always a journey, with no two books or journeys ever being the same. Although a clear destination is always in sight, the actual travel involves many different stops and detours, and where and when these occur is never predictable. That was the case in this book. Writing it was expected to be an enlightening experience, and that was the case regardless of how well versed I was on the topic at the beginning of the journey.

This chapter provides an opportunity to pause and share some of the unexpected detours and stops along the way, and some words of wisdom about this field, which is filled with tremendous promise. A total of five themes stand out and are worthy of being highlighted. Due to limited space, each theme is presented in summary form.

1. The performing arts as a call for innovation: Tapping performing arts in social justice youth practice is only the tip of the iceberg regarding innovation in this field. This observation does not surprise those actively involved in "innovative" programming in addressing youth social justice. Such a call does not come without its share of challenges from an evaluation or research perspective, however, not to mention funding for projects that do not look "typical" to uninformed funders. Such a call is essential if social justice youth practice is to continue its evolution.

This call for innovation is sufficiently flexible to take into account local circumstances and goals. It does not have to be bold to be classified as "innovative," as evidenced by the small scale of projects in our case studies before they evolved into significant organizations. Yet a program must seek to "push the envelope" for it to be labeled as innovative, and it must treat youth as equal partners, if not in charge, of these efforts.

Creativity is a trait that all youth possess and none more so than those who must successfully navigate difficult and dangerous terrain. No two social situations are ever the same; responses and solutions, too, fall into this perspective. There may be a core set of elements, but how each gets operationalized will differ according to local circumstances.

2. Is an outlet to express oneself sufficient?: Feeling trapped and without a dream of a future worth living for is a desperate state for youth when their future is all ahead of them. This sad but all too common situation results in frustration and anger, with few constructive individual and collective outlets. The performing arts are not just meant as an avenue for these feelings to be expressed without seeking solutions that redress social injustices. Is expressing these sentiments cathartic enough in itself? The answer is "no"!

We cannot dispute the value of finding a constructive and, hopefully, fun outlet for urban youth frustration and pain. Therapeutic results are integral to the use of the performing arts, as evidenced by how trauma can be expressed in a manner that resonates for all those involved. These youth also need to channel their energies and hopes in finding social change in their lives and surroundings.

3. Staff as the glue and inspiration: Finding staff who have the willingness and capabilities to deal with trauma, engage in the performing arts, and are youth-centered is not easy. Recruitment and screening of the "right" staff does not get enough attention in the professional literature. The generation of trust, respect, and hope on the part of participants is essential in making a program effective. This takes on even greater importance in innovative social justice youth practice.

Providing necessary supports (supervision, consultation, and training) will aid in attracting and keeping talented staff. Having a career ladder that facilitates program alumni staying with programs, as in the cases covered earlier, is an option that is viable and attractive and one that represents a return on investment on the part of youth and programs. Performing arts programs that have been in existence 20–30 years understand the value of the long view versus short-term gains.

4. If it takes a village, can we get a village?: The reader has undoubtedly picked up on the theme that it takes a collective effort ("it takes a village") to promote opportunities to advance the youth development field. Marshaling requisite commitment and resources to accomplish this goal, particularly in reaching urban marginalized youth, is a considerable challenge in this society.

For a village to take hold of this mission necessitates that the nation value youth of all backgrounds. That has not occurred, and, based on the current national climate, it does not seem to be in the stars. As the current presidential administration of President Trump takes hold as this book goes to press, youth in general, and not to mention those in urban centers, are not discussed unless related to violence and crime; this necessitates a counter-narrative to unfold, with subsequent social interventions.

Conclusion

I sincerely hope that this book has inspired readers to embrace the performing arts and social justice youth practice and has increased the thirst to make a contribution to this field. There is little dispute that advances will only be possible if we form collaborations among youth, providers, and academics and have the desire to be innovative and expand the boundaries of social justice youth practice. If so, we will make a significant and long-lasting contribution to the well-being of marginalized youth, their families, friends, and communities; society will be the ultimate beneficiary.

Social justice youth practice must continue to evolve if it is to remain relevant and expand in influence in the future. Part of what will fuel this evolution will be how well it responds to demographic changes in society, including newcomer youth, the increasing numbers of bi-racial youth, and the culture created by these youth.

The refugee crisis in Europe, in which youth and their families have been uprooted from countries torn by war or experiencing highly unstable economic conditions that make for an uncertain future find themselves in new homelands. How these new homelands welcome and support them will go a long way toward reshaping society and will determine how well they and their new homelands thrive in the immediate future. The performing arts have a role to play in shaping the future of countries receiving these refugees, including the United States.

REFERENCES

Abah, O. S., Okwori, J. Z., & Alubo, O. (2009). Participatory theatre and video: Acting against violence in northern Nigeria. *IDS Bulletin, 40* (3), 19–26.

Abrahams, F. (2012). Changing voices—voices of change: Young men in middle school choirs. In S. D. Harrison, G. F. Welch, & A. Adler (Eds.), *Perspectives on males and singing* (pp. 79–93). Rotterdam: Springer Netherlands.

Abramson, L., & Moore, D. B. (2014). Promoting positive peace one block at a time: Lessons from innovative community conferencing programs. In J. M. Fritz (Ed.), *Moving toward a just peace* (pp. 189–212). Rotterdam: Springer Netherlands.

Acevedo-Polakovich, I. D., Cousineau, J. R., Quirk, K. M., Gerhart, J. I., Bell, K. M., & Adomako, M. S. (2014). Toward an asset orientation in the study of US Latina/o youth biculturalism, ethnic identity, and positive youth development. *The Counseling Psychologist, 42* (2), 201–229.

Adachi, P. J., & Willoughby, T. (2013). Do video games promote positive youth development? *Journal of Adolescent Research, 28* (2), 155–165.

Adams, K. (2013). Like a bridge over troubled waters: The use of folk song in the intermediate music curriculum. *The Phenomenon of Singing, 1* (1), 1–10.

Adams-Taylor, S. (2014, November). *Racial disproportionality in school discipline and the school-to-prison pipeline*. 142nd APHA Annual Meeting and Exposition (November 15–November 19, 2014). APHA. Washington, DC.

Addams, J. (2010). *The spirit of youth and the city streets*. Urbana: University of Illinois Press.

Adderley, C. (2009). Music in motion: An overture to the student experience in the high-school marching band. In J. L. Kerchner & C. R. Abril (Eds.), *Musical experience in our lives: Things we learn and meanings we make* (pp. 239–253). Lanham, MD: Rowman & Littlefield.

Adejumo, C. O. (2010). Promoting artistic and cultural development through service learning and critical pedagogy in a low-income community art program. *Visual Arts Research, 36* (1), 23–34.

Adjapong, E. S., & Emdin, C. (2015). Rethinking pedagogy in urban spaces: Implementing hip-hop pedagogy in the urban science classroom. *Journal of Urban Learning, Teaching, and Research (JULTR), 11* (1), 66–77.

Agans, J. P., Champine, R. B., DeSouza, L. M., Mueller, M. K., Johnson, S. K., & Lerner, R. M. (2014). Activity involvement as an ecological asset: Profiles of participation and youth outcomes. *Journal of Youth and Adolescence, 43* (6), 919–932.

Agans, J. P., Champine, R. B., Johnson, S. K., Erickson, K., & Yalin, C. (2015). Promoting healthy lifestyles through youth activity participation: Lessons from research. In E. P. Bowers, G. L. Geldhof, S. K. Johnson, L. J. Hilliard, R. M. Herberg, J. V. Lerner, & R. M. Lerner (Eds.), *Promoting positive youth development: Lessons from the 4-H Study* (pp. 137–158). New York: Springer.

Agger, B. (2014). *Cultural studies as critical theory*. New York: Routledge.

Agosto, V., & Karanxha, Z. (2012). *Teacher leadership: Women (of African descent) enacting social justice*. Retrieved from http://works.bepress.com/cgi/viewcontent.cgi?article=1025&context=zorka_karanxha

Aidi, H. (2014). *Rebel music: Race, empire, and the new Muslim youth culture*. New York: Vintage.

Aisenberg, E., & Herrenkohl, T. (2008). Community violence in context risk and resilience in children and families. *Journal of Interpersonal Violence, 23* (3), 296–315.

Akom, A. A., Cammarota, J., & Ginwright, S. (2008). Youthtopias: Towards a new paradigm of critical youth studies. *Youth Media Reporter, 2* (4), 1–30.

Allen, D. (2012). *Toward participatory democracy*. Retrieved from http://ypp.dmlcentral.net/sites/all/files/publications/Boston_Review_DanielleAllen_Toward_Participatory_Democracy.pdf

Allen, N. M. T. (2005). Exploring hip-hop therapy with high-risk youth. *Praxis, 5* (1), 30–36.

Allsup, R. E., & Shieh, E. (2012). Social justice and music education: The call for apublic pedagogy. *Music Educators Journal, 98* (4), 47–51.

Alonso, A. D., & O'Shea, M. (2012). "You only get back what you put in": Perceptions of professional sport organizations as community anchors. *Community Development, 43* (5) 656–676.

Alrutz, M. (2011). Performative galleries: Integrating applied theatre and digital media into museum settings. *Youth Theatre Journal, 25* (2), 134–145.

Alrutz, M. (2013). Sites of possibility: Applied theatre and digital storytelling with youth. *Research in Drama Education: The Journal of Applied Theatre and Performance, 18* (1), 44–57.

Alrutz, M. (2014). *Digital storytelling, applied theatre, & youth: Performing possibility*. New York: Routledge.

Amanullah, S., Heneghan, J. A., Steele, D. W., Mello, M. J., & Linakis, J. G. (2014). Emergency department visits resulting from intentional injury in and out of school. *Pediatrics*, peds-2013.

Amin, S. (1989). *Eurocentrism*. New York; NYU Press.

Amin, S. (2009). *Eurocentrism*. New York: Monthly Review Press.

Amoabeng, S. (2012). *The pursuit and exploration of performance arts* (Doctoral dissertation). Kalamazoo College, Kalamazoo, MI.

Anaby, D., Korner-Bitensky, N., Law, M., & Cormier, I. (2015). Focus on participation for children and youth with disabilities: Supporting therapy practice through a guided knowledge translation process. *British Journal of Occupational Therapy, 79*, 7, 440–449.

Anderson, J. H. (2011). Situating Axel Honneth in the Frankfurt School Tradition. *Social and Critical Theory, 12* (1), 31–57.

Anderson, M., Cameron, D., & Sutton, P. (2012). Participation and creation in these brave new worlds: Technology and innovation as part of the landscape. *Research in Drama Education: The Journal of Applied Theatre and Performance, 17* (4), 469–476.

Anderson, M., Ewing, R., & Fleming, J. (2014). The role of family in young people's theatre attendance. *Youth Theatre Journal, 28* (1), 61–73.

Anderson, M. E., & Risner, D. (2012). A survey of teaching artists in dance and theater: Implications for preparation, curriculum, and professional degree programs. *Arts Education Policy Review, 113* (1), 1–16.

Antrop-González, R., & De Jesús, A. (2006). Toward a theory of critical care in urban small school reform: Examining structures and pedagogies of caring in two Latino community-based schools. *International Journal of Qualitative Studies in Education, 19* (4), 409–433.

Aponte, C. A. (2013). *When hip-hop and education converge: A look into hip-hop based education programs in the United States and Brazil* (Thesis). Carnegie Mellon University, Pittsburgh, PA.

Appert, C. M. (2015). To make song without singing: Hip hop and popular music in Senegal. *New Literary History, 46* (4), 759–774.

Aprile, A. (2012). Music-making with young children. In C. Korn-Bursztyn (Ed.), *Young children and the arts: Nurturing imagination and creativity* (pp. 173–194). Charlotte, NC: International Age Publishing.

Apsler, R. (2009). After-school programs for adolescents: A review of evaluation research. *Adolescence, 44* (173), 1–19.

Arbeit, M. R., Johnson, S. K., Champine, R. B., Greenman, K. N., Lerner, J. V., & Lerner, R. M. (2014). Profiles of problematic behaviors across adolescence: Covariations with indicators of positive youth development. *Journal of Youth and Adolescence, 43* (6), 971–990.

Armon, J., & Grassi, E. (2012). Developing justice-oriented teachers: Reciprocal mentoring in marginalized communities. *Jesuit Higher Education, 1* (2), 72–81.

Armstrong, A. E. (2006). Negotiating feminist identities and Theatre of the Oppressed. In J. Cohen-Cruz & M. Schutzman (Eds.). *A Boal companion: Dialogues on theatre and cultural politics* (pp. 173–184). New York: Routledge.

Atencio, M., & Wright, J. (2009). "Ballet it's too whitey": Discursive hierarchies of high school dance spaces and the constitution of embodied feminine subjectivities. *Gender and Education, 21* (1), 31–46.

Atkiss, K., Moyer, M., Desai, M., & Roland, M. (2011). Positive youth development: An integration of the developmental assets theory and the socio-ecological model. *American Journal of Health Education, 42* (3), 171–180.

Aujla, I. J., & Redding, E. (2014). The identification and development of talented young dancers with disabilities. *Research in Dance Education, 15* (1), 54–70.

Auslander, P. (1994). BOAL, BLAU, Brecht: The body. In M. Shutzman & J. Coen-Cruz (Eds.), *Playing Boal: Theatre, therapy, activism* (pp. 124–133). New York: Routledge.

Autry, C. E., & Anderson, S. C. (2007). Recreation and the Glenview neighborhood: Implications for youth and community development. *Leisure Sciences, 29* (3), 267–285.

Azmanova, A. (2012). De-gendering social justice in the 21st century: An immanent critique of neoliberal capitalism. *European Journal of Social Theory, 15* (2), 143–156.

Bada, X. (2014). *Mexican hometown associations in Chicagoacán.* New Brunswick, NJ: Rutgers University Press.

Baggetta, M. (2009). Civic opportunities in associations: Interpersonal interaction, governance experience and institutional relationships. *Social Forces, 88* (1), 175–199.

Bagley, C., & Castro-Salazar, R. (2012). Critical arts-based research in education: Performing undocumented historias. *British Educational Research Journal, 38* (2), 239–260.

Baim, C., & Brookes, S. (2002). *Geese theatre handbook: Drama with offenders and people at risk.* Hook, UK: Waterside Press.

Baker, A. M (2016). The process and product: Crafting community portraits with young people in feasible learning settings. *International Journal of Inclusive Education, 20* (1), 309–330.

Bakshi, A. J., & Joshi, J. (2014). The interface between positive youth development and youth career development: New avenues for career guidance practice. In G. Arulmani, A. J. Bakshi, F. T. L. Leong, & A. G. Watts (Eds.), *Handbook of career development* (pp. 173–201). New York: Springer.

Balcazar, F. E., Taylor-Ritzler, T., Dimpfl, S., Portillo-Peña, N., Guzman, A., Schiff, R., & Murvay, M. (2012). Improving the transition outcomes of low-income minority youth with disabilities. *Exceptionality, 20* (2), 114–132.

Baldridge, B. J. (2012). *(Re) Imagining black youth: Negotiating the social, political, and institutional dimensions of urban community-based educational spaces* (Doctoral dissertation). Columbia University, New York.

Baldridge, B. J. (2014). Relocating the deficit: Reimagining black youth in neoliberal times. *American Educational Research Journal, 51* (3), 440–472.

Balfour, M. (Ed.). (2004). *Theatre in prison: Theory and practice*. Bristol, UK: Intellect Books.

Balish, S. M., McLaren, C., Rainham, D., & Blanchard, C. (2014). Correlates of youth sport attrition: A review and future directions. *Psychology of Sport and Exercise, 15* (4), 429–439.

Ball, C. M. (2012). *"Bullets don't have names": The effects of social capital on adolescent African girls' integration into public space* (Master's thesis). Fordham University, New York.

Ballard, P. J., Malin, H., Porter, T. J., Colby, A., & Damon, W. (2015). Motivations for civic participation among diverse youth: More similarities than differences. *Research in Human Development, 12* (1), 63–83.

Ballivían, R. R., & Herrera, L. (2012). Schools of the street: Hip-hop as youth pedagogy in Bolivia. *International Journal of Critical Pedagogy, 4* (1), 172–184.

Balsano, A. B. (2005). Youth civic engagement in the United States: Understanding and addressing the impact of social impediments on positive youth and community development. *Applied Developmental Science, 9* (4), 188–201.

Balsano, A. B., Phelps, E., Theokas, C., Lerner, J. V., & Lerner, R. M. (2009). Patterns of early adolescents' participation in youth development programs having positive youth development goals. *Journal of Research on Adolescence, 19* (2), 249–259.

Banales, S. (2012). *Decolonizing being, knowledge, and power: Youth activism in California at the turn of the 21st century* (Doctoral dissertation). University of California at Berkeley.

Band, S. A., Lindsay, G., Neelands, J., & Freakley, V. (2011). Disabled students in the performing arts–are we setting them up to succeed? *International Journal of Inclusive Education, 15* (9), 891–908.

Banks, J. (2012). Storytelling to access social context and advance health equity research. *Preventive Medicine, 55* (5), 394–397.

Banks, S. (Ed.), (2010). *Ethical issues in youth work* (2nd ed). New York: Routledge.

Barber, B. L., Abbott, B. D., & Neira, C. J. B. (2014). Meaningful activity participation and positive youth development. In M. J. Furlong, R. Gilman, & E. S. Hueber (Eds.), *Handbook of positive psychology in schools* (2nd ed., pp. 227–244). New York: Routledge.

Barnett, L. A. (2008). Predicting youth participation in extracurricular recreational activities: Relationships with individual, parent, and family characteristics. *Journal of Park and Recreation Administration, 26* (2), 28–60.

Barron, B., Gomez, K., Pinkard, N., & Martin, C. K. (2014). *The Digital Youth Network: Cultivating digital media citizenship in urban communities*. Cambridge, MA: MIT Press.

Barton, W. H., & Butts, J. A. (2008). *Building on strength: Positive youth development in juvenile justice programs*. Chicago: Chapin Hall Center for Children at the University of Chicago.

Barz, G. (2014). *Singing for life: HIV/AIDS and music in Uganda*. New York: Routledge.

Basham, K. B. (2015). *Perspectives on the evolution of hip-hop music through themes of race, crime, and violence* (Honors thesis). Eastern Kentucky University, Richmond.

Baszile, D. T. (2009). Deal with it we must: Education, social justice, and the curriculum of hip hop culture. *Equity & Excellence in Education, 42* (1), 6–19.

Bateman, T. (2011). Punishing poverty: The Scaled Approach and youth justice practice. *The Howard Journal of Criminal Justice, 50* (2), 171–183.

Batsleer, J. (2012). Dangerous spaces, dangerous memories, dangerous emotions: Informal education and heteronormativity–a Manchester UK Youth Work vignette. *Discourse: Studies in the Cultural Politics of Education, 33* (3), 345–360.

Bazo, N. E. (2010). *Sharing the true colors: An exploration of theatre created by gay, lesbian, bisexual, and transgender youth* (Doctoral dissertation). University of Central Florida, Orlando.

Bean, C. N., Fortier, M., Post, C., & Chima, K. (2014). Understanding how organized youth sport may be harming individual players within the family unit: A literature review. *International Journal of Environmental Research and Public Health, 11* (10), 10226–10268.

Bean, E., Whitley, M. A., & Gould, D. (2014). Athlete impressions of a character-based sports program for underserved youth. *Journal of Sport Behavior, 37* (1), 3–23.

Beck, D., & Purcell, R. (2010). *Popular education practice for youth and community development*. Thousand Oaks, CA: Sage Learning Matters Ltd.

Becker, E., & Dusing, S. (2010). Participation is possible: A case report of integration into a community performing arts program. *Physiotherapy Theory and Practice, 26* (4), 275–280.

Becker, J. (2012). *Campaigning for justice: Human rights advocacy in practice*. Palo Alto, CA: Stanford University Press.

Becker, K. (2016). *Fighting segregation with song: Then, music inspired and united a movement. Now, we need to sing more than ever*. Boston University. http://www.bu.edu/research/articles/civil-rights-movement-freedom-songs/

Bell, L. A., & Desai, D. (Eds.). (2014). *Social justice and the arts*. New York: Routledge.

Bell, L. A., Desai, D., & Irani, K. (2013). Storytelling for social justice: Creating arts-based counterstories to resist racism. In M. S. Hanley, G. W. Nobit, G. L. Sheppard, & T. Barone (Eds.), *Culturally relevant arts education for social justice: A way out* (pp. 15–24). New York: Routledge.

Bell, P., Bricker, L., Reeve, S., Zimmerman, H. T., & Tzou, C. (2013). Discovering and supporting successful learning pathways of youth in and out of school: Accounting for the development of everyday expertise across settings. In B. Bevan, L. Brecker, S. Reeve, H. T. Zimmerman, & C. Tzou (Eds.), *Lost opportunities* (pp. 119–140). Rotterdam: Springer Netherlands.

Belliveau, G. (2015). Using drama to build community in Canadian schools. In *Creating together: Participatory, community-based, and collaborative arts practices and scholarship across Canada* (pp. 131–144). Waterloo, ON, Canada: Wilfred Laurier University Press.

Benedict, C., Schmidt, P., Spruce, G., & Woodford, P. (Eds.). (2013). *The Oxford handbook of social justice in music education*. New York: Oxford University Press.

Bennett, A. (2013). *Music, style, and aging: Growing old disgracefully?* Philadelphia, PA: Temple University Press.

Bennett, A. (2015). Youth culture, ageing and identity. In J. Twigg & W. Martin (Eds.), *Routledge handbook of cultural gerontology* (pp. 353–360). New York: Routledge.

Bennett, A., & Janssen, S. (2016). Popular music, cultural memory, and heritage. *Popular Music and Society, 39* (1), 1–7.

Bensimon, M. (2012). The sociological role of collective singing during intense moments of protest: The disengagement from the Gaza Strip. *Sociology, 40* (2), 241–257.

Benson, P. L., & Roehlkepartain, E. C. (2008). Spiritual development: A missing priority in youth development. *New Directions for Youth Development, 2008* (118), 13–28.

Benson, P. L., & Scales, P. C. (2012). Developmental assets. In B. B. Brown & P. J. Prinstein (Eds.), *Encyclopedia of adolescence* (pp. 667–683). New York: Springer.

Benson, P. L., Scales, P. C., Hamilton, S. F., & Sesma, A. (2006). *Positive youth development: Theory, research, and applications*. New York: John Wiley & Sons.

Berihun, G., Kumsa, M. K., Hussein, A., Jackson, J., Baksh, A., Crutchley, J., . . . Ma, Y. (2015). Reflections on using physical objects as data generation strategies: An example from a study of youth violence and healing. *Qualitative Social Work, 14* (3), 338–355.

Bermudez, A. (2012). Youth civic engagement: Decline or transformation? A critical review. *Journal of Moral Education, 41* (4), 529–542.

Bernstein, J. S. (2011). *Arts marketing insights: The dynamics of building and retaining performing arts audiences*. New York: John Wiley & Sons.

Bers, M. U. (2010). Beyond computer literacy: Supporting youth's positive development through technology. *New Directions for Youth Development, 2010* (128), 13–23.

Bers, M. U. (2012). *Designing digital experiences for positive youth development: From playpen to playground*. New York: Oxford University Press.

Besley, T. (2009). Governmentality of youth: Beyond cultural studies. *Contemporary Readings in Law and Social Justice, 2,* 36–83.

Bessant, J. (2004). Mixed messages: Youth participation and democratic practice. *Australian Journal of Political Science, 39* (2), 387–404.

Beyerlein, K., & Hipp, J. R. (2006). From pews to participation: The effect of congregation activity and context on bridging civic engagement. *Social Problems, 53* (1), 97–117.

Biggs-El, C. (2012). Spreading the indigenous gospel of rap music and spoken word poetry: Critical pedagogy in the public sphere as a stratagem of empowerment and critique. *Western Journal of Black Studies, 36* (2), 161–168.

Bintliff, A. V. (2011). *Re-engaging disconnected youth: Transformative learning through restorative and social justice education. Adolescent cultures, school and society* (Vol. 51). New York: Peter Lang.

Bischoff, S. A. (2012). *Expressions of resistance: Intersections of Filipino American identity, hip hop culture, and social justice* (Doctoral dissertation). Washington State University, Pullman, WA.

Black, J., Castro, J. C., & Lin, C. C. (2015). *Youth practices in digital arts and new media: Learning in formal and informal settings*. New York: Palgrave Macmillan.

Blake, A. L. (2012). *Bagunçaço: Music for social change in Salvador, Brazil* (Doctoral dissertation). University of Texas, Austin.

Blake, S. N. W. (2016). *(Re)building grandmother's house: The work of queer youth theatre facilitators, their goals, methods, and practice* (Doctoral dissertation). University of Texas, Austin.

Blanchet-Cohen, N., & Cook, P. (2014). The transformative power of youth grants: Sparks and ripples of change affecting marginalized youth and their communities. *Children & Society, 28* (5), 392–403.

Blatterer, H. (2010). The changing semantics of youth and adulthood. *Cultural Sociology, 4* (1), 63–79.

Blomfield, C. J., & Barber, B. L. (2009). Brief report: Performing on the stage, the field, or both? Australian adolescent extracurricular activity participation and self-concept. *Journal of Adolescence, 32* (3), 733–739.

Boal, A. (1992). *Games for actors and non-actors.* London: Routledge.

Boal, A. (1994). *The rainbow of desire: The Boal method of theatre and therapy.* London: Routledge.

Boal, A. (1997). Theater of the Oppressed. *UNESCO Courier, 50* (11), 32–37.

Boal, A. (1998). *The legislative theatre: Using performance to make politics.* London: Routledge.

Boal, A. (2000). *Theater of the Oppressed.* London: Pluto Press.

Boal, A. (2001). *Hamlet and the baker's son: My life in theatre and politics.* London: Routledge.

Boal, A. (2009). Augusto Boal (C. & M.-O. Leal McBride, Trans.): Theatre of the oppressed. In K. Prentki & S. Preston (Eds.), *The applied theatre reader* (pp. 130–137). New York: Routledge.

Bodén, A. (2013). *Street dance stories.* Retrieved from http://www.diva-portal.org/smash/get/diva2:628217/FULLTEXT01.pdfMay

Bohnert, A., Fredricks, J., & Randall, E. (2010). Capturing unique dimensions of youth organized activity involvement theoretical and methodological considerations. *Review of Educational Research, 80* (4), 576–610.

Bond, K. E., & Stinson, S. W. (2016). "It's work, work, work, work": Young people's experiences of effort and engagement in dance (2007). In S. W. Stinson (Ed.), *Embodied curriculum theory and research in arts education* (pp. 269–295). New York: Springer International.

Borden, L., & Serido, J. (2009). From program participant to engaged citizen: A developmental journey. *Journal of Community Psychology, 37* (4), 423–438.

Borden, L. M., Perkins, D. F., Villarruel, F. A., Carleton-Hug, A., Stone, M. R., & Keith, J. G. (2006). Challenges and opportunities to Latino youth development increasing meaningful participation in youth development programs. *Hispanic Journal of Behavioral Sciences, 28* (2), 187–208.

Borgeson, K., & Valeri, R. (2015). Gay skinheads negotiating a gay identity in a culture of traditional masculinity. *Journal of Men's Studies, 23* (1), 44–62.

Bose, M., Horrigan, P., Doble, C., & Shipp, S. C. (2014). *Community matters: Service-learning in engaged design and planning.* New York: Routledge.

Bourdieu, P. (1993). Youth is just a word. *Sociology in question,* 94–102.

Bourke, L., & Hunter, M. A. (2011). Not just an audience: Young people transforming our theatre. *Platform Papers, 26,* i–vi, 1–63, 65–69.

Bower, J. M., & Carroll, A. (2015). Benefits of getting hooked on sports or the arts: Examining the connectedness of youth who participate in sport and creative arts activities. *International Journal of Child and Adolescent Health, 8* (2), 169–178.

Bowers, E. P., Geldhof, G. J., Johnson, S. K., Hilliard, L. J., Hershberg, R. M., Lerner, J. V., & Lerner, R. M. (Eds.). (2015). Applying research about adolescence in real-world settings: The sample case of the 4-H Study of Positive Youth Development. In E. P. Bowers, G. L. Geldhof, S. K. Johnson, L. J. Hilliard, R. M. Herberg, J. V. Lerner, & R. M. Lerner (Eds.), *Promoting positive youth development: Lessons from the 4-H Study* (pp. 1–20). New York: Springer.

Bowers, E. P., Johnson, S. K., Warren, D. J., Tirrell, J. M., & Lerner, J. V. (2015). Youth–adult relationships and positive youth development. In E. P. Bowers, G. L. Geldhof, S. K. Johnson, L. J. Hilliard, R. M. Herberg, J. V. Lerner, & R. M. Lerner (Eds.), *Promoting positive youth development: Lessons from the 4-H Study* (pp. 97–120). New York: Springer.

Bowles, N., & Nadon, D. R. (2013). *Staging social justice: Collaborating to create activist theatre.* Carbondale: Southern Illinois University Press.

Boydell, K. M., Jackson, S., & Strauss, J. S. (2012). Help seeking experiences of youth with first episode psychosis: A research-based dance production. In K. M. Boydell & H. B. Ferguson (Eds.), *Hearing voices: Qualitative inquiry in early psychosis* (pp. 25–44). Waterloo, ON, CAN: Wilfred Laurier University Press.

Boyes-Watson, C. (2008). *Peacemaking circles & urban youth: Bringing justice home.* St. Paul, MN: Living Justice Press.

Bozlak, C. T., & Kelley, M. A. (2015). Participatory action research with youth. In H. A. Larson, J. Caringi, L. Pyles, & J. Jurkowski (Eds.), *Participatory action research* (pp. 67–90). New York: Oxford University Press.

Brader, A., & Luke, A. (2013). Re-engaging marginalized youth through digital music production: Performance, audience and evaluation. *Pedagogies: An International Journal, 8* (3), 197–214.

Bradley, B. S., Deighton, J., & Selby, J. (2004). The 'Voices' project: Capacity-building in community development for youth at risk. *Journal of Health Psychology, 9* (2), 197–212.

Bradley, D. (2006). *Global song, global citizens? Multicultural choral music education and the community youth choir: Constituting the multicultural human subject.* Online Submission. Retrieved from http://eric.ed.gov/?id=ED518074

Bradshaw, C. P., Brown, J. S., & Hamilton, S. F. (2006). Applying positive youth development and life-course research to the treatment of adolescents involved with the judicial system. *Journal of Addictions & Offender Counseling, 27* (1), 2–16.

Brandellero, A., & Janssen, S. (2014). Popular music as cultural heritage: Scoping out the field of practice. *International Journal of Heritage Studies, 20* (3), 224–240.

Brass, T. (2014). *Class, culture and the agrarian myth.* Boston: Brill.

Braun, B., & Williams, S. (2002). We the people: Renewing commitment to civic engagement. *Journal of Family and Consumer Sciences, 94* (3), 8–19.

Bresler, L. (2010). Teachers as audiences: Exploring educational and musical values in youth performances. *Journal of New Music Research, 39* (2), 135–145.

Brinner, B. (2009). *Playing across a divide: Israeli-Palestinian musical encounters.* New York: Oxford University Press.

Bronk, K. C. (2011). A grounded theory of the development of noble youth purpose. *Journal of Adolescent Research, 27* (1), 78–109.

Brooks, C. M., Daschuk, M. D., Poudrier, J., & Almond, N. (2015). First Nations youth redefine resilience: Listening to artistic productions of "Thug Life" and hip-hop. *Journal of Youth Studies, 18* (6), 706–725.

Brooks-Gunn, J., & Roth, J. (2014). Invited commentary: Promotion and prevention in youth development: Two sides of the same coin? *Journal of Youth and Adolescence, 43* (6), 1004–1007.

Brown, A. A. (2016). *"Healing spaces of refuge": Social justice youth development, radical healing, and artistic expression for black youth* (Doctoral dissertation). Texas A & M University, College Station).

Brown, R. N., & Kwakye, C. J. (2012). *Wish to live: The hip-hop feminism pedagogy reader* (3rd ed). New York: Peter Lang.

Brown, S., & James, J. (2004). Event design and management: Ritual sacrifice? In I. Yeoman, M. Robertson, J. Ali-Knight, S. Drummond, & U. McMahan-Beattle, (Eds.), *Festival and events management: An international arts and culture perspective* (pp. 53–64). Oxford: Butterworth-Heinemann.

Browning, C. R., & Soller, B. (2014). Moving beyond neighborhood: Activity spaces and ecological networks as contexts for youth development. *Cityscape* (Washington, DC), *16* (1), 165.

Broyles-González, Y. (1994). *El teatro campesino: Theater in the Chicano movement.* Austin: University of Texas Press.

Bruening, J. E., Clark, B. S., & Mudrick, M. (2015). Sport-based youth development in practice: The long-term impacts of an urban after-school program for girls. *Journal of Park & Recreation Administration, 33* (2) 87–103.

Brugués, A. O. (2011). Music performance anxiety-Part 1. A review of its epidemiology. *Medical Problems of Performing Artists, 26* (2), 102–105.

Bryant, Y. (2008). Relationships between exposure to rap music videos and attitudes toward relationships among African American youth. *Journal of Black Psychology, 34* (3), 356–380.

Bryderup, I., & Frorup, A. K. (2011). Social pedagogy as relational dialogic work. In C. Cameron & P. Moss (Eds.), *Social pedagogy and working with children and young people: Where care and education meet* (pp. 85–104). Philadelphia, PA: Jessica Kingsley.

Bucholtz, M. (2002). Youth and cultural practice. *Annual Review of Anthropology, 31* (202), 525–552.

Buchroth, I., & Parkin, C. (Eds.). (2010). *Using theory in youth and community work practice.* Thousand Oaks, CA:SAGE.

Buck, R., & Rowe, N. (Eds.). (2015). *Moving oceans: Celebrating dance in the South Pacific.* New York: Routledge.

Buckley, M., & Saarni, C. (2009). Implications for positive youth development. In R. Gilman, E. S. Huebner, & M. J. Furlong (Eds.), *Handbook of positive psychology in schools* (pp. 107–118). New York: Routledge.

Buis, J. S., & dA, M. M. (2013). Music and dance make me feel alive: from Mandela's prison songs and dances to public policy. *Torture: quarterly journal on rehabilitation of torture victims and prevention of torture, 23*(2), 55–67.

Bundick, M. J. (2011). Extracurricular activities, positive youth development, and the role of meaningfulness of engagement. *The Journal of Positive Psychology, 6* (1), 57–74.

Bunt, L., & Stige, B. (2014). *Music therapy: An art beyond words.* New York: Routledge.

Burkemper, E., Hutchison, W. J., Wilson, J., & Stretch, J. J. (2013). *Practicing social justice.* New York: Routledge.

Burt, R. (2007). *The male dancer: Bodies, spectacle, sexualities.* New York: Routledge.

Butler, L. (2014). Something larger than ourselves: Redefining the young artists at work program as an art-as-activism residency for teens. *Journal of Museum Education, 39* (3), 262–275.

Butler, P. (2010). *Let's get free: A hip-hop theory of justice.* New York: The New Press.

Cahill, H. (2008). *Resisting risk and rescue as the raison d'etre for arts interventions* (Doctoral dissertation). University of Melbourne, Parkville Vic, Australia.

Cain, M., Lakhani, A., & Istvandity, L. (2016). Short and long term outcomes for culturally and linguistically diverse (CALD) and at-risk communities in participatory music programs: A systematic review. *Arts & Health, 8* (2), 105–124.

Caldwell, L. L., & Witt, P. A. (2011). Leisure, recreation, and play from a developmental context. *New Directions for Youth Development, 2011* (130), 13–27.

Callina, K. S., Johnson, S. K., Buckingham, M. H., & Lerner, R. M. (2014). Hope in context: Developmental profiles of trust, hopeful future expectations, and civic engagement across adolescence. *Journal of Youth and Adolescence, 43* (6), 869–883.

Callina, K. S., Mueller, M. K., Buckingham, M. H., & Gutierrez, A. S. (2015). Building hope for positive youth development: Research, practice, and policy. In E. P. Bowers, G. L. Geldhof, S. K. Johnson, L. J. Hilliard, R. M. Herberg, J. V. Lerner, & R. M. Lerner (Eds.), *Promoting positive youth development: Lessons from the 4-H Study* (pp. 71–96). New York: Springer

Calvert, S. L. (2013). Children's media: The role of music and audio features. In S-L. Tan & A. J. Cohen (Eds.), *The psychology of music in multimedia* (pp. 267–288). New York: Oxford University Press

Camangian, P. (2008). Untempered tongues: Teaching performance poetry for social justice. *English Teaching: Practice and Critique, 7* (2), 35–55.

Camiré, M., Trudel, P., & Forneris, T. (2014). Examining how model youth sport coaches learn to facilitate positive youth development. *Physical Education and Sport Pedagogy, 19* (1), 1–17.

Cammarota, J., & Romero, A. (2011). Participatory action research for high school students: Transforming policy, practice, and the personal with social justice education. *Educational Policy, 25* (3), 488–506.

Campbell, D., Trzesniewski, K., Nathaniel, K., Enfield, R., & Erbstein, N. (2013). Positive youth development merits state investment. *California Agriculture, 67* (1), 38–46.

Campbell, P. A. (2010). *Songs in their hearts: Music and its meaning in children's lives* (2nd ed.). New York: Oxford University Press.

Campbell, P. S. (2015). Music in the culture of children. In V. Lindsay Levine & P. V. Bohlman (Eds.), *This thing called music: Essays in honor of Bruno Nettl* (pp. 15–27). Lanham, MD: Rowman & Little Publishers.

Capila, A., & Bhalla, P. (2010). *"Street theatre for edutainment": A participatory research with youth in Delhi.* ERIC Online Submission. https://eric.ed.gov/?id=ED516877

Caprara, G. V., Kanacri, B. P. L., Gerbino, M., Zuffianò, A., Alessandri, G., Vecchio, G., . . . Bridglall, B. (2014). Positive effects of promoting prosocial behavior in early adolescence: Evidence from a school-based intervention. *International Journal of Behavioral Development, 38* (4), 386–396.

Carter, E. W., Brock, M. E., & Trainor, A. A. (2014). Transition assessment and planning for youth with severe intellectual and developmental disabilities. *The Journal of Special Education, 47* (4), 245–255.

Carter, E. W., Ditchman, N., Sun, Y., Trainor, A. A., Swedeen, B., & Owens, L. (2010). Summer employment and community experiences of transition-age youth with severe disabilities. *Exceptional Children, 76* (2), 194–212.

Carter, J. (2016). The physics of the mola: Writing indigenous resurgence on the contemporary stage. *Modern Drama, 59* (1), 26–48.

Casteran, H., & Roederer, C. (2013). Does authenticity really affect behavior? The case of the Strasbourg Christmas Market. *Tourism Management, 36* (2), 153–163.

Castrillo, P. D. R. (2012). Karl Gaspar and the Mindanao Theater: 1970–1990. *Philippine Studies: Historical and Ethnographic Viewpoints, 44* (1), 39–51.

Cater, M., & Jones, K. Y. (2014). Measuring perceptions of engagement in teamwork in youth development programs. *Journal of Experiential Education, 37* (2), 176–186.

Catherwood, J., & Leonard, R. H. (2015). Rivers and bridges: Theatre in regional planning. In M. O. Stephenson, Jr., & S. Tate (Eds.), *Arts and community change: Exploring cultural development policies, practices, and dilemmas* (pp. 28–53). New York: Routledge.

Cauce, A. M., Cruz, R., Corona, M., & Conger, R. (2011). The face of the future: Risk and resilience in minority youth. In G. Carlo & L. J. Crockett (Eds.), *Health disparities in youth and families* (pp. 13–32). New York: Springer.

Chacko, E., & Menon, R. (2013). Longings and belongings: Indian American youth identity, folk dance competitions, and the construction of 'tradition'. *Ethnic and Racial Studies, 36* (1), 97–116.

Chahine, I. C. (2011). Beyond Eurocentrism: Situating ethnomathematics within the history of mathematics narrative. *Journal Internacional de Estudos em Educação Matemática, 4* (2), 35–48.

Chan, Y. L. P. (2009). In their own words: How do students relate drama pedagogy to their learning in curriculum subjects? *RiDE: The Journal of Applied Theatre and Performance, 14* (2), 191–209.

Chappell, S. V., & Cahnmann-Taylor, M. (2013). No child left with crayons: The imperative of arts-based education and research with language 'minority' and other minoritized communities. *Review of Research in Education, 37* (1), 243–268.

Chappell, S. V., & Faltis, C. J. (2013). *The arts and emergent bilingual youth: Building culturally responsive, critical and creative education in school and community contexts.* New York: Routledge.

Chase, P. A., Warren, D. J., & Lerner, R. M. (2015). Schoole engagement, academic achievement and positive youth development. In E. P. Bowers, G. L. Geldhof, S. K. Johnson, L. J. Hilliard, R. M. Herberg, J. V. Lerner, & R. M. Lerner (Eds.), *Promoting positive youth development: Lessons from the 4-H Study* (pp. 57–70). New York: Springer

Chau, C. (2010). YouTube as a participatory culture. *New Directions for Youth Development, 2010* (128), 65–74.

Chávez, M. S. (2012). Autoethnography, a Chicana's methodological research tool: The role of storytelling for those who have no choice but to do critical race theory. *Equity & Excellence in Education, 45* (2), 334–348.

Chavez, V. (2014, November). *Cultural humility: People, principles & practices.* Presented at the 142nd APHA annual meeting and exposition, Washington, DC.

Checkoway, B. (2011). What is youth participation? *Children and Youth Services Review, 33* (2), 340–345.

Checkoway, B., & Aldana, A. (2013). Four forms of youth civic engagement for diverse democracy. *Children and Youth Services Review, 35* (11), 1894–1899.

Checkoway, B., & Richards-Schuster, K. (2006). Youth participation for educational reform in low-income communities of color. In S. Ginwright, P. Noguera, & J. Cammarota (Eds.), *Beyond resistance* (pp. 319–332). New York: Routledge.

Cheesman, S. (2011). Facilitating dance making from a teacher's perspective within a community integrated dance class. *Research in Dance Education, 12* (1), 29–40.

Chen, K. K., Lune, H., & Queen, E. L. (2013). How values shape and are shaped by nonprofit and voluntary organizations: The current state of the field. *Nonprofit and Voluntary Sector Quarterly, 42* (5), 856–885.

Chen, Q. (2015). Discussion on role and functions of props in dance. *Cross-Cultural Communication, 11* (3), 110–112.

Cheon, J. W., & Canda, E. (2010). The meaning and engagement of spirituality for positive youth development in social work. *Families in Society: The Journal of Contemporary Social Services, 91* (2), 121–126.

Cherng, H. Y. S. (2015). Social isolation among racial/ethnic minority immigrant youth. *Sociology Compass, 9* (6), 509–518.

Chhabra, D. (2010). Branding authenticity. *Tourism Analysis, 15* (6), 735–740.

Chhuon, V., & Wallace, T. L. (2014). Creating connectedness through being known: Fulfilling the need to belong in US high schools. *Youth & Society, 46* (3), 379–401.

Childers, J. P. (2012). *The evolving citizen: American youth and the changing norms of democratic engagement* (Vol. 4). University Park, PA: Penn State Press.

Chimurenga, T. (2015, August 13). The Watts uprising @ 50. *Los Angeles Watts Times.*

Cho, S., Crenshaw, K. W., & McCall, L. (2013). Toward a field of intersectionality studies: Theory, applications, and praxis. *Signs, 38* (4), 785–810.

Christens, B. D. (2012). Targeting empowerment in community development: A community psychology approach to enhancing local power and well-being. *Community Development Journal, 47* (4), 538–554.

Christens, B. D., & Dolan, T. (2011). Interweaving youth development, community development, and social change through youth organizing. *Youth & Society, 43* (2), 528–548.

Christens, B. D., & Speer, P. W. (2015). Community organizing: Practice, research, and policy implications. *Social Issues and Policy Review, 9* (1), 193–222.

Christensen, M. C. (2012). *Using theatre for social change to address sexual violence against college women* (Doctoral dissertation). University of Utah, Salt Lake City.

Chua, J. (2014). Dance talent development across the lifespan: A review of current research. *Research in Dance Education, 15* (1), 23–53.

Chung, S. K. (2007). Media/visual literacy art education: Sexism in hip-hop music videos. *Art Education, 60* (3), 33–38.

Clark, J. (2009). Acting up and speaking out: Using Theatre of the Oppressed and collective memory work as alternative research methods and empowerment in work with girls. *Agenda, 23* (79), 49–64.

Clary, E. G., & Rhodes, J. E. (Eds.). (2006). *Mobilizing adults for positive youth development: Strategies for closing the gap between beliefs and behaviors.* New York: Springer Publisher.

Clay, A. (2006). "All I need is one mic": Mobilizing youth for social change in the post-civil rights era. *Social Justice, 33* (2), 105–121.

Clay, A. (2012). *The hip-hop generation fights back: Youth, activism and post-civil rights politics.* New York: New York University Press.

Clemons, K. A., & Clemons, K. M. (2013). What the music said: Hip hop as a transformative educational tool. In M. S. Hanley, G. W. Nobit, G. L. Sheppard & T. Barone (Eds.), *Culturally relevant arts education for social justice: A way out* (pp. 58–70). New York: Routledge.

Clift, S. (2012). Creative arts as a public health resource: Moving from practice-based research to evidence-based practice. *Perspectives in Public Health*, 132 (3), 120–127.

Clift, S., Hancox, G., Morrison, I., Shipton, M., Page, S., Skingley, A., & Vella-Burrows, T. (2015). Group singing as a public health resource. In S. Clift & P. M. Camic (Eds.), *Oxford textbook of creative arts, health, and wellbeing: International perspectives on practice, policy and research* (pp. 251–257). New York: Oxford University Press.

Clonan-Roy, K., Jacobs, C. E., & Nakkula, M. J. (2016). Towards a model of positive youth development specific to girls of color: Perspectives on development, resilience, and empowerment. *Gender Issues*, 33 (2), 96–121.

Coakley, J. (2011). Youth sports what counts as 'positive development'? *Journal of Sport & Social Issues*, 35 (3), 306–324.

Cocke, D. (2015). Community cultural development as a site of joy, structure, and transformation. In M. O. Stephenson Jr., & S. Tate (Eds.), *Arts and community change: Exploring cultural development policies, practices and dilemmas* (pp. 136–165). New York: Routledge.

Coffey, J., & Farrugia, D. (2014). Unpacking the black box: The problem of agency in the sociology of youth. *Journal of Youth Studies*, 17 (4), 461–474.

Cohen, E., & Cohen, S. A. (2015). Beyond Eurocentrism in tourism: A paradigm shift to mobilities. *Tourism Recreation Research*, 40 (2), 157–168.

Cohen, L. (2014). *Fostering racial and economic diversity in performing arts organizations: Identifying sociodemographic and administrative barriers to inclusion* (Doctoral dissertation). University of Delaware, Newark, DE.

Cohen, M. L., Silber, L. H., Sangiorgio, A., & Iadeluca, V. (2012). At-risk youth: Music-making as a means to promote positive relationships. G. E. McPherson & G. F. Welch (Eds.), *The Oxford handbook of music education* (Vol. 2, pp. 185–202). New York: Oxford University Press.

Cohen-Cruz, J. (2006). Introduction: The ecology of theater-in-community. In R. H. Leonard & A. Kilkelly (Eds.), *Performing communities: Grassroots ensemble theaters deeply rooted in eight U. S. communities* (pp. 3–24). Oakland, CA: New Village Press.

Cohen-Cruz, J., & Schutzman, M. (Eds.). (2006). *A Boal companion: Dialogues on theatre and cultural politics.* New York: Routledge.

Collins, P. H. (2012). Looking back, moving ahead: Scholarship in service to social justice. *Gender & Society*, 26 (1), 14–22.

Collins, P. H., & Bilge, S. (2016). *Intersectionality.* Cambridge, UK: Polity Press.

Conner, J. (2012).*The value of youth organizing.* Research Publication, (2013-12). Cambridge, MA: Harvard University Berkman Center.

Conner, J. O. (2016). Pawns or power players: The grounds on which adults dismiss or defend youth organizers in the USA. *Journal of Youth Studies*, 19 (3), 403–420.

Connolly, M. K., Quin, E., & Redding, E. (2011). Dance 4 your life: Exploring the health and well-being implications of a contemporary dance intervention for female adolescents. *Research in Dance Education*, 12 (1), 53–66.

Conrad, D. (2004). Popular theatre: Empowering pedagogy for youth. *Youth Theatre Journal, 18* (1), 87–106.

Conrad, D. (2005). Rethinking 'at-risk' in drama education: Beyond prescribed roles. *Research in Drama Education, 10* (1), 27–41.

Conrad, D. (2006). Entangled (in the) sticks: Ethical conundrums of popular theater as pedagogy and research. *Qualitative Inquiry, 12* (3), 437–458.

Conrad, D. (2008). Exploring risky youth experiences: Popular theatre as a participatory, performative research method. *International Journal of Qualitative Methods, 3* (1), 12–24.

Conrad, D., Smyth, P., & Kendal, W. (2015). *Participatory arts based research with youth. Creating together: Participatory, community-based, and collaborative arts practices and scholarship across Canada.* Waterloo, ON, CAN: Wilfrid Laurier University Press.

Conrad, D. H. (2015). Education and social innovation: The youth uncensored project—a case study of youth participatory research and cultural democracy in action. *Canadian Journal of Education/Revue canadienne de l'éducation, 38* (1), 1–25.

Conroy, C. (2009). Disability: Creative tensions between drama, theatre and disability arts. *Research in Drama Education: The Journal of Applied Theatre and Performance, 14* (1), 1–14.

Coppens, N. M., Page, R., & Thou, T. C. (2006). Reflections on the evaluation of a Cambodian youth dance program. *American Journal of Community Psychology, 37* (3-4), 321–331.

Cormier, P., & Gorman, E. (2014). Unpacking the Backpack: A Dance-Based Inquiry of the Trail. The Qualitative Report Conference. http://nsuworks.nova.edu/tqrc/fifth/day2/36/

Corrarino, M. (2015, October 15). U. S. stands alone: Not signing U. N. Child Rights Treaty leaves migrant children vulnerable. *Huffington Post.* Retrieved from http://www.huffingtonpost.com/b-shaw-drake/children-migrants-rights_b_8271874.html

Cote, J. E., & Allahar, A. L. (2006). *Critical youth studies: A Canadian focus.* Toronto, ON, CAN: Person Prentice Hall.

Coulter, R. (2015, November). Sexual-orientation differences in positive youth development. Presented at the *143rd APHA annual meeting and exposition*, Chicago, IL.

Countryman, J., Gabriel, M., & Thompson, K. (2015). Children's spontaneous vocalisations during play: Aesthetic dimensions. *Music Education Research, 18* (1), 1–19.

Cox, K. (2008). Tools for building on youth strengths. *Reclaiming Children and Youth, 16* (4), 19–24.

Craps, S. (2013). Beyond Eurocentrism. In G. Buelens, S. Durrant, & R. Eaglestone (Eds.), *The future of trauma theory: Contemporary literary and cultural criticism* (pp. 45–62). New York: Routledge.

Crean, M. (2013, June). Once upon a time in the Bronx: Working with youth to address violence through performance and play. In *Proceedings of the 12th International Conference on Interaction Design and Children* (pp. 443–446). New York: ACM.

Creasap, K. (2012). Social movement scenes: Place-based politics and everyday resistance. *Sociology Compass, 6* (2), 182–191.

Cremin, T., Goouch, K., Blakemore, L., Goff, E., & Macdonald, R. (2006). Connecting drama and writing: Seizing the moment to write. *Research in Drama Education, 11* (3), 273–291.

Crnic, M. (2012). *Social capital and neighbourhood centres in Queensland: Qualitative case studies of three neighbourhood centres* (Doctoral dissertation). Queensland University of Technology.

Crosnoe, R., & Johnson, M. K. (2011). Research on adolescence in the twenty-first century. *Annual Review of Sociology, 37* (August), 439–460.

Crowley, K., Barron, B. J., Knutson, K., & Martin, C. K. (2015). Interest and the development of pathways to science. In *Handbook of Interest in mathematics and science learning and related activities* (pp. 297–313). Washington, DC: American Educational Research Association.

Crowther, G. J., McFadden, T., Fleming, J. S., & Davis, K. (2016). Leveraging the power of music to improve science education. *International Journal of Science Education, 38* (1), 73–95.

Cuervo, H., & Wyn, J. (2014). Reflections on the use of spatial and relational metaphors in youth studies. *Journal of Youth Studies, 17* (7), 901–915.

Cushing, D. F., Love, E. W., & van Villet, W. (2012). Through the viewfinder: Using multimedia techniques to engage Latino youth in community planning. In M. Rios, L. Vasques & L. Miranda, L. (Eds.), *Dialogos: Placemaking in Latino communities* (pp. 172–185). New York: Routledge.

Dadsetan, P., Anari, A., & Sedghpour, B. S. (2008). Social anxiety disorders and drama-therapy. *Journal of Iranian Psychologists, 4,* 115–123.

Daley, A., Solomon, S., Newman, P. A., & Mishna, F. (2008). Traversing the margins: Intersectionalities in the bullying of lesbian, gay, bisexual and transgender youth. *Journal of Gay & Lesbian Social Services, 19* (3-4), 9–29.

D'Amico, M., Lalonde, C., & Snow, S. (2015). Evaluating the efficacy of drama therapy in teaching social skills to children with Autism Spectrum Disorders. *Drama Therapy Review, 1* (1), 21–39.

Damon, W., Bronk, K. C., & Porter, T. (2015). *Youth entrepreneurship. Emerging trends in the social and behavioral sciences: An interdisciplinary, searchable, and linkable resource.* Retrieved from http://onlinelibrary.wiley.com/doi/10.1002/9781118900772.etrds0391/abstract;jsessionid=F4D93457AB727BFB0EDBFB521BE8EA38.f02t04?userIsAuthenticated=false&deniedAccessCustomisedMessage=

Daniel, E., Dys, S. P., Buchmann, M., & Malti, T. (2016). Developmental trajectories of social justice values in adolescence: Relations with sympathy and friendship quality. *Social Development, 25* (3), 548–564.

Darrow, A. A., Johnson, C. M., Ollenberger, T., & Miller, A. M. (2001). The effect of an intergenerational choir performance on audience members' attitudinal statements toward teens and older persons. *International Journal of Music Education, 38* (1), 43–50.

Datoo, A. K., & Chagani, Z. (2011). Street theatre: Critical pedagogy for social studies education. *Social Studies Research and Practice, 6* (2), 21–30.

Dávila, A. M. (2012). *Culture works: Space, value, and mobility across the neoliberal Americas.* New York: New York University Press.

Davis, N. Y., Yuval-Davis, N., Kaptani, E., & Kaptani, E. (n.d.). *Identity, performance and social action: Participatory theatre among refugees.* Retrieved from https://www.researchgate.net/profile/Nira_Yuval-Davis/publication/237120226_Identity_performance_and_social_action_Participatory_theatre_among_refugees/links/54d1fd-090cf25ba0f04228f0.pdf

Dawes, N. P., & Larson, R. (2011). How youth get engaged: Grounded-theory research on motivational development in organized youth programs. *Developmental Psychology, 47* (1), 259–269.

Dawes, N. P., Modecki, K. L., Gonzales, N., Dumka, L., & Millsap, R. (2015). Mexican-origin youth participation in extracurricular activities: Predicting trajectories of involvement from 7th to 12th grade. *Journal of Youth and Adolescence, 44* (11), 2172–2188.

Daykin, N., De Viggiani, N., Pilkington, P., & Moriarty, Y. (2013). Music making for health, well-being and behavior change in youth justice settings: A systematic review. *Health Promotion International, 28* (2), 197–210.

Daykin, N., Orme, J., Evans, D., Salmon, D., McEachran, M., & Brain, S. (2008). The impact of participation in performing arts on adolescent health and behavior: A systematic review of the literature. *Journal of Health Psychology, 13* (2), 251–264.

Deane, K. L., & Harré, N. (2014). Program theory-driven evaluation science in a youth development context. *Evaluation and Program Planning, 45* (1), 61–70.

Debies-Carl, J. S. (2013). Are the kids alright? A critique and agenda for taking youth cultures seriously. *Social Science Information, 52* (1), 110–133.

Debnam, K. J., Johnson, S. L., Waasdorp, T. E., & Bradshaw, C. P. (2014). Equity, connection, and engagement in the school context to promote positive youth development. *Journal of Research on Adolescence, 24* (3), 447–459.

DeCarlo, A. (2013). The rise and call of group rap therapy: A critical analysis from its creator. *Group Analysis, 46* (2), 225–238.

DeCarlo, A., & Hockman, E. (2004). RAP therapy: A group work intervention method for urban adolescents. *Social Work with Groups, 26* (3), 45–59.

DeJaeghere, J. G., & McCleary, K. S. (2010). The making of Mexican migrant youth civic identities: Transnational spaces and imaginaries. *Anthropology & Education Quarterly, 41* (3), 228–244.

De Kloet, J. (2010). *China with a cut: Globalisation, urban youth and popular music* (Vol. 3). Amsterdam, Holland: Amsterdam University Press.

Delgado, M. (1999). *Community social work practice in an urban context: The potential of a capacity enhancement perspective.* New York: Oxford University Press.

Delgado, M. (2000). *New arenas for community social work practice with urban youth: The use of the arts, humanities, and sports.* New York: Columbia University Press.

Delgado, M. (2002). *New frontiers for youth development in the twenty-first century: Revitalizing and broadening youth development.* New York: Columbia University Press.

Delgado, M. (2012). *Prisoner re-entry and work: Adding business to the mix.* Boulder, CO: Lynne Rienner Publisher.

Delgado, M. (2013). *Social justice and the urban obesity crisis: Implications for social work.* New York: Columbia University Press.

Delgado, M. (2015). *Urban youth and photovoice: Visual ethnography in action.* New York: Oxford University Press.

Delgado, M. (2016a). *Celebrating urban community life: Fairs, festivals, parades and community practice.* Toronto: University of Toronto Press.

Delgado, M. (2016b). *Community practice and urban youth: Social justice service-learning and civic engagement.* New York: Routledge Ltd.

Delgado, M. (2017). *Urban youth friendships and community social work practice.* New York: Oxford University Press.

Delgado, M., & Humm-Delgado, D. (2013). *Asset assessments and community social work practice.* New York: Oxford University Press.

Delgado, M., Jones, L. K., & Rohani, M. (2005).*Social work practice with immigrant and refugee youth in the United States.* Boston: Allyn & Bacon.

Delgado, M., & Staples, L. (2008). *Youth-led community organizing: Theory and action.* New York: Oxford University Press.

DeLorenzo, L. C., & Silverman, M. (2016). *From the margins: The underrepresentation of black and latino students/teachers in music education.* Retrieved from http://webcache.googleusercontent.com/search?q=cache:http://www-usr.rider.edu/~vrme/v27n1/visions/DeLorenzo_Silverman_Underrepresentation_Black_Latino_Students-Teachers_Music_Education.pdf

DePass, C. (2012). 'Freedom songs' in selected Caribbean-Canadian contexts: Retrospective fragments. *Journal of Contemporary Issues in Education, 7* (1). Retrieved from http://ejournals.library.ualberta.ca/index.php/JCIE/article/view/18075

Derby, J. (2012). Art education and disability studies. *Disability Studies Quarterly, 32* (1). Retrieved from http://dsq-sds.org/article/view/3027/3054

Deutsch, N. L., & Jones, J. N. (2008). "Show me an ounce of respect": Respect and authority in adult-youth relationships in after-school programs. *Journal of Adolescent Research, 23* (6), 667–688.

Dewhurst, M. (2013). Narrowing in on the answers: Dissecting social justice art education. In M. S. Hanley, G. W. Nobit, G. L. Sheppard & T. Barone (Eds.), *Culturally relevant arts education for social justice: A way out* (pp. 143–153). New York: Routledge.

Diaz-Strong, D., Gomez, C., Lance-Duarte, M., & Meiners, E. R. (2014). Out for immigration justice: Thinking through social and political change. In E. Tuck & K. W. Yang (Eds.), *Youth resistance research and theories of change* (pp. 218–229). New York: Routledge.

Dill, L. J. (2015). Poetic justice: Engaging in participatory narrative analysis to find solace in the 'killer corridor'. *American Journal of Community Psychology, 55* (1-2), 128–135.

Dill, L. J., & Ozer, E. J. (2016). "I'm not just runnin' the streets": Exposure to neighborhood violence and violence management strategies among urban youth of color. *Journal of Adolescent Research, 31* (5), 536–556.

Dimitriadis, G. (2008). *Studying urban youth culture primer.* New York: Peter Lang.

Dimitriadis, G. (2014). Resistance: The anatomy of an idea. In E. Tuck & K. W. Yang (Eds.). (2014). *Youth resistance research and theories of change* (pp. 29–45). New York: Routledge.

Disegna, M., Osti, L., & Brida, J. G. (2011). *Authenticity perception of cultural events: A host-tourist analysis.* Rochester, NY: Social Science Research Network.

Dixon-Román, E. J. (2013). The forms of capital and the developed achievement of Black males. *Urban Education, 48* (6), 828–862.

Doane, R. (2006). The habitus of dancing notes on the swing dance revival in New York City. *Journal of Contemporary Ethnography, 35* (1), 84–116.

Donlan, A. E., Lynch, A. D., & Lerner, R. M. (2015). Peer relationships and positive youth development. In E. P. Bowers, G. L. Geldhof, S. K. Johnson, L. J. Hilliard, R. M. Herberg, J. V. Lerner, & R. M. Lerner (Eds.), *Promoting positive youth development: Lessons from the 4-H Study* (pp. 121–136). New York: Springer.

Dover, A. G. (2013). Teaching for social justice: From conceptual frameworks to classroom practices. *Multicultural Perspectives, 15* (1), 3–11.

Dowdy, C. S. (2012). *Youth, music, and agency: Undoing race, poverty and violence in Rio de Janeiro, Brazil* (Doctoral dissertation). American University, Washington, DC.

Downey, G., Dalidowicz, M., & Mason, P. H. (2015). Apprenticeship as method: Embodied learning in ethnographic practice. *Qualitative Research, 15* (2), 183–200.

Duckworth, A. (2016). *Grit: The power of passion and perseverance.* London: Vermillion.

Duke, N. N., Borowsky, I. W., & Pettingell, S. L. (2012). Adult perceptions of neighborhood: Links to youth engagement. *Youth & Society, 44* (3), 408–430.

Dunn, K. (2013). School-to-prison pipeline. *Faulkner Law Review, 5*, 115.

Dupree, D., Spencer, T. R., & Spencer, M. B. (2015). Stigma, stereotypes and resilience identities: The relationship between identity processes and resilience processes among Black American adolescents. In L. Theron, L. Liebenberg, M. Ungar. *Youth resilience and culture* (pp. 117–129). Rotterdam: Springer Netherlands.

Durlak, J. A., Mahoney, J. L., Bohnert, A. M., & Parente, M. E. (2010). Developing and improving after-school programs to enhance youth's personal growth and adjustment: A special issue of AJCP. *American Journal of Community Psychology, 45* (3-4), 285–293.

Durlak, J. A., Weissberg, R. P., & Pachan, M. (2010). A meta-analysis of after-school programs that seek to promote personal and social skills in children and adolescents. *American Journal of Community Psychology, 45* (3-4), 294–309.

Dutton, S. E. (2001). Urban youth development–Broadway style: Using theatre and group work as vehicles for positive youth development. *Social Work with Groups, 23* (4), 39–58.

Dworkin, J., & Larson, R. (2006). Adolescents' negative experiences in organized youth activities. *Journal of Youth Development, 1* (3), 1–19.

Dwyer, P. (2004). Making bodies talk in Forum Theatre. *Research in Drama Education, 9* (2), 199–210.

Dyer, R. (2013). *In the space of a song: The uses of song in film.* New York: Routledge.

Eales, L., & Goodwin, D. (2015). "We all carry each other, sometimes": Care-sharing as social justice practice in integrated dance. *Leisure/Loisir, 39* (2), 277–298.

Eccles, J. S., & Gootman, J. A. (2002). *Community programs to promote youth development.* Washington, DC: National Academy Press.

Eccles, J. S., & Roeser, R. W. (2011). Schools as developmental contexts during adolescence. *Journal of Research on Adolescence, 21* (1), 225–241.

Edell, D. (2013). "Say it how it is": Urban teenage girls challenge and perpetuate stereotypes through writing and performing theatre. *Youth Theatre Journal, 27* (1), 51–62.

Edelman, J., & Šorli, M. (2015). Measuring the value of theatre for Tyneside audiences. *Cultural Trends, 24* (3), 232–244.

Edge, S., Newbold, K. B., & McKeary, M. (2014). Exploring socio-cultural factors that mediate, facilitate, & constrain the health and empowerment of refugee youth. *Social Science & Medicine, 117* (1), 34–41.

Edmonds, A. (2013). *Well-being, participation and young citizens shaping place* (Doctoral dissertation). University of South Australia, Adelaide.

Edwards, J. (2014*). Local actors achieving positive youth development: A case study of movimiento comunal Nicaragüense* (Doctoral dissertation). University of Guelph, Guelph, CAN.

Einarsdottir, S. L., & Gudmundsdottir, H. R. (2016). The role of choral singing in the lives of amateur choral singers in Iceland. *Music Education Research, 18* (1), 39–56.

Ekstrom, J. E. (2015). *The end that crowned our work: My experience and growth as a musician and future educator with the Blue Stars Drum and Bugle Corps* (Undergraduate senior honors thesis). Ball State University, Muncie, IN).

Elam, H. J. (2001). *Taking it to the streets: The social protest theater of Luis Valdez and Amiri Baraka.* Ann Arbor, MI: University of Michigan Press.

Eliasoph, N. (2014). Measuring the grassroots: Puzzles of cultivating the grassroots from the top down. *The Sociological Quarterly, 55* (3), 467–492.

Emdin, C. (2010). Affiliation and alienation: Hip-hop, rap, and urban science education. *Journal of Curriculum Studies, 42* (1), 1–25.

Emmons, S., & Thomas, A. (2008). Understanding performance anxiety. *Journal of Singing, 64* (4), 461–465.

Enciso, P., Cushman, C., Edmiston, B., Post, R., & Berring, D. (2011). Is that what you really want?': A case study of intracultural ensemble-building within the paradoxes of 'urbanicity'. *RIDE: The Journal of Applied Theatre and Performance, 16* (2), 215–233.

Engdahl, E. (2012). The East Bay Center for the Performing Arts: A model for community-based multicultural arts education. *Multicultural Education, 19* (2), 43–48.

Engels, H. J., Gretebeck, R. J., Gretebeck, K. A., & Jiménez, L. (2005). Promoting healthful diets and exercise: Efficacy of a 12-week after-school program in urban African Americans. *Journal of the American Dietetic Association, 105* (3), 455–459.

Epstein, W. M. (2013). *Empowerment as ceremony.* New Brunswick, NJ: Transaction Publishers.

Erevelles, N. (2014). Crippin' Jim Crow: Disability, dis-location, and the school-to-prison pipeline. In L. Ben-Moshe, C. Chapman & A. Carey (Eds.), *Disability incarcerated: Imprisonment and disability in the United States and Canada* (pp. 81–100). New York: Palgrave Macmillan.

Ergler, C. R., & Wood, B. E. (2014). Re-imagining youth participation in the 21st century. In P. Kelley & A. Kamp (Eds.), *A critical youth studies for the 21st century* (pp. 394–413). Boston: Brill.

Ersing, R. L. (2009). Building the capacity of youths through community cultural arts. *Best Practices in Mental Health, 5* (1), 26–43.

Erstad, O., & Sefton-Green, J. (2013). *Identity, community, and learning lives in the digital age.* Cambridge University Press.

Etherton, M., & Prentki, T. (2006). Drama for change? Prove it! Impact assessment in applied theatre. *Research in Drama Education, 11* (2), 139–155.

Evans, A. B., Banerjee, M., Meyer, R., Aldana, A., Foust, M., & Rowley, S. (2012). Racial socialization as a mechanism for positive development among African American youth. *Child Development Perspectives, 6* (3), 251–257.

Evans, S. D. (2007). Youth sense of community: Voice and power in community contexts. *Journal of Community Psychology, 35* (6), 693–709.

Fader, J. J. (2013). *Falling back: Incarceration and transitions to adulthood among urban youth.* New Brunswick, NJ: Rutgers University Press.

Fairman, S. (2014, April 10). *Reframe: The Unusual Suspects Theatre Company.* KCET. Retrieved from http://www.kcet.org/arts/artbound/counties/los-angeles/change-together.html

Farb, A. F., & Matjasko, J. L. (2012). Recent advances in research on school-based extracurricular activities and adolescent development. *Developmental Review, 32* (1), 1–48.

Farrugia, D. (2016). Introduction: Understanding youth homelessness. In D. Farrugia (Ed.), *Youth homelessness in late modernity* (pp. 1–16). Singapore: Springer.

Feagan, R., & Rossiter, K. (2011). University-community engagement: A case study using popular theatre. *Education + Training, 53* (2/3), 140–154.

Ferguson, G. M., Boer, D., Clobert, M., Prade, C., & Saroglou, V. (2016). "Get up, stand up, stand up for your rights!": The Jamaicanization of youth across 11 countries through reggae music? *Journal of Cross-Cultural Psychology, 47* (4), 581–604.

Ferrare, J. J., & Apple, M. W. (2012). Youth marginalized and the city. *Pedagogy, Culture & Society, 20* (1), 163–172.

Ferreira, M. L., & Devine, D. (2012). Theater of the Oppressed as a rhizome acting for the rights of indigenous peoples today. *Latin American Perspectives, 39* (2), 11–26.

Ferreira, P. D., Coimbra, J. L., & Menezes, I. (2012). Diversity within diversity-exploring connections between community, participation and citizenship. *JSSE- Journal of Social Science Education, 11* (3), 118–132.

Ferrer-Wreder, L., Adamson, L., Kumpfer, K. L., & Eichas, K. (2012). Advancing intervention science through effectiveness research: A global perspective. *Child & Youth Care Forum, 41* (2), 109–117.

Ferrer-Wreder, L., Lorente, C. C., Kurtines, W., Briones, E., Bussell, J., Berman, S., & Arrufat, O. (2002). Promoting identity development in marginalized youth. *Journal of Adolescent Research, 17* (2), 168–187.

Ferrera, M. (2015, November). *Chicago Area Youth Health Service Corps: A youth led, health promotion program within the immigrant community.* Presented at the 143rd APHA annual meeting and exposition, Chicago, IL.

Ferro, S., & Watts, M. W. (2011). *Dance Performance and Community Memory in Service-Learning.* Retrieved from http://www.simoneferro.com/wp-content/uploads/2011/12/Dance_CSL.pdf

Fields, A., Snapp, S., Russell, S. T., Licona, A. C., & Tilley, E. H. (2014). Youth voices and knowledges: Slam poetry speaks to social policies. *Sexuality Research and Social Policy, 11* (4), 310–321.

Fine, M. (2012). Youth participatory action research. In N. Lesko & S. Talburt (Eds.), *Keywords in youth studies: Tracing affects, movements, knowledges* (pp. 318–323). New York: Routledge.

Fine, M., & Jaffe-Walter, R. (2007). Swimming: On oxygen, resistance, and possibility for immigrant youth under siege. *Anthropology & Education Quarterly, 38* (1), 76–96.

Fine, M., & Torre, M. E. (2004). Re-membering exclusions: Participatory action research in public institutions. *Qualitative Research in Psychology, 1* (1), 15–37.

Fischer, R. L., Craven, M. A., & Heilbron, P. (2011). Putting youth development into practice: Learning from an innovative fellowship program. *New Directions for Youth Development, 2011* (S1), 77–105.

Fisher, A. S. (2009). Bearing witness: The position of theatre makers in the telling of trauma. In K. Prentki & S. Preston (Eds.), *The applied theatre reader* (pp. 108–115). New York: Routledge.

Fisher, S., Reynolds, J. L., Hsu, W. W., Barnes, J., & Tyler, K. (2014). Examining multiracial youth in context: Ethnic identity development and mental health outcomes. *Journal of Youth and Adolescence, 43* (10), 1688–1699.

Fisher, T. A. (2009). *If obesity is so bad, why are so many people fat? Interrogating, exploring, and understanding obesity through theatre.* Retrieved from http://steinhardt.nyu.edu/scmsAdmin/media/users/ch1097/TAFisher_obesity_topic_proposal.pdf

Flanagan, C. A., & Christens, B. D. (2011). Youth civic development: Historical context and emerging issues. *New Directions for Child and Adolescent Development, 2011* (134), 1–9.

Flanagan, C. A., Martínez, M. L., Cumsille, P., & Ngomane, T. (2011). Youth civic development: Theorizing a domain with evidence from different cultural contexts. *New Directions for Child and Adolescent Development, 2011* (134), 95–109.

Flenaugh, T. (2012). *Youth Orchestra Los Angeles (YOLA): Creating access to excellent music education for underrepresented students of color* (Doctoral dissertation). UCLA, Los Angeles.

Fleming, D., Durham, S. G., Lewis, M., & Leonard, A. (2015). *Art field experiences within after school programs: A university/school partnership.* Poster presentation at the National Youth At Risk Conference, Savannah, GA.

Fleming, M., Merrell, C., & Tymms, P. (2004). The impact of drama on pupils' language, mathematics, and attitude in two primary schools. *Research in Drama Education, 9* (2), 177–197.

Fletcher-Watson, B., Fletcher-Watson, S., McNaughton, M. J., & Birch, A. (2014). From cradle to stage: How early years performing arts experiences are tailored to the developmental capabilities of babies and toddlers. *Youth Theatre Journal, 28* (2), 130–146.

Flicker, S. (2008). Who benefits from community-based participatory research? A case study of the Positive Youth Project. *Health Education & Behavior, 35* (1), 70–86.

Flint, K., Graves, W., & Morong, J. (2015). ICivic engagement: In and outside the classroom. In *Students' pathway to success: A faculty guide* (pp. 202–218). Retrieved from https://journals.uncc.edu/facultyguide/article/view/389/390

Flora, P. K., & Faulkner, G. E. (2007). Physical activity: An innovative context for intergenerational programming. *Journal of Intergenerational Relationships, 4* (4), 63–74.

Flores, K. S. (2007). *Youth participatory evaluation: Strategies for engaging young people* (Vol. 14). New York: John Wiley & Sons.

Flores-Gonzalez, N., Rodriguez, M., & Rodriguez-Muniz, M. (2006). From hip-hop to humanization: Batey Urbano as a space for Latino youth culture and community action. In S. Ginwright, P. Noguera & J. Cammarota (Eds.), *Beyond resistance* (pp. 175–196). New York: Routledge.

Fogarty, M. (2015). The body and dance. In J. Shepherd & K. Devine (Eds.), *The Routledge reader on the sociology of music* (pp. 245–253). New York: Routledge.

Forkby, T., & Kiilakoski, T. (2014). Building capacity in youth work: Perspective and practice of youth clubs in Finland and in Sweden. *Youth & Policy, 112*, 1–17.

Forneris, T., Bean, C., & Halsall, T. (2016). Positive youth development programming with marginalized populations. In N. L. Holt (Ed.), *Positive youth development through sport* (pp. 168–179). New York: Routledge.

Forrest, L. (2014). Your song, my song, our song: Developing music therapy programs for a culturally diverse community in home-based paediatric palliative care. *Australian Journal of Music Therapy, 25* (1), 15–27.

Forrest-Bank, S., Nicotera, N., Anthony, E., & Jenson, J. (2015). Finding their way: Perceptions of risk, resilience, and positive youth development among adolescents and young adults from public housing neighborhoods. *Children and Youth Services Review, 55* (Aug), 147–158.

Forsyth, M. (2012). Lifting the lid on 'the community': Who has the right to control access to traditional knowledge and expressions of culture? *International Journal of Cultural Property, 19* (1), 1–31.

Foster, K. R., & Spencer, D. (2011). At risk of what? Possibilities over probabilities in the study of young lives. *Journal of Youth Studies, 14* (1), 125–143.

Foster, V. (2012). What if? The use of poetry to promote social justice. *Social Work Education, 31* (6), 742–755.

Fox, H. (2007). Playback theatre: Inciting dialogue and building community through personal story. *TDR/The Drama Review, 51* (4), 89–105.

Franklin, K. (2013). Engaging youth through African-derived dance and culture. *Journal of Physical Education, Recreation & Dance, 84* (7), 28–30.

Fraser, A. (2012). The spaces, politics, and cultural economies of electronic dance music. *Geography Compass, 6* (8), 500–511.

Frazier, I. (2015, December 7). Bronx dreams: A community project to change the world with art. *The New Yorker*, pp. 38–45.

Fredricks, J. A., & Simpkins, S. D. (2012). Promoting positive youth development through organized after-school activities: Taking a closer look at participation of ethnic minority youth. *Child Development Perspectives, 6* (3), 280–287.

Freebody, K., & Finneran, M. (Eds.). (2015). *Drama and social justice: Theory, research and practice in international contexts.* New York: Routledge.

Freer, P. K. (2009). Boys' voices: Inside and outside choral music. In J. L. Kerchner & C. R. Abril (Eds.), *Musical experience in our lives: Things we learn and meanings we make* (pp. 217–237). Lanham, MD: Rowman & Littlefield.

Freer, P. K., & Tan, L. (2014). The self-perceptions of young men as singers in Singaporean pre-university schools. *Research Studies in Music Education, 36* (2), 165–178.

Freire, K. E., Perkinson, L., Morrel-Samuels, S., & Zimmerman, M. A. (2015). Three Cs of translating evidence-based programs for youth and families to practice settings. *New Directions for Child and Adolescent Development, 2015* (149), 25–39.

Freire, P. (2009). Pedagogy of the oppressed. In K. Prentki & S. Preston (Eds.), *The applied theatre reader* (pp. 310–313). New York: Routledge.

French, K. (2015). *Youth empowerment as demonstrated by the Jóvenes en Acción program.* Capstone Collection, Paper 2771. Retrieved from http://digitalcollections.sit.edu/capstones/2771

Fürst, J. (2015). Swinging across the Iron Curtain and Moscow's Summer of Love: How western youth culture went east. In R. Jobs & D. Pomfret (Eds.), *Transnational histories of youth in the twentieth century* (pp. 236–259). Basingstoke, UK: Palgrave Macmillan.

Furstenberg, F. F. (2000). The sociology of adolescence and youth in the 1990s: A critical commentary. *Journal of Marriage and Family, 62* (4), 896–910.

Fusco, C. (2007). 'Healthification' and the promises of urban space a textual analysis of place, activity, youth (PLAY-ing) in the city. *International Review for the Sociology of Sport, 42* (1), 43–63.

Futch, V. A. (2011). (Re) presenting spaces of/for 'at-opportunity' urban youth. *Curriculum Inquiry, 41* (1), 98–109.

Gal, T., & Duramy, B. F. (Eds.). (2015). *International perspectives and empirical findings on child participation: From social exclusion to child inclusive policies.* New York: Oxford University Press.

Gallagher, K. (2014). *Why theatre matters: Urban youth, engagement, and a pedagogy of the real.* Toronto: University of Toronto Press.

Gallagher, K. (2015). Responsible art and unequal societies. In K. Freebody & M. Finneran (Eds.), *Drama and social justice: Theory, research and practice in international contexts* (pp. 53–72). New York: Routledge.

Gallagher, K., & Booth, D. (Eds.). (2015). *How theatre educates: Convergences and counterpoints with artists, scholars, and advocates.* Toronto: University of Toronto Press.

Gallardo, M. E. (2014). .*Developing cultural humility: Embracing race, privilege and power.* Thousand Oaks, CA:SAGE.

Gao, Z., Huang, C., Liu, T., & Xiong, W. (2012). Impact of interactive dance games on urban children's physical activity correlates and behavior. *Journal of Exercise Science & Fitness, 10* (2), 107–112.

Gao, Z., Zhang, T., & Stodden, D. (2013). Children's physical activity levels and psychological correlates in interactive dance versus aerobic dance. *Journal of Sport and Health Science, 2* (3), 146–151.

Garcia, M. (2014). *Spanish-English code switching in slam poetry.* https://scholarship.tricolib.brynmawr.edu/handle/10066/12514

Garlock, M. (2012). The performance and expansion of global storytelling in "It is In You". *Storytelling, Self, Society, 8* (3), 138–166.

Garoian, C. R. (1999). Performance art as critical pedagogy in studio art education. *Art Journal, 58* (1), 57–62.

Garst, B. A., Browne, L. P., & Bialeschki, M. D. (2011). Youth development and the camp experience. New directions for youth development, *2011* (130), 73–87.

Garzon, N. S. (2014). *Applied theater: Giving voice to low-income teenage immigrants through theater* (Master's thesis). Paper 56. Retrieved from http://scholarship.rollins.edu/mls/56

Gastic, B., & Johnson, D. (2009). Teacher-mentors and the educational resilience of sexual minority youth. *Journal of Gay & Lesbian Social Services, 21* (2-3), 219–231.

Gavin, L. E., Catalano, R. F., David-Ferdon, C., Gloppen, K. M., & Markham, C. M. (2010). A review of positive youth development programs that promote adolescent sexual and reproductive health. *Journal of Adolescent Health, 46* (3), S75-S91.

Gazzah, M. (2008). *Rhythms and rhymes of life: Music and identification processes of Dutch-Moroccan youth.* Amsterdam, Holland: Amsterdam University Press.

Geiser, K. E., & Quinn, B. P. (2012). *Oakland kids first: Peers advising students to succeed: Implementation study.* Stanford, CA: John W. Gardner Center for Youth and their Communities.

Geldhof, G. J., Bowers, E. P., Boyd, M. J., Mueller, M. K., Napolitano, C. M., Schmid, K. L., . . . Lerner, R. M. (2014). Creation of short and very short measures of the five Cs of positive youth development. *Journal of Research on Adolescence, 24* (1), 163–176.

Geldhof, G. J., Bowers, E. P., Mueller, M. K., Napolitano, C. M., Callina, K. S., Walsh, K. J., . . . Lerner, R. M. (2015). The Five Cs model of positive youth development. In E. P. Bowers, G. L. Geldhof, S. K. Johnson, L. J. Hilliard, R. M. Herberg, J. V. Lerner & R. M. Lerner (Eds.), *Promoting positive youth development: Lessons from the 4-H Study,* 161–186. New York: Springer.

George-Graves, N. (Ed.). (2015). *The Oxford handbook of dance and theater.* New York: Oxford University Press.

Gerber, B. L., & Horoschak, L. (2012). An attack on the Tower of Babel: Creating a national arts/special education resource center. In *The intersection of arts education and special education: Exemplary programs and approaches* (pp. 113–128). Washington, DC. Retrieved from http://education.kennedy-center.org//education/vsa/resources/Finalprofessionialpapersbook2013.pdf#page=113

Gerdes, E. V., & VanDenend Sorge, T. (2015). Building humans and dances: Exploring cultural relevancy as teaching artists. *Journal of Dance Education, 15* (2), 72–76.

Gibbs, L., Mutch, C., O'Connor, P., & MacDougall, C. (2013). Research with, by, for and about children: Lessons from disaster contexts. *Global Studies of Childhood, 3* (2), 129–141.

Giguere, M. (2011). Dancing thoughts: An examination of children's cognition and creative process in dance. *Research in Dance Education, 12* (1), 5–28.

Gilbert, A. G. (2015). *Creative dance for all ages* (2nd ed.). Champaign, IL: Human Kinetics.

Ginwright, S. (2011). Hope, healing, and care: Pushing the boundaries of civic engagement for African American youth. *Liberal Education, 97* (2), 34–39.

Ginwright, S. (2015). *Hope and healing in urban education: How urban activists and teachers are reclaiming matters of the heart.* New York: Routledge.

Giroux, H. A. (2011). Fighting for the future: American youth and the global struggle for democracy. *Cultural Studies, Critical Methodologies, 11* (4), 328–340.

Giroux, H. A. (2012). *Disposable youth, racialized memories, and the culture of cruelty.* New York: Routledge.

Giroux, H. (2014). Class casualties: Disappearing youth in the age of George W. Bush. *Workplace: A Journal for Academic Labor,* (11). Retrieved from http://ices.library.ubc.ca/index.php/workplace/article/view/184697

Giroux, H. A. (2015). Totalitarian paranoia in the post-Orwellian surveillance state. *Cultural Studies, 29* (2), 108–140.

Gitonga, P. N., & Delport, A. (2015). Exploring the use of hip hop music in participatory research studies that involve youth. *Journal of Youth Studies, 18* (9), 984–896.

Glick Schiller, N., & Schmidt, G. (2016). Envisioning place: Urban sociabilities within time, space and multiscalar power. *Identities, 23* (1), 1–16.

Glik, D., Nowak, G., Valente, T., Sapsis, K., & Martin, C. (2002). Youth performing arts entertainment-education for HIV/AIDS prevention and health promotion: Practice and research. *Journal of Health Communication, 7* (1), 39–57.

Goffman, E. (1963). *Stigma: Notes on the management of spoiled identity.* New York: Touchstone Book.

Goldbard, A. (2006). *New creative community: The art of cultural development.* Oakland, CA: New Village Press.

Goldman, S., Booker, A., & McDermott, M. (2008). Mixing the digital, social, and cultural: Learning, identity, and agency in youth participation. D. Buckingham (Ed.), *Youth, identity, and digital media* (pp. 185–206). Cambridge, MA: MIT Press.

González, A. (2004). *Jarocho's soul: Cultural identity and Afro-Mexican dance*. Lanham, MD: University Press of America.

Goodall, H. L., Jr. (2012). *Counter-narrative: How progressive academics can challenge extremists and promote social justice*. Walnut Cree, CA: Left Coast Press, Inc.

Goodman, E. (2002).Ensemble performance. In J. Rick (Ed.), *Musical performance: A guide to understanding* (pp. 153–162). New York: Cambridge University Press.

Googins, B., Capoccia, V. A., & Kaufman, N. (1983). The interactional dimension of planning: A framework for practice. *Social Work, 28* (4), 273–277.

Gormally, S. (2015)."I've been there, done that . . . ": A study of youth gang desistance. *Youth Justice, 15* (2), 148–165.

Gormally, S., & Coburn, A. (2014). Finding nexus: Connecting youth work and research practices. *British Educational Research Journal, 40* (5), 869–885.

Gorter, J. W., Stewart, D., Smith, M. W., King, G., Wright, M., Nguyen, T., . . . Swinton, M. (2014). Pathways toward positive psychosocial outcomes and mental health for youth with disabilities: A knowledge synthesis of developmental trajectories. *Canadian Journal of Community Mental Health, 33* (1), 45–61.

Gosa, T., & Fields, T. (2012). Is hip-hop education another hustle? The (ir) responsible use of hip-hop as pedagogy. In *Hip-hop I: The cultural practice and critical pedagogy of international hip-hop* (pp. 195–210). Retrieved from file:///C:/Users/delgado/Downloads/gosa_fields_hip_hop_education-04-28-2011%20(1).pdf

Grady, J., Marquez, R., & Mclaren, P. (2012). A critique of neoliberalism with fierceness: Queer youth of color creating dialogues of resistance. *Journal of homosexuality, 59* (7), 982–1004.

Gray, N., de Boehm, C. O., Farnsworth, A., & Wolf, D. (2010). Integration of creative expression into community based participatory research and health promotion with Native Americans. *Family & community health, 33* (3), 186–192.

Grazer, J. M. (2012). *A tempest in the halls: Intersections of social justice, student collaboration, and devised theatre* (Doctoral dissertation). Kennesaw State University, Kennesaw, GA.

Green, G. P., & Haines, A. (2015). *Asset building & community development*. Thousand Oaks, CA:SAGE.

Green, K. L. (2013). "The way we hear ourselves is different from the way others hear us": Exploring the literate identities of a Black radio youth collective. *Equity & Excellence in Education, 46* (3), 315–326.

Greenberg, M. T., & Lippold, M. A. (2013). Promoting healthy outcomes among youth with multiple risks: Innovative approaches. *Annual Review of Public Health, 34*, 253–270.

Greene, J. P. (2015). Learning from live theater: Students realize gains in knowledge, tolerance, and more. *Education Next, 15* (1), 55. http://ostrc.org/newsletter/documents/LearningfromLiveTheater_000.pdf

Greene, S., Burke, K., & McKenna, M. (2013). Forms of voice: Exploring the empowerment of youth at the intersection of art and action. *The Urban Review, 45* (3), 311–334.

Greenfader, C. M., Brouillette, L., & Farkas, G. (2015). Effect of a performing arts program on the oral language skills of young English learners. *Reading Research Quarterly, 50* (2), 185–203.

Grewe, M. E., Taboada, A., Dennis, A., Chen, E., Stein, K., Watson, S., . . . Lightfoot, A. F. (2015). "I learned to accept every part of myself": The transformative impact of a theatre-based sexual health and HIV prevention programme. *Sex Education, 15* (3), 303–317.

Griffin, C. (2013). *Representations of youth: The study of youth and adolescence in Britain and America.* New York: John Wiley & Sons.

Grills, C., Cooke, D., Douglas, J., Subica, A., Villanueva, S., & Hudson, B. (2016). Culture, racial socialization, and positive African American youth Development. *Journal of Black Psychology, 42* (4), 343–373.

Grodach, C. (2011). Art spaces in community and economic development: Connections to neighborhoods, artists, and the cultural economy. *Journal of Planning Education and Research, 31* (1), 74–85.

Guerrero, L. R., Dudovitz, R., Chung, P. J., Dosanjh, K. K., & Wong, M. D. (2016). Grit: A potential protective factor against substance use and other risk behaviors among Latino adolescents. *Academic pediatrics, 16* (3), 275–281.

Guèvremont, A., Findlay, L., & Kohen, D. (2008). Organized extracurricular activities of Canadian children and youth. *Health Rep, 19* (3), 65–69.

Guhrs, T., Rihoy, L., & Guhrs, M. (2006). Using theatre in participatory environmental policy making. *Participatory Learning and Action, 55,* 87–93.

Gundlach, H., & Neville, B. (2012). Authenticity: Further theoretical and practical development. *Journal of Brand Management, 19* (4), 484–499.

Gutierrez, L., Gant, L. M., & Richards-Schuster, K. (2014). Community organization in the twenty-first century: Scholarship and practice directions for the future. *Journal of Community Practice, 22* (1-2), 1–9.

Hackney, M. E., & Earhart, G. M. (2010). Recommendations for implementing tango classes for persons with Parkinson disease. *American Journal of Dance Therapy, 32* (1), 41–52.

Haddix, M., & Sealey-Ruiz, Y. (2012). Cultivating digital and popular literacies as empowering and emancipatory acts among urban youth. *Journal of Adolescent & Adult Literacy, 56* (3), 189–192.

Hall, L. E. C. (2014). *It's the singer, not the song: A critical investigation into perceptions of the benefits of singing in daily life* (Dissertation). University of Chester, Chester, England).

Hall, R. (2011). Eurocentrism and the postcolonial implications of skin color among Latinos. *Hispanic Journal of Behavioral Sciences, 33* (1), 105–117.

Hall, R. (2013). Eurocentrism as psychological colonization: Race versus culture in the manufacture of 'knowledge' vis-á-vis Filipino populations. *Budhi: A Journal of Ideas and Culture, 6* (2 & 3), 257–269.

Halpern, R. (2005). Instrumental relationships: A potential relational model for inner-city youth programs. *Journal of Community Psychology, 33* (1), 11–20.

Halpern, R. (2006). After-school matters in Chicago apprenticeship as a model for youth programming. *Youth & Society, 38* (2), 203–235.

Halse, C., Hanley, M., Pippa, C., Finnerty, D., Thornton, L. B., Acevedo, A. D., . . . Iverson, S. V. (2013). *Staging social justice: Collaborating to create activist theatre.* Carbondale, IL: SIU Press.

Halverson, E. R. (2009). Artistic production processes as venues for positive youth development. *Revista Interuniversitaria de Formacion del Profesorado [Interuniversity Journal of Teacher Education], 23* (3), 181–202.

Halverson, E. R., Lowenhaupt, R., Gibbons, D., & Bass, M. (2009). Conceptualizing identity in youth media arts organizations: A comparative case study. *E-Learning and Digital Media, 6* (1), 23–42.

Hamada, D., & Stavridi, S. (2014). Required skills for children's and youth librarians in the digital age. *IFLA Journal, 40* (2), 102–109.

Hämäläinen, J. (2003). The concept of social pedagogy in the field of social work. *Journal of Social Work, 3* (1), 69–80.

Hamby, A., Pierce, M., Daniloski, K., & Brinberg, D. (2011). The use of participatory action research to create a positive youth development program. *Social Marketing Quarterly, 17* (3), 2–17.

Hamilton, S. F. (2015a). Linking research to the practice of youth development. *Applied Developmental Science, 19* (2), 57–59.

Hamilton, S. F. (2015b). Translational research and youth development. *Applied Developmental Science, 19* (2), 60–73.

Hammett, D. (2012). Reworking and resisting arginalize influences: Cape Town hip-hop. *GeoJournal, 77* (3), 417–428.

Hammond, W. (2010). *Principles of strength-based practice. Calgary, Alberta: Resiliency Initiatives.* Retrieved from http://www.ayscbc.org/Principles%20of%20Strength-2.pdf

Hankey, J. (2014). Youth, education, and marginality: Local and global expressions. *Alberta Journal of Educational Research, 60* (1), 241–244.

Hanley, M. S., Sheppard, G. L., Noblit, G. W., & Barone, T. (2013). *Culturally relevant arts education for social justice: A way out of no way.* New York: Routledge.

Hanlon, T. E., Simon, B. D., O'Grady, K. E., Carswell, S. B., & Callaman, J. M. (2009). The effectiveness of an after-school program targeting urban African American youth. *Education and Urban Society, 42* (1), 96–118.

Hanna, J. L. (2008). A nonverbal language for imagining and learning: Dance education in K–12 curriculum. *Educational Researcher, 37* (8), 491–506.

Hansen, D. M., & Larson, R. W. (2007). Amplifiers of developmental and negative experiences in organized activities: Dosage, motivation, lead roles, and adult-youth ratios. *Journal of Applied Developmental Psychology, 28* (4), 360–374.

Hari, B. (2009). Songs of belonging: Musical interactions in early life. In J. L. Kerchner & C. R. Abril (Eds.), *Musical experience in our lives: Things we learn and meanings we make,* 21–37. Lanham, MD: Rowman & Littlefield.

Harlop, Y., & Aristizabal, H. (2013). Using theater to promote social justice in communities: Pedagogical approaches to community and individual learning. In M. S. Hanley, G. W. Nobit, G. L. Sheppard & T. Barone (Eds.), *Culturally relevant arts education for social justice: A way out.* (pp. 25–35). New York: Routledge.

Harrell, S. P., & Bond, M. A. (2006). Listening to diversity stories: Principles for practice in community research and action. *American Journal of Community Psychology, 37* (3-4), 365–376.

Harris, A., & Lemon, A. (2012). Bodies that shatter: Creativity, culture and the new pedagogical imaginary. *Pedagogy, Culture & Society, 20* (3), 413–433.

Harris, A., Wyn, J., & Younes, S. (2010). Beyond apathetic or activist youth: 'Ordinary' young people and contemporary forms of participation. *Young, 18* (1), 9–32.

Harrison, G. (2010). Community music in Australia. *International Journal of Community Music, 3* (3), 337–342.

Harrison, K. (2012). Epistemologies of applied ethnomusicology. *Ethnomusicology, 56* (3), 505–529.

Hart, R. (2009). Charting change in the participatory settings of childhood. Children, politics and communication: In Z. Blair (Ed.), *Participation at the margins*. (pp. 7–29). Saarbrucken, Germany: Lambert Academic Publishers.

Hart, R. A. (2013). *Children's participation: The theory and practice of involving young citizens in community development and environmental care*. New York: Routledge.

Harvey, L., Roberts, S., & Dillabough, J. A. (2016). Youth rising? The politics of youth in the global economy. *British Journal of Sociology of Education, 37* (3), 465–480.

Haskett, B. L. (2013). They came for the kids and stayed for the teacher: The Desert Winds Community Steel Orchestra. *International Journal of Community Music, 6* (2), 175–182.

Hastings, T. H. (2012). *Giving voice to the peace and justice challenger intellectuals: Counterpublic development as civic engagement* (Doctoral dissertation). Portland State University, Oregon.

Hayes, C. J. (2007). Community music and the GLBT chorus. *International Journal of Community Music, 1* (1), 63–67.

Hayes-Bautista, D. E. (2012). *El Cinco de Mayo: An American tradition*. Los Angeles, CA: University of California Press.

Head, B. W. (2011). Why not ask them? Mapping and promoting youth participation. *Children and Youth Services Review, 33* (4), 541–547.

Heath, S. (2001). Three's not a crowd: Plans, roles, and focus in the arts. *Educational Researcher, 30* (7), 10–17.

Heath, S. B. (2015). Museums, theaters, and youth orchestras advancing creative arts and sciences within underresourced communities. In W. G. Tierney (Ed.), *Rethinking education and poverty*. (pp. 177–198). Baltimore, MD: Johns Hopkins University Press.

Heathcote, D. (2009). Drama as a process for change. In K. Prentki & S. Preston (Eds.), *The applied theatre reader* (pp. 200–206). New York: Routledge.

Hedden, D. (2012). An overview of existing research about children's singing and the implications for teaching children to sing. *Update: Applications of Research in Music Education, 30* (2), 52–62.

Heggestad, A. K. T., & Slettebø, Å. (2015). How individuals with dementia in nursing homes maintain their dignity through life storytelling–a case study. *Journal of Clinical Nursing, 24* (15-16), 2323–2330.

Heinze, H. J. (2013). Beyond a bed: Support for positive development for youth residing in emergency shelters. *Children and Youth Services Review, 35* (2), 278–286.

Heltzel, P. G. (2015). The church as a Theatre of the Oppressed. In T. Hart & W. Vander Lugt (Eds.), *Theatrical theology: Explorations in performing the faith*. (pp. 241–262). Eugene, OR: Cascade Publishers.

Heppner, M. J., & Jung, A. K. (2012). When the music changes, so does the dance: With shifting US demographics, how do career centers need to change. *Asian Journal of Counselling, 19* (1), 2–27.

Hershberg, R. M., Johnson, S. K., DeSouza, L. M., Hunter, C. J., & Zaff, J. (2015). Promoting contribution among youth: Implications from positive youth development research for youth development programs. In E. P. Bowers, G. L. Geldhof, S. K. Johnson, L. J.

Hilliard, R. M. Herberg, J. V. Lerner & R. M. Lerner (Eds.), *Promoting positive youth development: Lessons from the 4-H Study.* (pp. 211–228). New York: Springer.

Hickey, M. (2009). At-risk teens: Making sense of life through music composition. In J. L. Kerchner & C. R. Abril (Eds.), *Musical experience in our lives: Things we learn and meanings we make.* (pp. 199–215). Lanham, MD: Rowman & Littlefield.

Hickey-Moody, A. (2013). *Youth, arts and education: Reassembling subjectivity through affect.* New York: Routledge.

Hickey-Moody, A. (2015). 6 Little publics and youth arts as cultural pedagogy. In M. Watkins, G. Noble, & C. Driscoll (Eds.), *Cultural pedagogies and human conduct.* (pp. 78–91). New York: Routledge.

Hickling-Hudson, A. (2013). Theatre-arts pedagogy for social justice: Case study of the Area Youth Foundation in Jamaica. *Current Issues in Comparative Education, 15* (2), 15–34.

Higgins, L. (2012). *Community music: In theory and in practice.* New York: Oxford University Press, USA.

Hill, A. J., & Donaldson, L. P. (2012). We shall overcome: Promoting an agenda for integrating spirituality and community practice. *Journal of Religion & Spirituality in Social Work: Social Thought, 31* (1-2), 67–84.

Hill, M. L., & Petchauer, E. (Eds.). (2012). *Schooling hip-hop: Expanding hip-hop based education across the curriculum.* New York: Teachers College Press.

Hirsch, B. J., Deutsch, N. L., & DuBois, D. L. (2011). *After-school centers and youth development: Case studies of success and failure.* New York: Cambridge University Press.

Hlagala, R. B., & Delport, C. S. (2014). Ideologies and theories for youth practice work. *Commonwealth Youth and Development, 12* (1), 59–74.

Ho, E., Clarke, A., & Dougherty, I. (2015). Youth-led social change: Topics, engagement types, organizational types, strategies, and impacts. *Futures, 67* (1), 52–62.

Hoang, D. (2012). *Taking youth engagement to the next generation: Lessons from best youth engagement practices toward food sustainability* (Major research paper). Ryerson University, Toronto, Canada.

Hodkinson, P., & Bennett, A. (Eds.). (2013). *Ageing and youth cultures: Music, style and identity.* London: A & C Black.

Hofstadter, R. (1955). *The age of reform.* New York: Alfred A. Knopf.

Holdsworth, N. (2013). Boys don't do dance, do they? *Research in Drama Education: The Journal of Applied Theatre and Performance, 18* (2), 168–178.

Holloway, S., & Valentine, G. (2014). *Cyberkids: Youth identities and communities in an online world.* New York: Routledge.

Holt, N. L. (Ed.). (2007). *Positive youth development through sport.* New York: Routledge.

Holt, N. L., Sehn, Z. L., Spence, J. C., Newton, A. S., & Ball, G. D. (2012). Physical education and sport programs at an inner city school: Exploring possibilities for positive youth development. *Physical Education & Sport Pedagogy, 17* (1), 97–113.

Honneth, A., & Reitz, C. (2013). Herbert Marcuse and the Frankfurt School. *Radical Philosophy Review, 16* (1), 49–57.

Hostettler, N. (2013). *Eurocentrism.* New York: Routledge.

Howard, K. A., Budge, S. L., Gutierrez, B., Owen, A. D., Lemke, N., Jones, J. E., & Higgins, K. (2011). Future plans of urban youth: Influences, perceived barriers, and coping strategies. *Journal of Career Development, 37* (4), 655–676.

Howard, S., Carroll, J., Murphy, J., & Peck, J. (2002). Using 'endowed props' in scenario-based design. In *Proceedings of the second Nordic Conference on Human-Computer Interaction* (pp. 1–10). ACM.

Hoxie, A. M. E., & Debellis, L. M. (2014). Engagement in out-of-school time: How youth become engaged in the arts. In David J. Shernoff, Janine Bempechat, (Eds.), *Engaging youth in schools: Evidence- based models to guide future innovations*. New York: NSSE Yearbook by Teachers College Record.

Huang, L.-L., & Hsu, J.-Y. (2011). From cultural building, economic revitalization to local partnership? The changing nature of community mobilization in Taiwan. *International Planning Studies, 16* (2), 131–150.

Hughes, C., Jackson, A., & Kidd, J. (2007). The role of theater in museums and historic sites: Visitors, audiences, and learners. In L. Bresler (Ed.), *International handbook of research in arts education.* (pp. 679–699). Rotterdam: Springer Netherlands.

Hughes, D., Rodriguez, J., Smith, E. P., Johnson, D. J., Stevenson, H. C., & Spicer, P. (2006). Parents' ethnic-racial socialization practices: A review of research and directions for future study. *Developmental Psychology, 42* (5), 747–770.

Hughes, J. & Ruding, S. (2009). Made to measure? A critical interrogation of applies theatre as intervention with young officials in the U.K. In. T. Premski & S. Preston (Eds.). *The applied reader*, (pp. 217–225). London, UK: Routledge.

Hughes, J., & Wilson, K. (2004). Playing a part: The impact of youth theatre on young people's personal and social development. *Research in Drama Education, 9* (1), 57–72.

Hull, G. A., & Katz, M. (2006). Crafting an agentive self: Case studies of digital storytelling. *Research in the Teaching of English, 41* (1), 43–81.

Humphreys, B. R., Ruseski, J. E., & Soebbing, B. P. (2014). Sport participation among us high school students: Trends and directions. *Journal of Contemporary Athletics, 8* (3), 179–195.

Hunter, M. A., & Milne, G. (2005). Young people and performance in Australia and New Zealand. *Australasian Drama Studies*, (47), 3–13.

Hutchinson, S. (2013). Dancing in place. In S. Hutchinson (Ed.), *Salsa world: A global dance in local contexts* (pp. 1–25). Philadelphia, PA: Temple University Press.

Hytten, K. (2006). Education for social justice: Provocations and challenges. *Educational Theory, 56* (2), 221–236.

Hytten, K., & Bettez, S. C. (2011). Understanding education for social justice. *Educational Foundations, 25* (1), 7–24.

Ibrahim, A., & Steinberg, S. R. (Eds.). (2014). *Critical youth studies reader.* Switzerland, New York: Peter Lang.

Ife, J. (2004). *Linking community development and human rights.* Melbourne, AUS: Deakin University, Community Development, Human Rights and the Grassroots Conference.

Imani, N. (2014). The incarcerative mentality of Eurocentrism: Prisoner identification and jailing the imperfect body. In S. M. Bowman (Ed.), *Color behind bars: Racism in the US prison system* (Vol. 1, pp. 153–169). Santa Barbara, CA: Praeger.

Intrator, S. M., & Siegel, D. (2014). *The quest for mastery: Positive youth development through out-of-school programs.* Cambridge, MA: Harvard Education Press.

Irazábal, C., & Huerta, C. (2016). Intersectionality and planning at the margins: LGBTQ youth of color in New York. *Gender, Place & Culture, 23* (5), 714–732.

Isaacson, M. (2014). Clarifying concepts: Cultural humility or competency. *Journal of Professional Nursing, 30* (3), 251–258.

Iwasaki, Y. (2016). The role of youth engagement in positive youth development and social justice youth development for high-risk, marginalised youth. *International Journal of Adolescence and Youth, 21* (3), 267–278.

Jackson, C. J., Mullis, R. M., & Hughes, M. (2010). Development of a theater-based nutrition and physical activity intervention for low-income, urban, African American adolescents. *Progress in community health partnerships: Research, Education, and Action, 4* (2), 89–98.

Jackson, W. C. (2014). The circle of courage: The socialization of youth in the 21st century. *Reclaiming Children and Youth, 23* (3), 16–20.

Jacquez, F., Vaughn, L. M., & Wagner, E. (2013). Youth as partners, participants or passive recipients: A review of children and adolescents in community-based participatory research (CBPR). *American Journal of Community Psychology, 51* (1-2), 176–189.

James, C. D. (2016). *Painting pictures: Reframing the world of inner-city youth.* Newark, NJ: Painting Pictures, Inc.

James, C. E. (2012). Students 'at risk': Stereotypes and the schooling of black boys. *Urban Education, 47* (2), 464–494.

James, N. (2005). *"Actup!" Theatre as education and its impact on young people's learning.* Retrieved from https://lra.le.ac.uk/handle/2381/8512

Jamsari, E. A., & Talib, N. M. (2015). Eurocentrism in Reinhart Dozy's Spanish Islam: A history of the Muslims in Spain. *Mediterranean Journal of Social Sciences, 5* (29), 74–80. Retrieved from http://www.mcser.org/journal/index.php/mjss/article/view/5424

Jeffs, T., & Smith, M. K. (Eds.). (2010a). *Youth work practice.* New York: Palgrave Macmillan.

Jeffs, T., & Smith, M. K. (2010a). Youth workers as controllers: Issues of method and purpose. In T. Jeffs & M. K. Smith (Eds.), *Youth work practice* (pp. 106–122). New York: Palgrave Macmillan.

Jennings, L. (2014). Do men need empowering too? A systematic review of entrepreneurial education and microenterprise development on health disparities among inner-city Black male youth. *Journal of Urban Health, 91* (5), 836–850.

Jennings, L. B., Parra-Medina, D. M., Hilfinger-Messias, D. K., & McLoughlin, K. (2006). Toward a critical social theory of youth empowerment. *Journal of Community Practice, 14* (1-2), 31–55.

Jensen, A. P. (2011). Convergence culture, learning, and participatory youth theatre performance. *Youth Theatre Journal, 25* (2), 146–158.

Jensen, A. P., & Lazarus, J. (2014). Theatre teacher beliefs about quality practice in the secondary theatre classroom: An ethnographic study. *Youth Theatre Journal, 28* (1), 44–60.

Jenson, J. M. (2012). *Risk, resilience, and positive youth development: Developing effective community programs for at-risk youth: Lessons from the Denver Bridge Project.* New York: Oxford University Press.

Jiang, X., & Peterson, R. D. (2012). Beyond participation: The association between school extracurricular activities and involvement in violence across generations of immigration. *Journal of Youth and Adolescence, 41* (3), 362–378.

Jocson, K. M. (2008). *Youth poets: Empowering literacies in and out of schools* (Vol. 304). New York: Peter Lang.

Johansson, O. (2010). The limits of community-based theatre: Performance and HIV prevention in Tanzania. *TDR/The Drama Review, 54* (1), 59–75.

Johnson, S. L., Jones, V., & Cheng, T. L. (2015). Promoting 'healthy futures' to reduce risk behaviors in urban youth: A randomized controlled trial. *American Journal of Community Psychology, 56* (1-2), 36–45.

Johnston-Goodstar, K., Richards-Schuster, K., & Sethi, J. K. (2014). exploring critical youth media practice: Connections and contributions for social work. *Social Work, 59* (4), 339–346.

Johnston-Goodstar, K., & Sethi, J. (2013). Native youth media as social justice youth development. *Journal of American Indian Education, 52* (3), 65–80.

Jones, D., & Skogrand, L. (2014). Positive youth development as shared among cultures. *Reclaiming Children and Youth, 23* (3), 26–29.

Jones, D., & Skogrand, L. (2015). Informing 4-H youth development in Southeast Alaska native villages. *Assessing Resilience, 8* (1) 36–44.

Jones, G. (2009). *Youth.* Cambridge, UK: Polity Press.

Jones, H. M. F. (2014). 'Counting young people is not youth work': The tensions between values, targets and positive activities in neighbourhood-based work. *Journal of Youth Studies, 17* (2), 220–235.

Jones, K., & Perkins, D. (2005). Determining the quality of youth-adult relationships within community-based youth programs. *Journal of Extension, 43* (5) Article 5FEA5. Retrieved from http://www.joe.org/joe/2005october/a5.php

Jones, L. M., & Mitchell, K. J. (2016). Defining and measuring youth digital citizenship. *New Media & Society, 18* (9), 2063–2079.

Jones, M. I., Dunn, J. G. H., Holt, N. L., Sullivan, P. J., & Bloom, G. A. (2011). Exploring the '5 Cs' of positive youth development in sport. *Journal of Sport Behavior, 34* (3), 250–267.

Jones, S., Hall, C., Thomson, P., Barrett, A., & Hanby, J. (2013). Re-presenting the 'forgotten estate': Participatory theatre, place and community identity. *Discourse: Studies in the Cultural Politics of Education, 34* (1), 118–131.

Jordan, G., & Weedon, C. (2015). The celebration of difference and the cultural politics of racism. In B. Adam & S. Allan (Eds.), *Theorizing culture: An interdisciplinary critique after postmodernism* (pp. 149–164). London: UCL Press.

Jupp, E. (2007). Participation, local knowledge and empowerment: Researching public space with young people. *Environment and Planning A, 39* (12), 2832–2844.

Kabir, N., & Rickards, T. (2006). Students at risk: Can connections make a difference? *Youth Studies Australia, 25* (4), 17–24.

Kajner, T., Chovanec, D., Underwood, M., & Mian, A. (2013). Critical community service learning: Combining critical classroom pedagogy with activist community placements. *Michigan Journal of Community Service Learning, 19* (2), 36–49.

Kane, K. M. (2014). Transformative performing arts and mentorship pedagogy: Nurturing developmental relationships in a multidisciplinary dance theatre program for youth. *Journal of Education and Training Studies, 2* (2), 224–232.

Kanyako, V. (2015). Arts and war healing: Peacelinks Performing Arts in Sierra Leone. *African Conflict & Peacebuilding Review, 5* (1), 106–122.

Kao, T. S. A., & Huang, B. (2015). Bicultural straddling among immigrant adolescents: A concept analysis. *Journal of Holistic Nursing, 33* (3), 269–281.

Kapucu, N. (2011). Social capital and civic engagement. *International Journal of Social Inquiry, 4* (1), 23–43.

Karabanow, J., & Naylor, T. (2015). Using art to tell stories and build safe spaces: Transforming academic research into action. *Canadian Journal of Community Mental Health, 34* (1), 1–19.

Karoblis, G. (2010). Dance. In *Handbook of phenomenological aesthetics* (pp. 67–70). Rotterdam: Springer Netherlands.

Kauzlarich, D. (2012). 12 Music as resistance to state crime and violence. In E. Stanley & J. M. Culloch (Eds.), *State crime and resistance* (pp. 154–169). New York: Routledge.

Kearney, W. B. (2014). *Equipping quality youth development professionals: Improving child and youth program experiences.* Bloomington, IN: Iuniverse.

Keeney, K. P., & Korza, P. (2015). Assessing arts-based social change endeavors: Controversies and complexities. In M. O. Stephenson, Jr., & S. Tate (Eds.), *Arts and community change: Exploring cultural development policies, practices and dilemmas* (pp. 186–211). New York: Routledge.

Kehily, M. J. (2014). Sex'n'drugs'n'rock'n'roll: Young people as consumers. In W. Taylor, R. Earle & R. Hester (Eds.), *Youth justice handbook: Theory, policy and practice* (pp. 41–49). New York: Routledge.

Keller, A. (2014). *A rowing and group counseling positive youth development summer program for adolescent girls* (Master's Thesis). Saint Mary's College of California, Los Angeles, CA.)

Kelly, A. L. (2015). Voices from Roosevelt: Community-based devised theatre as a youth rite of passage. *Theatre Symposium, 23* (1) 95–105.

Kelly, B. L., & Doherty, L. (2016). A historical overview of art and music-based activities in social work with groups: Nondeliberative practice and engaging young people's strengths. *Social Work with Groups,* 1–15.

Kelly, P., & Kamp, A. (2014). *A critical youth studies for the 21st century.* Boston, MA: Brill.

Kelman, C., & Warnick, D. (1978). The ethics of social interventions: Goals, means and consequences. In Bermant & H. C. Kelman (Eds.), *The ethics of social interventions* (pp. 33–44). New York: John Wiley & Sons.

Kelsey, T. W. (1994). The agrarian myth and policy responses to farm safety. *American Journal of Public Health, 84* (7), 1171–1177.

Kemp, S. P. (2011). "Leaders of today, builders of tomorrow": Transforming youth and communities in urban youth programs. In S. Sutton & S. Kemp (Eds.), *The paradox of urban space* (pp. 135–156). New York: Palgrave Macmillan.

Kenny, C., & Fraser, T. N. (Eds.). (2012). *Living indigenous leadership: Native narratives on building strong communities.* Vancouver, BC: UBC Press.

Kenny, D. (2011). *The psychology of music performance anxiety.* New York: Oxford University Press.

Kenyon, D. B., & Hanson, J. D. (2012). Incorporating traditional culture into positive youth development programs with American Indian/Alaska Native youth. *Child Development Perspectives, 6* (3), 272–279.

Kerchner, J. L., & Abril, C. R. (Eds.). (2009). *Musical experience in our lives: Things we learn and meanings we make.* Lanham, MD: R&L Education.

Kerr-Berry, J. A. (2012). Dance education in an era of racial backlash: Moving forward as we step backwards. *Journal of Dance Education, 12* (2), 48–53.

Keuroghlian, A. S., Shtasel, D., & Bassuk, E. L. (2014). Out on the street: A public health and policy agenda for lesbian, gay, bisexual, and transgender youth who are homeless. *American Journal of Orthopsychiatry, 84* (1), 66–72.

Khan, B. (2014). *Come and become: Investigating how youth development is facilitated at the Fusion Youth Activity and Technology Centre* (Doctoral dissertation). School of Environmental Design and Rural Development, University of Guelph, Canada.

Kim, H. E. (2014). *The school of performing arts at Bellevue Baptist Church as a model of the church-based arts academy.* (Doctoral dissertation, The Southern Baptist Theological Seminary, Lousivlle, KY).

Kindall-Smith, M. (2012). What a difference in 3 years! Risking social justice content in required undergraduate music education curricula. *Journal of Music Teacher Education, 22* (3), 34–50.

King, G., Kingsnorth, S., Sheffe, S., Vine, R., Crossman, S., Pinto, M., . . . Savage, D. (2015). An inclusive arts-mediated program for children with and without disabilities: Establishing community and an environment for child development through the arts. *Children's Health Care, 45* (2), 204–226.

King, J. E., & Swartz, E. E. (2015). *The Afrocentric praxis of teaching for freedom: Connecting culture to learning.* New York: Routledge.

King, P. E. (2008). Spirituality as fertile ground for positive youth development. In R. M. Lerner, R. W. Roeser & E. Phelps (Eds.), *Positive youth development & spirituality: From theory to research* (pp. 55–73). West Conshohocken, PA: Templeton Foundation Press.

King, P. E., Clardy, C. E., & Ramos, J. S. (2014). Adolescent spiritual exemplars: Exploring spirituality in the lives of diverse youth. *Journal of Adolescent Research, 29* (2), 186–212.

Kinloch, V. (2012). *Crossing boundaries-teaching and learning with urban youth.* New York: Teachers College Press.

Kirova, A., & Emme, M. (2008). Fotonovela as a research tool in image-based participatory research with immigrant children. *International Journal of Qualitative Methods, 7* (2), 35–57.

Kirschman, K. J. B., Roberts, M. C., Shadlow, J. O., & Pelley, T. J. (2010). An evaluation of hope following a summer camp for inner-city youth. *Child & Youth Care Forum, 39* (6), 385–396.

Kirshner, B. (2009). "Power in numbers": Youth organizing as a context for exploring civic identity. *Journal of Research on Adolescence, 19* (3), 414–440.

Kirshner, B. (2015). *Youth activism in an era of education inequality.* New York: New York University Press.

Kiruthu, F. (2014). Music as a strategy of youth resilience in Dadaab Refugee Camp, Kenya. *Research on Humanities and Social Sciences, 4* (17), 7–16.

Kisiel, C., Blaustein, M., Spinazzola, J., Schmidt, C. S., Zucker, M., & van der Kolk, B. (2006). Evaluation of a theater-based youth violence prevention program for elementary school children. *Journal of School Violence, 5* (2), 19–36.

Kitchen, J. (2015). The ensemble domesticated: Mapping issues of autonomy and power in performing arts projects in schools. *Power and Education, 7* (1), 90–105.

Kivnick, H. Q., & Lymburner, A. M. (2009). CitySongs: Primary prevention in the field. *The Journal of Primary Prevention, 30* (1), 61–73.

Klau, M. (2006). Exploring youth leadership in theory and practice. *New Directions for Youth Development, 2006* (109), 57–87.

Kleinerman, K. (2010). Singing for leadership: Fostering the development of female leaders through voice. *Advancing Women in Leadership, 30* (1), 1–23.

Knight, H. (2015). Social justice and the arts. *Journal of Education for Teaching, 41* (1), 102–105.

Korman, C. (2015, December 23). December players stand up to gun violence. *USA Today*, p. 5C.

Kornbeck, J. (2009). "Important but widely misunderstood": The problem of defining social pedagogy in Europe. In J. Kornbeck & N. R. Jensen (Eds.), *The diversity of social pedagogy in Europe* (pp. 211–231). Breman, Germany: Hoech Schul Verlag.

Kornbeck, J., & Jensen, N. R. (2009). *The diversity of social pedagogy in Europe* (Vol. 7). Bremen, Germany: BoD–Books on Demand.

Kraus, R. (2012). Spiritual origins and belly dance: How and when artistic leisure becomes spiritual. *Journal of Dance & Somatic Practices, 4* (1), 59–77.

Kress, T. M., Degennaro, D., & Paugh, P. (2013). Introduction: Critical pedagogy 'under the radar' and 'off the grid'. *The International Journal of Critical Pedagogy, 4* (2), 1–13.

Krieger, J. L., Coveleski, S., Hecht, M. L., Miller-Day, M., Graham, J. W., Pettigrew, J., & Kootsikas, A. (2013). From kids, through kids, to kids: Examining the social influence strategies used by adolescents to promote prevention among peers. *Health Communication, 28* (7), 683–695.

Krinsky, C. (Ed.), (2008). *Moral panics over contemporary children and youth*. Farnham, UK: Ashgate Publishing.

Krogstad, J. M. (2014, July 8). *A view of the future through kindergarten demographics*. Washington, DC: Pew Hispanic Center.

Krogstad, J. M., & Passel, J. S. (2015, July 24). *5 facts about illegal immigration in the U. S.* Washington, DC: Pew Hispanic Center.

Kronick, R. F. (2013). *At-risk youth: Theory, practice, reform*. New York: Routledge.

Krossa, S. (2012). Europeon society. In G. Ritzer (Ed.), *The Wiley-Blackwell encyclopedia of globalization*. New York: John Wiley & Sons.

Kuftinec, S. (2003). *Staging America: Cornerstone and community-based theater*. Carbondale, IL: Southern Illinois University Press.

Kultti, A. (2013). Singing as language learning activity in multilingual toddler groups in preschool. *Early Child Development and Care, 183* (12), 1955–1969.

Kumasi, K. D. (2012). Roses in the concrete: A critical race perspective on urban youth and school libraries. *Knowledge Quest, 40* (5), 32–37.

Kuper, L. E. (2015). *Gender development and suicidality among transgender and gender nonconforming youth and young adults* (Doctoral dissertation). Northwestern University, Evansville, IL.

Kupersmidt, J. B., & Rhodes, J. E. (2014). Mentor training. In D. L. DuBois & M. J. Kracher (Eds.), *Handbook of youth mentoring* (pp. 439–456). Thousand Oaks, CA: Sage Publications.

Kurtines, W. M., Ferrer-Wreder, L., Berman, S. L., Lorente, C. C., Briones, E., Montgomery, M. J., . . . Arrufat, O. (2008). Promoting positive youth development: The Miami Youth Development Project (YDP). *Journal of Adolescent Research, 23* (3), 256–267.

Kuwor, S. K. (2015). *The holistic nature of dance and its therapeutic dimensions in health care delivery*. Retrieved from http://sonam2015.mywapblog.com/files/uhas-lecture-2015.pdf

Kwon, S. A. (2013). *Uncivil youth: Race, activism, and affirmative governmentality*. Durham, NC: Duke University Press.

Laing, J., & Mair, J. (2015). Music festivals and social inclusion–the festival organizers' perspective. *Leisure Sciences, 37* (3), 252–268.

Lal, S., Donnelly, C., & Shin, J. (2015). Digital storytelling: An innovative tool for practice, education, and research. *Occupational therapy in health care, 29* (1), 54–62.

Lal, V. (2012). The politics and consequences of eurocentrism in university disciplines. In A. Curaj, P. Scott, L. Viasceanu & L. Wilson (Eds.), *European higher education at the crossroads* (pp. 1039–1055). Rotterdam: Springer Netherlands.

Lam, C. B., & McHale, S. M. (2015). Time use as cause and consequence of youth development. *Child Development Perspectives, 9* (1), 20–25.

Lambert, J. (2011). *Digital storytelling: Capturing lives, creating community* (4th ed). New York: Routledge.

Landy, R. J., & Montgomery, D. T. (2012). *Theatre for change: Education, social action and therapy.* New York: Palgrave Macmillan.

Langeveld, C., Belme, D., & Koppenberg, T. (2014). *Collaboration in performing arts.* Retrieved from http://repub.eur.nl/pub/77498/

Lansford, J. E. (2006). Peer effects in community programs. Deviant peer influences in programs for youth. K. A. Dodge & T. J. Dishion (Eds.), *Problems and solutions* (pp. 215–233). New York: Guilford Press.

Lanspery, S. C., & Hughes, D. M. (2015). Homegrown partnerships that make a difference for youth. *Journal of Applied Developmental Psychology, 40* (1), 38–46.

Larson, R. W., Hansen, D. M., & Moneta, G. (2006). Differing profiles of developmental experiences across types of organized youth activities. *Developmental Psychology, 42* (5), 849–863.

Larson, R. W., Pearce, N., Sullivan, P. J., & Jarrett, R. L. (2007). Participation in youth programs as a catalyst for negotiation of family autonomy with connection. *Journal of Youth and Adolescence, 36* (1), 31–45.

Larson, R. W., & Tran, S. P. (2014). Invited commentary: Positive youth development and human complexity. *Journal of Youth and Adolescence, 43* (6), 1012–1017.

Larson, R. W., & Walker, K. C. (2010). Dilemmas of practice: Challenges to program quality encountered by youth program leaders. *American Journal of Community Psychology, 45* (3-4), 338–349.

Larson, R. W., Walker, K. C., Rusk, N., & Diaz, L. B. (2015). Understanding youth development from the practitioner's point of view: A call for research on effective practice. *Applied Developmental Science, 19* (2), 74–86.

Lesko, N. (2001). *Act your age! A cultural construction of adolescence.* New York: Routledge Falmer.

Laughey, D. (2006). *Music and youth culture.* Edinburgh, Scotland: Edinburgh University Press.

Lauver, S. C., & Little, P. (2005). Recruitment and retention strategies for out-of-school-time programs. *New Directions for Youth Development,* (105), 71–89.

Lauzon, A., Christie, S., Cross, H., Khan, B., & Khan, B. (2015). Youth learning in after-school programs: Exploring learning outcomes. In V. C. X. Wang (Ed.), *Handbook of research on learning outcomes and opportunities in the digital age* (pp. 376–400). Hersey, PA: Information Science Reference.

Lavie-Ajayi, M., & Krumer-Nevo, M. (2013). In a different mindset: Critical youth work with marginalized youth. *Children and Youth Services Review, 35* (10), 1698–1704.

Law, B. M., Siu, A. M., & Shek, D. T. (2012). Recognition for positive behavior as a critical youth development construct: Conceptual bases and implications on youth service development. *The Scientific World Journal*. Retrieved from http://www.hindawi.com/journals/tswj/2012/809578/abs/

Lawson, M. A., & Lawson, H. A. (2013). New conceptual frameworks for student engagement research, policy, and practice. *Review of Educational Research, 83* (3), 432–479.

Lea, G. W., Belliveau, G., Wager, A., & Beck, J. L. (2011). A loud silence: Working with research-based theatre and a/r/tography. *International Journal of Education & the Arts, 12* (16), 1–18.

Leccardi, C., & Ruspini, E. (Eds.). (2012). *A new youth?: Young people, generations and family life*. London: Ashgate Publishing.

Lee, J. A., & Finney, S. D. (2005). Using popular theatre for engaging racialized minority girls in exploring questions of identity and belonging. *Child & Youth Services, 26* (2), 95–118.

Lee, T. Y., Cheung, C. K., & Kwong, W. M. (2012). Resilience as a positive youth development construct: A conceptual review. *The Scientific World Journal*. Retrieved from http://www.hindawi.com/journals/tswj/2012/390450/abs/

Lefebvre, H. (1991). *The production of space*. Cambridge, MA: Blackwell.

Leland, J. (2016, August 28). Grandmaster flash beats back time: As a nerdy Bronx teenager with a pair of turntables, he helped change the course of pop culture. *The New York Times*, pp. 20–21.

Lenette, C., & Ingamells, A. (2015). Mind the gap! The growing chasm between funding-driven agencies, and social and community knowledge and practice. *Community Development Journal, 50* (1), 88–103.

Leonard, R. H., & Kilkelly, A. (2006a). Findings: Knowing the secrets behind the laughter. In R. H. Leonard, R. H., & A. Kilkelly (Eds.), *Performing communities: Grassroots ensemble theaters deeply rooted in eight U. S. communities* (pp. 25–43). Oakland, CA: New Village Press.

Leonard, R. H., & Kilkelly, A. (2006b). Findings: Knowing the secrets behind the laughter. In R. H. Leonard, R. H., & A. Kilkelly (Eds.), *Performing communities: Grassroots ensemble theaters deeply rooted in eight U. S. communities* (pp. 25–43). Oakland, CA: New Village Press.

Leong, S. (2016). A planetary perspective. In P. Burnard, E. Mackinlay & K. Powell (Eds.), *The Routledge international handbook of intercultural arts research* (pp. 344–357). New York: Routledge.

Lerman, L., & Zollar, J. W. J. (2015). A dialogue on dance and community practice. In M. O. Stephenson, Jr. & S. Tate (Eds.), *Arts and community change: Exploring cultural development policies, practices and dilemmas* (pp. 166–185). New York: Routledge.

Lerner, R. M., Buckingham, M. H., Champine, R. B., Greenman, K. N., Warren, D. J., & Weiner, M. B. (2015). Positive development among diverse youth. *Emerging Trends in the Social and Behavioral Sciences: An Interdisciplinary, Searchable, and Linkable Resource*. Retrieved from http://works.bepress.com/roslynn_brain/118/

Lerner, R. M., Lerner, J. V., P Bowers, E., & John Geldhof, G. (2015). *Positive youth development and relational-developmental-systems*. New York: John Wiley & Sons, Inc.

Lerner, R. M., Roeser, R. W., & Phelps, E. (Eds.). (2008). *Positive youth development & spirituality: From theory to research*. West Conshohocken, PA: Templeton Foundation Press.

Lesko, H., & Soundarajan, T. (2015). Digital storytelling in Appalachia: Gathering and sharing community voices and values. In M. O. Stephenson, Jr. & S. Tate (Eds.), *Arts and community change: Exploring cultural development policies, practices and dilemmas* (pp. 99–107). New York: Routledge.

Levesque, R. J. (2014). Dance. In R. J. Levesque (Ed.), *Encyclopedia of adolescence* (pp. 599–600). New York: Springer.

Levine, P. (2008). A public voice for youth: The audience problem in digital media and civic education. In W. L. Bennett (Ed.), *Civic life online: Learning how digital media can engage youth* (pp. 119–138). Cambridge, MA: MIT Press.

Levy, D. (2011). Participatory eco-drama. *Green Teacher*, (91), 40–43.

Levy, D. L., & Byrd, D. C. (2011). Why can't we be friends? Using music to teach social justice. *Journal of the Scholarship of Teaching and Learning, 11* (2), 64–75.

Lewis, K. M., Vuchinich, S., Ji, P., DuBois, D. L., Acock, A., Bavarian, N., . . . Flay, B. R. (2016). Effects of the Positive Action Program on indicators of positive youth development among urban youth. *Applied Developmental Science, 20* (1), 16–28.

Lewis, T. T. (2014). *Using creativity as a form of intervention for at-risk-youth: The development of Creativity2Day* (Masters thesis). Buffalo State University, Buffalo, New York.

Liao, L. C., & Sánchez, B. (2015). An exploratory study of the role of mentoring in the acculturation of Latino/a youth. *Journal of Community Psychology, 43* (7), 868–877.

Liebenberg, L., & Theron, L. C. (2015). Innovative qualitative explorations of culture and resilience. In L. C. Theron & L. Liebenberg (Eds.), *Youth resilience and culture* (pp. 203–215). Rotterdam: Springer Netherlands.

Lightfoot, A. F., Taboada, A., Taggart, T., Tran, T., & Burtaine, A. (2015). "I learned to be okay with talking about sex and safety": Assessing the efficacy of a theatre-based HIV prevention approach for adolescents in North Carolina. *Sex Education, 15* (4), 348–363.

Lin, A., & Man, E. (2011). Doing-hip-hop in the transformation of youth identities. In C. Higgins (Ed.), *Social class, habitus, and cultural capital: Identity formation in globalizing contexts* (pp. 201–220). Berlin, Germany: Mouton de Gruyter.

Lim, M., Chang, E., & Song, B. (2013). Three initiatives for community-based art education practices. *Art Education, 66* (4), 7–13.

Lima, A. C. (2016). "Once upon a time in Bronx" and the current urban challenges of the Theater of the Oppressed. Combination of participatory art and theater in public spaces in Bronx, New York City, USA. *Urban*, (08-09), 39–49.

Lind, C., Prinsloo, I., Wardle, M. L., & Pyrch, T. (2010). Social justice: Hearing voices of marginalized girls expressed in theatre performance. *Advances in Nursing Science, 33* (3), E12-E23.

Ling, P. J., & Monteith, S. (Eds.). (2014). *Gender in the Civil Rights Movement.* New York: Routledge.

Linton, J. M., Choi, R., & Mendoza, F. (2016). Caring for children in immigrant families: Vulnerabilities, resilience, and opportunities. *Pediatric Clinics of North America, 63* (1), 115–130.

Lipman, T. H., Schucker, M. M., Ratcliffe, S. J., Holmberg, T., Baier, S., & Deatrick, J. A. (2011). Diabetes risk factors in children: A partnership between nurse practitioner and high school students. *MCN: The American Journal of Maternal/Child Nursing, 36* (1), 56–62.

Lippman, J. R., & Greenwood, D. N. (2012). A song to remember emerging adults recall memorable music. *Journal of Adolescent Research, 27* (6), 751–774.

List, G. (1963). The boundaries of speech and song. *Ethnomusicology, 7* (1), 1–16.

Lobman, C. (2015). Performance, theater, and improvisation. In J. E. Johnson, S. G. Eberle, T. S. Henricks & D. Kuschner (Eds.), *The handbook of the study of play* (Vol. 2, pp. 349–364). Thousand Oaks, CA: SAGE.

Lobo, Y. B., & Winsler, A. (2006). The effects of a creative dance and movement program on the social competence of Head Start preschoolers. *Social Development, 15* (3), 501–519.

Lonie, D., & Dickens, L. (2016). Becoming musicians: Situating young people's experiences of musical learning between formal, informal and non-formal spheres. *Cultural Geographies, 23* (1), 87–101.

Lopez, A., Yoder, J. R., Brisson, D., Lechuga-Pena, S., & Jenson, J. M. (2015). Development and validation of a positive youth development measure the bridge-positive youth development. *Research on Social Work Practice, 25* (6), 726–738.

Lopez, G., & Patten, E. (2015). *The impact of slowing immigration: Foreign-born share falls among 14 largest U. S. Hispanic origin groups.* Washington, DC: Hispanic Research Center.

Lopez Castillo, M. A., Carlson, J. A., Cain, K. L., Bonilla, E. A., Chuang, E., Elder, J. P., & Sallis, J. F. (2015). Dance class structure affects youth physical activity and sedentary behavior: A study of seven dance types. *Research Quarterly for Exercise and Sport, 86* (3), 225–232.

Lorenzo-Laza, R., Ideishi, R. I., & Ideishi, S. K. (2007). Facilitating preschool learning and movement through dance. *Early Childhood Education Journal, 35* (1), 25–31.

Love, B. L. (2015). What is hip-hop-based education doing in *nice* fields such as early childhood and elementary education? *Urban Education, 50* (1), 106–131.

Low, B. (2011). *Slam school: Learning through conflict in the hip-hop and spoken word classroom.* Palo Alto, CA: Stanford University Press.

Lower, L. M., Newman, T. J., & Anderson-Butcher, D. (2015). Validity and reliability of the teamwork scale for youth. *Research on Social Work Practice.* doi: 1049731515589614

Lacy, S. (2006). Art and everyday lives: Activism in feminist performance art. In J. Cohen-Cruz & M. Schulzman (Eds.), *A Boal companion: Dialogues on theatre and cultural politics* (pp. 91–102). New York: Routledge.

Luthar, S. S., & Barkin, S. H. (2012). Are affluent youth truly 'at risk'? Vulnerability and resilience across three diverse samples. *Development and Psychopathology, 24* (02), 429–449.

Lytra, V. (2011). Negotiating language, culture and pupil agency in complementary school classrooms. *Linguistics and Education, 22* (1), 23–36.

Macías, A. (2008). *Mexican American mojo: Popular music, dance, and urban culture in Los Angeles, 1935–1968.* Durham, NC: Duke University Press.

Madsen, K. A., Hicks, K., & Thompson, H. (2011). Physical activity and positive youth development: Impact of a school-based program. *Journal of School Health, 81* (8), 462–470.

Maeso, S. R., & Araújo, M. (2015). Eurocentrism, political struggles and the entrenched will-to-ignorance: An introduction. In M. Araújo & M. Maeso (Eds.), *Eurocentrism, racism and knowledge: Debates on history and power in Europe and the Americas* (pp. 1–22). New York: Palgrave.

Magaña, J. E. (2015). *Worth the weight: The sustainability of breaking culture in Phoenix, Arizona* (Doctoral dissertation). Arizona State University, Tempe, AZ.

Mahoney, J. L., Harris, A. L., & Eccles, J. S. (2006). Organized activity participation, positive youth development, and the over-scheduling hypothesis. Social policy report. *Society for Research in Child Development, 20* (4). Retrieved from http://eric.ed.gov/?id=ED521752

Mahoney, J. L., Larson, R. W., Eccles, J. S., & Lord, H. (2005). Organized activities as developmental contexts for children and adolescents. In J. L. Mahoney & R. W. Larson (Eds.), *Organized activities as contexts of development: Extracurricular activities, after-school and community programs* (pp. 3–22). Malwah, NJ: Lawrence Erlbaum Associates.

Maira, S. (2012). *Desis in the house: Indian American youth culture in NYC*. Philadelphia, PA: Temple University Press.

Maira, S., & Shihade, M. (2012). Hip hop from '48 Palestine youth, music, and the present/absent. *Social Text, 30* (3 112), 1–26.

Maley, M. (2012). An ecological approach to adolescent obesity: Working together to support healthy youth. *ACT for Youth Center of Excellence,* 1–8. Retrieved from http://www.actforyouth.net/resources/rf/rf_obesity_0212.pdf

Malin, H. (2015). Arts participation as a context for youth purpose. *Studies in Art Education, 56* (3), 268–280.

Malin, H., Ballard, P. J., & Damon, W. (2015). Civic purpose: An integrated construct for understanding civic development in adolescence. *Human Development, 58* (2), 103–130.

Mallett, C. A. (2012). Delinquent youth with disabilities. In R. Levesque (Ed.), *Encyclopedia of adolescence* (pp. 633–638). New York: Springer US.

Malloy, A. (2016). *Scripting resistance: Governance through Theatre of the Oppressed* (Dissertation). University of Waterloo, Canada.

Malone, M. L., & Malone, H. L. (2015). Housing segregation and the prison industrial complex: Looking at the roots of today's school-to-prison pipeline. In L. Dowdell Drakeford (Ed.), *The race controversy in American education* (Vol. 1, pp. 149–168). Santa Barbara, CA: Praeger.

Manchester, H., & Pett, E. (2015). Teenage kicks: Exploring cultural value from a youth perspective. *Cultural Trends, 24* (3), 223–231.

Maposa, J. F., & Louw-Potgieter, J. (2014). An outcome evaluation of a youth development programme. *Social Work/Maatskaplike Werk, 48* (2). Retrieved from http://socialwork.journals.ac.za/pub/article/view/97

María, H. L. (2015). *Towards new forms of learning. Exploring the potential of participatory theatre in sustainability science* (Doctoral dissertation). Universitat Autònoma de Barcelona. Institut de Ciència i Tecnologia Ambientals Retrieved from https://dialnet.unirioja.es/servlet/dctes?codigo=73550

Marin, C. (2014). Enacting engagement: Theatre as a pedagogical tool for human rights education. *Youth Theatre Journal, 28* (1), 32–43.

Marks, A. K., Ejesi, K., & García Coll, C. (2014). Understanding the US immigrant paradox in childhood and adolescence. *Child Development Perspectives, 8* (2), 59–64.

Markusen, A., & Brown, A. (2014). From audience to participants: New thinking for the performing arts. *Análise Social, 49* (213), 866–883.

Marsh, K., & Dieckmann, S. (2016). Music as shared space for young immigrant children and their mothers. In P. Burnard, E. Mackinlay & K. Powell (Eds.), *The Routledge international handbook of intercultural arts research* (pp. 358–368). New York: Routledge.

Martin, R. (2006). *Staging the political. A Boal companion: Dialogues on theatre and cultural politics.* New York: Taylor & Francis.

Martin, A. K. (2013). *A singing sanctuary: Identity and resiliency construction in underserved youth through vocal expression* (Master's thesis). University of British Columbia, Vancouver, BC, Canada.

Martinek, T. (2005). Promoting positive youth development through a values-based sport program. RICYDE. *Revista Internacional de Ciencias del Deporte, 1*(1), 1–13.

Masten, A. S. (2011). Resilience in children threatened by extreme adversity: Frameworks for research, practice, and translational synergy. *Development and Psychopathology, 23* (2), 493–506.

Masten, A. S. (2014). Invited commentary: Resilience and positive youth development frameworks in developmental science. *Journal of Youth and Adolescence, 43* (6), 1018–1024.

Masten, A. S. (2014a). Global perspectives on resilience in children and youth. *Child Development, 85* (1), 6–20.

Masten, A. S. (2014b). Invited commentary: Resilience and positive youth development frameworks in developmental science. *Journal of Youth and Adolescence, 43* (6), 1018–1024.

Matloff-Nieves, S., Fusco, D. Connolly, J., & Maulik, N. (2016). Democratizing urban spaces: A social justice approach to youth work. In M. Heathfield & D. Fusco (Eds.), *Youth and inequality in education: Global actions in youth work* (pp. 175–194). New York: Routledge.

Matsuba, M. K., Elder, G., Petrucci, F., & Reimer, K. S. (2010). Re-storying the lives of at-risk youth: A case study approach. In K. C. McLean & M. Pasupathi (Eds.), *Narrative development in adolescence* (pp. 131–149). New York: Springer US.

Maynes, M. J., Pierce, J. L., & Laslett, B. (2012). *Telling stories: The use of personal narratives in the social sciences and history.* Ithaca, NY: Cornell University Press.

Mayor, C. (2012). Playing with race: A theoretical framework and approach for creative arts therapists. *The Arts in Psychotherapy, 39* (3), 214–219.

Mbembe, A. J. (2016). Decolonizing the university: New directions. *Arts and Humanities in Higher Education, 15* (1), 29–45.

McAvinehey, C. (2011). *Theatre prison.* Hampshire, UK: Palgrave Macmillan.

McBride, A. M., Johnson, E., Olate, R., & O'Hara, K. (2011). Youth volunteer service as positive youth development in Latin America and the Caribbean. *Children and Youth Services Review, 33* (1), 34–41.

McCammon, L. A. (2007). Research on drama and theater for social change. In *International handbook of research in arts education* (pp. 945–964). Rotterdam: Springer Netherlands.

McCammon, L. A., Saldaña, J., Hines, A., & Omasta, M. (2012). Lifelong impact: Adult perceptions of their high school speech and/or theatre participation. *Youth Theatre Journal, 26* (1), 2–25.

McCarthy-Brown, N. (2009). The need for culturally relevant dance education. *Journal of Dance Education, 9* (4), 120–125.

McCollum, I. (2015). The benefits of theater participation on child and adolescent development and academic performance. In *Kalamazoo College psychology VanLiere Symposium Collection*. Kalamazoo, MI: Kalamazoo College. https://cache.kzoo.edu/handle/10920/29672

McCready, L. T. (2004). Understanding the marginalization of gay and gender non- conforming Black male students. *Theory into Practice, 43* (2), 136–143.

McDonald, J. (2006). Balancing the 'town and gown': The risky business of creating youth theatre in regional Queensland. *International Journal of Pedagogies and Learning, 2* (2), 6–13.

McDonnell, E. (2015). Rebel music: Race, empire, and the new Muslim youth culture. By Hisham D. Aidi. *Journal of the American Academy of Religion, 83* (1), 288–291.

McFerran, K. (2011). Music therapy with bereaved youth: Expressing grief and feeling better. *Prevention Researcher, 18* (3), 17–20.

McGough, B. L., & Salomon, D. (2014). *Engaging students through social media*. San Francisco, CA: Jossey-Bass.

McHale, S. M., Dotterer, A., & Kim, J. Y. (2009). An ecological perspective on the media and youth development. *American behavioral scientist, 52* (8), 1186–1203.

McLaughlin, M. W., Irby, M. A., & Langman, J. (1994). *Urban sanctuaries: Neighborhood organizations in the lives and futures of inner-city youth*. San Francisco, CA: Jossey-Bass.

McLean, H. E. (2014). Cracks in the Creative City: The contradictions of community arts practice. *International Journal of Urban and Regional Research, 38* (6), 2156–2173.

McMains, J. (2016). Salsa steps toward intercultural education. *Journal of Dance Education, 16* (1), 27–30.

Meer, L. F. (2007). Playback theatre in Cuba: The politics of improvisation and free expression. *TDR/The Drama Review, 51* (4), 106–120.

Meiners, E. R. (2010). *Right to be hostile: Schools, prisons, and the making of public enemies*. New York: Routledge.

Melchior, E. (2011). Culturally responsive dance pedagogy in the primary classroom. *Research in Dance Education, 12* (2), 119–135.

Menke, S. (2015). *Your story matters: Theatre for community in practice with the Boys and Girls Club of Bloomington-Normal*. Retrieved from http://digitalcommons.iwu.edu/cgi/viewcontent.cgi?article=1020&context=theatre honproj

Metzger, A., Crean, H. F., & Forbes-Jones, E. L. (2009). Patterns of organized activity participation in urban, early adolescents: Associations with academic achievement, problem behaviors, and perceived adult support. *The Journal of Early Adolescence, 29* (3), 426–442.

Mienczakowski, J. (2009). Pretending to know: Ethnography, artistry and audience. *Ethnography and Education, 4* (3), 321–333.

Milton, T. (2011). *Overcoming the magnetism of street life: Crime-engaged youth and the programs that transform them*. Lanham, MD: Lexington Books.

Miranda, D. (2013). The role of music in adolescent development: Much more than the same old song. *International Journal of Adolescence and Youth, 18* (1), 5–22.

Mitchell, C. (2009). "This has nothing to do with us—or does it?" Youth as knowledge producers in addressing HIV and AIDS in a Canadian preservice education program. *Counterpoints, 334*, 83–92.

Mitchell, C., & de Lange, N. (2012). *Handbook of participatory video*. Landham, MD: AltaMira Press.

Mitra, D. (2006). Student voice or empowerment? Examining the role of school-based youth-adult partnerships as an avenue toward focusing on social justice. *IEJLL: International Electronic Journal for Leadership in Learning, 10* (22). http://iejll.journalhosting.ucalgary.ca/iejll/index.php/ijll/article/viewFile/622/284

Mitra, D., Serriere, S., & Kirshner, B. (2014). Youth participation in US contexts: Student voice without a national mandate. *Children & Society, 28* (4), 292–304.

Mmari, K. N., Blum, R. W., & Teufel-Shone, N. (2010). What increases risk and protection for delinquent behaviors among American Indian youth? Findings from three tribal communities. *Youth & Society, 41* (3), 382–413.

Modirzadeh, L. (2013). Documentary theater in education: Empathy building as a tool for social change. In M. S. Hanley, G. W. Nobit, G. L. Sheppard & T. Barone (Eds.), *Culturally relevant arts education for social justice: A way out* (pp. 47–57). New York: Routledge.

Mohammadzadeh, M. (2015). Deconstructing placemaking: Needs, opportunities, and assets. *Urban Policy and Research, 33* (3), 370–373.

Mohler, C. E. (2012a). Unusual Suspects Company. http://theunusualsuspects.org/

Mohler, C. E. (2012b). How to turn "a bunch of gang-bangin' criminals into big kids having fun": Empowering incarcerated and at-risk youth through ensemble theatre. *Theatre Topics, 22* (1), 89–102.

Mohr, E. (2014). Posttraumatic growth in youth survivors of a disaster: An arts-based research project. *Art Therapy, 31* (4), 155–162.

Moje, E. B. (2015). Youth cultures, literacies, and identities in and out of school. In J. Flood, S. B. Heath, & D. Lapp (Eds.), *Handbook of research on teaching literacy through the communicative and visual arts. Volume II: A project of the international reading association* (pp. 207–220). New York: Routledge.

Moldavanova, A., & Goerdel, H. T. (2014). *The community-based pathways to achieving sustainability for public and nonprofit arts organizations in an urban context.* Retrieved from http://wpsa.research.pdx.edu/papers/docs/maldavanovaandgoerdel.pdf

Moletsane, R., Mitchell, C., Stuart, J., Walsh, S., & Taylor, M. (2008, March). *Ethical issues in using participatory video in addressing gender violence in and around schools: The challenges of representation.* In *Annual American Educational Research Association Conference.* New York (pp. 24–28).

Molnár, V. (2014). Reframing public space through digital mobilization flash mobs and contemporary urban youth culture. *Space and Culture, 17* (1), 43–58.

Moloney, M. (2005, September 1). "Those who suffer write the songs": Remembering Frank Harte, 1933–2005. *The Journal of Music.* Retrieved from http:journalofmusic.com/focus/those-who-suffer-write-songs

Monchalin, R., Flicker, S., Wilson, C., Prentice, T., Oliver, V., Jackson, R., . . . Restoule, J. P. (2016). "When you follow your heart, you provide that path for others": Indigenous models of youth leadership in HIV prevention. *International Journal of Indigenous Health, 11*(1), 135–158.

Moore, E. A., & Mertens, D. M. (2015). Deaf culture and youth resilience in diverse American communities. In L. C. Theron & l. Liebenberg (Eds.), *Youth resilience and culture* (pp. 143–155). Rotterdam: Springer Netherlands.

Moore, M. C. (2009). Creation to performance: The journey of an African American community gospel-jazz ensemble. In J. L. Kerchner & C. R. Abril (Eds.), *Musical experience in our lives: Things we learn and meanings we make* (pp. 277–296). Lanham, MD: Rowman & Littlefield.

Moore, S. E., Robinson, M. A., Adedoyin, A. C., Brooks, M., Harmon, D. K., & Boamah, D. (2016). Hands up—Don't shoot: Police shooting of young Black males: Implications for social work and human services. *Journal of Human Behavior in the Social Environment, 26* (3-4), 254–266.

Morad, M. (2016). Queering the macho grip: Transgressing and subverting gender in Latino music and dance. *Ethnologie française, 1* (1), 103–114.

Moran, S. (2014). What 'purpose' means to youth: Are there cultures of purpose? *Applied Developmental Science, 18* (3), 163–175.

Morgan, C., Sibthorp, J., & Wells, M. S. (2014). Fun, activities, and social context: *Journal of Park and Recreation Administration, 32* (3). Retrieved from http://www.cabdirect. org/abstracts/20143356986.html;jsessionid=EB7C1EFABA62903AF7243614F7F08 EEB

Morillo, S. (2014). Bullets in motion. In D. Northrop (Ed.), *A companion to world history* (pp. 375–388). New York: John Wiley & Sons.

Morrel-Samuels, S., Hutchison, P., Perkinson, L., Bostic, B., & Zimmerman, M. (2015). *Selecting, implementing and adapting youth empowerment solutions.* Retrieved from http://deepblue.lib.umich.edu/bitstream/handle/2027.42/110221/YES%20Ada pta-tion%20Guide%20FINAL.pdf?sequence=1&isAllowed=y

Morris, A. A. (2012). *Playing with possibilities: Facilitation of theatre collective creation for social justice in the secondary drama classroom* (Doctoral dissertation). Mount Saint Vincent University, Halifax, Canada.

Morris, C. B. (2012). Critical race, multicultural art education. In N. Addison & L. Burgess (Eds.), *Debates in art and design education* (pp. 43–50). New York: Routledge.

Morrissey, K. M., & Werner-Wilson, R. J. (2005). The relationship between out-of-school activities and positive youth development: An investigation of the influences of communities and family. *Adolescence, 40* (157), 66–85.

Morton, M. H., & Montgomery, P. (2013). Youth empowerment programs for improving adolescents' self-efficacy and self-esteem a systematic review. *Research on Social Work Practice, 23* (1), 22–33.

Mosavel, M., & Thomas, T. (2010). Project REECH: Using theatre arts to authenticate local knowledge. *New Solutions: A Journal of Environmental and Occupational Health Policy, 19* (4), 407–422.

Moxley, D. P., & Abbas, J. M. (2016). Envisioning libraries as collaborative community anchors for social service provision to vulnerable populations. *Practice,* 1–20.

Moxley, D. P., & Calligan, H. F. (2015). Positioning the arts for intervention design research in the human services. *Evaluation and program planning, 53* (1), 34–43.

Moxley, D. P., Feen-Calligan, H., & Washington, O. G. (2012). Lessons learned from three projects linking social work, the arts, and humanities. *Social Work Education, 31* (6), 703–723.

Munsell, S. E., & Bryant Davis, K. E. (2015). Dance and special education. *Preventing School Failure: Alternative Education for Children and Youth, 59* (3), 129–133.

Musil, P. S. (2010). Perspectives on an expansive postsecondary dance. *Journal of Dance Education, 10* (4), 111–121.

Nakkula, M. J., Foster, K. C., Mannes, M., & Bolstrom, S. (2010). *Building healthy communities for positive youth development* (Vol. 7). New York: Springer Science & Business Media.

Nasir, K. M. (2015). The September 11 generation, hip-hop and human rights. *Journal of Sociology, 51* (4), 1039–1051.

Neblett, E. W., Rivas-Drake, D., & Umaña-Taylor, A. J. (2012). The promise of racial and ethnic protective factors in promoting ethnic minority youth development. *Child Development Perspectives, 6* (3), 295–303.

Neelands, J. (2009). Acting together: Ensemble as a democratic process in art and life. *RiDE: The Journal of Applied Theatre and Performance, 14* (2), 173–189.

Nelson, B. (2011). "I made myself": Playmaking as a pedagogy of change with urban youth. *RiDE: The Journal of Applied Theatre and Performance, 16* (2), 157–172.

Nelson, M. E., Hull, G., & Roche -Smith, J. (2008). Challenges of multimedia self—presentation: Taking, and mistaking, the show on the road. *Written Communication, 25* (4), 415–440.

Nembhard, G. N. (2012). *Storying for social justice: A professional learning journey* (Doctoral dissertation). University of Toronto, Canada.

Nenga, S. K. (2012). Not the community, but a community: Transforming youth into citizens through volunteer work. *Journal of Youth Studies, 15* (8), 1063–1077.

Newell, M. L., & Coffee, G. (2012). A social justice approach to assessment. In D. Shriberg & S. Y. Song (Eds.), *School psychology and social justice: Conceptual foundations and tools for practice* (pp. 173–188). New York: Routledge.

Newman, J. L., & Dantzler, J. (2015). Fostering individual and school resilience: When students at risk move from receivers to givers. *Assessing Resilience, 8* (1), 80–89.

Newman, T. J., & Alvarez, M. A. G. (2015). Coaching on the wave: An integrative approach to facilitating youth development. *Journal of Sport Psychology in Action, 6* (3), 127–140.

Ngo, B. (2009). Ambivalent urban, immigrant identities: The incompleteness of Lao American student identities. *International Journal of Qualitative Studies in Education, 22* (2), 201–220.

Nicholas, D. B., Newton, A. S., Calhoun, A., Dong, K., Hamilton, F., Kilmer, C., . . . Shankar, J. (2016). The experiences and perceptions of street-involved youth regarding emergency department services. *Qualitative Health Research, 26,* 6, 851–862.

Nicolas, G., & DeSilva, A. M. (2008). Application of the ecological model: Spirituality research with ethnically diverse youths. In R. M. Lerner, R. W. Roeser & E. Phelps (Eds.), *Positive youth development & spirituality: From theory to research* (pp. 305–321). West Conshohocken, PA: Templeton Foundation Press.

Nicholls, A. (Ed.), (2006). *Social entrepreneurship: New models of sustainable social change.* New York: Oxford University Press.

Nielsen, C. S., & Burridge, S. (2015a). Introduction. *Dance education around the world: Perspectives on dance, young people and change* (pp.ix-xx). New York: Routledge.

Nielsen, C. S., & Burridge, S. (Eds.). (2015b). *Dance education around the world: Perspectives on dance, young people and change.* New York: Routledge.

Ní Laoire, C. (2016). Making space for ambiguity: The value of multiple and participatory methods in researching diasporic youth identities. *Identities, 21* (4), 470–484.

Noam, G. G., & Bernstein-Yamashiro, B. (2013). Youth development practitioners and their relationships in schools and after-school programs. *New Directions for Youth Development,* (137), 57–68.

Noble-Carr, D., Barker, J., McArthur, M., & Woodman, E. (2014). Improving practice: The importance of connections in establishing positive identity and meaning in the lives of vulnerable young people. *Children and Youth Services Review, 47,* (Part 3), 389–396.

Noddings, N. (1995). Teaching themes of care. *Phi Delta Kappan, 76* (9), 675–679.

Nolas, S. M. (2014). Exploring young people's and youth workers' experiences of spaces for 'youth development': Creating cultures of participation. *Journal of Youth Studies, 17* (1), 26–41.

Noone, J., Castillo, N., Allen, T. L., & Esqueda, T. (2015). Latino teen theater: A theater intervention to promote Latino parent–adolescent sexual communication. *Hispanic Health Care International, 13* (4), 209–216.

Nordin-Bates, S. M. (2012). Performance psychology in the performing arts. In S. Murphy (Ed.), *The Oxford handbook of sport and performance psychology* (pp. 81–114). New York: Oxford University Press.

Nordkvelle, Y. T. (2015). Pedagogy and education in the context of globalisation: A historical reconstruction of Eurocentrism in pedagogy. *Radical Pedagogy, 12* (1), 1524–6345.

Nortier, J., & Svendsen, B. A. (Eds.), (2015*). Language, youth and identity in the 21st century: Linguistic practices across urban spaces.* New York: Cambridge University Press.

Norton, C. L., & Watt, T. T. (2014). Exploring the impact of a wilderness-based positive youth development program for urban youth. *Journal of Experiential Education, 37* (4), 335–350.

Novick, S. R. (2015). *Advisory as an ecological asset: The role of advisory in fostering the positive youth development of adolescents transitioning to high school* (Doctoral dissertation). Boston University, Boston, MA).

Numrich, P., & Kniss, F. (2007). *Sacred assemblies and civic engagement: How religion matters for America's newest immigrants.* New Brunswick, NJ: Rutgers University Press.

Nurmi, A. M., & Kokkonen, M. (2015). Peers as teachers in physical education hip hop classes in Finnish high school. *Journal of Education and Training Studies, 3* (3), 23–32.

Nybell, L. M., Shook, J. J., & Finn, J. L. (2013). *Childhood, youth, and social work in transformation: Implications for policy and practice.* New York: Columbia University Press.

Nzinga, F. (2012). "Growing the size of the black woman": Feminist activism in Havana hip hop. In C. Morrow & T. A. Fredrick (Eds.), *Getting in is not enough: Women and the global workplace* (pp. 282–298). Baltimore, MD: The Johns Hopkins University Press.

O'Connor, C., Hill, L. D., & Robinson, S. R. (2009). Who's at risk in school and what's race got to do with it? *Review of Research in Education, 33* (1), 1–34.

O'Connor, M., & Colucci, E. (2016). Exploring domestic violence and social distress in Australian-Indian migrants through community theater. *Transcultural Psychiatry, 53* (1), 24–44.

Oberg, C. M. (2008). Performance ethnography: Scholarly inquiry in the here and now. *Transformative Dialogues: Teaching & Learning Journal, 2* (1), 1–4.

Odello, D. (2016). Performing tradition: History, expression, and meaning in drum corps shows. *Popular Music and Society, 39* (2), 241–258.

Ohmer, M. L., & Owens, J. (2013). Using photovoice to empower youth and adults to prevent crime. *Journal of Community Practice, 21* (4), 410–433.

Oldenburg, R. (1999). *The great good place.* New York: Marlowe & Co.

Olsen, H. M., & Dieser, R. B. (2012). "I am hoping you can point me in the right direction regarding playground accessibility": A case study of a community which lacked social policy toward playground accessibility. *World Leisure Journal, 54* (3), 269–279.

O'Neill, J. R., Pate, R. R., & Liese, A. D. (2011). Descriptive epidemiology of dance participation in adolescents. *Research Quarterly for Exercise and Sport, 82* (3), 373–380.

Opara, R. S. (2012). *Art as a media for social commentary: A case study of Igbo Bongo musicians, south-eastern Nigeria* (Doctoral dissertation). University of Louisville, KY.

Orleans, P. K. N. (2012). Using the arts and new media in community organizing and community building. In M. Minkler (Ed.), *Community organizing and community building for health and welfare* (3rd ed., pp. 288–307). New Brunswick, NJ: Rutgers University Press.

Osborne, M. S., & Kenny, D. T. (2008). The role of sensitizing experiences in music performance anxiety in adolescent musicians. *Psychology of Music, 36* (4), 447–462.

Osei-Kaft, N. (2013). Exploring arts-based inquiry for social justice in graduate education. In M. S. Hanley, G. W. Nobit, G. L. Sheppard & T. Barone (Eds.), *Culturally relevant arts education for social justice: A way out* (pp. 130–140). New York: Routledge.

Osman, C. A., Rahim, H. L., Yusof, M. M., Zikrul, M., Noor, H., & Lajin, N. F. M. (2014). Empowering disabled youth with entrepreneurial values. In *2nd Asian Entrepreneurship Conference proceeding* (pp. 103–112). Singapore: Springer.

Page, R. D. (2012). *Dance: The stepchild of the Black Arts Movement* (Doctoral dissertation). California State University, Long Beach, CA).

Palidofsky, M. (2010). If I cry for you. Turning unspoken trauma into song and musical theatre. *International Journal of Community Music, 3* (1), 121–128.

Palidofsky, M., & Stolbach, B. C. (2012). Dramatic healing: The evolution of a trauma-informed musical theatre program for incarcerated girls. *Journal of Child & Adolescent Trauma, 5* (3), 239–256.

Pane, D. M., & Rocco, T. S. (2014). School-to-prison pipeline revisited/looking to the future. In *Transforming the school-to-prison pipeline* (pp. 301–310). Rotterdam, Netherlands: Sense Publishers.

Papacharisis, V., Goudas, M., Danish, S. J., & Theodorakis, Y. (2005). The effectiveness of teaching a life skills program in a sport context. *Journal of Applied Sport Psychology, 17* (3), 247–254.

Papinczak, Z. E., Dingle, G. A., Stoyanov, S. R., Hides, L., & Zelenko, O. (2015). Young people's uses of music for well-being. *Journal of Youth Studies, 18* (9) 1119–1134.

Parchment, T. M., Jones, J., Del-Villar, Z., Small, L., & McKay, M. (2016). Integrating positive youth development and clinical care to enhance high school achievement for young people of color. *Journal of Public Mental Health, 15* (1), 50–62.

Paris, D., & Winn, M. T. (2013). *Humanizing research: Decolonizing qualitative inquiry with youth and communities.* Thousand Oaks: SAGE.

Park, J. H., & 朴宰亨. (2015). *Soviet Korean youth in post-Soviet Kyrgyzstan: Their education and mobility.* Retrieved from http://repository.lib.eduhk.hk/jspui/handle/2260.2/16827

Pascale, L. M. (2013). The power of simply singing together in the classroom. *The Phenomenon of Singing, 2,* 177–183. Passell, J. S. (2011). Demography of immigrant youth: Past, present, and future. *Future Child, 21* (1):19–41.

Passell, J. S., & Lope, M. H. (2012, August 14). *Up to 1.7 million unauthorized immigrant youth may benefit from new deportation rules.* Washington, DC: Pew Hispanic Center.

Pearrow, M. M. (2008). A critical examination of an urban-based youth empowerment strategy: The teen empowerment program. *Journal of Community Practice, 16* (4), 509–525.

Peck, C. (2015). "I want to play too": Why today's youth are resisting the rules of the theatre. *Theatre Symposium, 23* (1), 124–136.

Peddie, I. (Ed.), (2006). *The resisting muse: Popular music and social protest*. Farnham, UK: Ashgate Publishing.

Pellegrino, A. M., Zenkov, K., & Aponte-Martinez, G. (2014). Middle school students, slam poetry and the notion of citizenship. *Journal of Educational Controversy, 8* (1), Article 8.

Pennington, J. L., Brock, C. H., & Ndura, E. (2012). Unraveling the threads of white teachers' conceptions of caring: Repositioning white privilege. *Urban Education, 47* (4), 743–775.

Pente, E., Ward, P., Brown, M., & Sahota, H. (2015). The co-production of historical knowledge: Implications for the history of identities. *Identity Papers: A journal of British and Irish Studies, 1* (1), 32–53.

Peterson, D. J., Newman, M. E., Leatherman, J., & Miske, S. (2014). Engaging youth, serving community. *Reclaiming Children and Youth, 23* (3), 37–40.

Peterson, G. T., & Anderson, E. (2012). The performance of softer masculinities on the university dance floor. *The Journal of Men's Studies, 20* (1), 3–15.

Pew Hispanic Research Center. (2015, September 28). *Modern immigration wave brings 59 million to U. S., driving population growth and change through 2065: Views of immigration's impact on U. S. society mixed*. Author.

Phillips, L. (2012). Emergent motifs of social justice storytelling as pedagogy. *Storytelling, Self, Society, 8* (2), 108–125.

Pica-Smith, C., & Veloria, C. (2012). "At risk means a minority kid": Deconstructing deficit discourses in the study of risk in education and human services. *Pedagogy and the Human Sciences, 1* (2), 33–48.

Picher, M. C. (2007). Democratic process and the Theater of the Oppressed. *New Directions for Adult and Continuing Education, 2007* (116), 79–88.

Picower, B. (2012). *Practice what you teach: Social justice education in the classroom and the streets* (Vol. 13). New York: Routledge.

Pine, J. B., & Gilmore J. H. (2007). *Authenticity: What consumers really want?* Cambridge, MA: Harvard Business School.

Pitzer, R. (2013). Youth music at the Yakama nation tribal school. In P. S. Campbell & T. Wiggins (Eds.), *The Oxford handbook of children's musical cultures* (pp. 46–60). New York: Oxford University Press.

Pokhrel, A. K. (2011). Eurocentrism. In D. K. Chatterjee (Ed.), *Encyclopedia of global justice* (pp. 321–325). Rotterdam: Springer Netherlands.

Porfilio, B., Gardner, L. M., & Roychoudhury, D. (2013). Ending the 'war against youth': Social media and hip-hop culture as sites of resistance, transformation and (re) conceptualization. *Journal for Critical Education Policy Studies, 11* (4). Retrieved from http://jceps.com/wp-content/uploads/PDFs/11-4-05.pdf

Poteet, M., & Simmons, A. (2016). Not boxed in: Acculturation and ethno-social identities of Central American male youth in Toronto. *Journal of International Migration and Integration, 17* (3), 867–885.

Powell, J. L. (2014). Risk, welfare, education and youth. *International Letters of Social and Humanistic Sciences, (07),* 22–30.

Prentki, T., & Preston, S. (2009). Applied theatre: An introduction. In K. Prentki & S. Preston (Eds.), *The applied theatre reader* (pp. 9–15). New York: Routledge.

Preston, S. (2009a). Introduction to participation. In K. Prentki & S. Preston (Eds.), *The applied theatre reader* (pp.127–129). New York: Routledge.

Preston, S. (2009b). Introduction to transformation. In T. Preston & S. Preston (Eds.), *The applied theatre reader* (pp. 301–302). New York: Routledge.

Preston, S. (2011). Back on whose track? Reframing ideologies of inclusion and misrecognition in a participatory theatre project with young people in London. *RiDE: The Journal of Applied Theatre and Performance, 16* (2), 251–264.

Price, E. G., III. (Ed.). (2011). *The Black church and hip hop culture: Toward bridging the generational divide.* Lanham, MD: Scarecrow Press.

Prinsloo, E. H. (2016). The role of the humanities in decolonising the academy. *Arts and Humanities in Higher Education, 15* (1), 164–168.

Prior, R. W. (2010). Using forum theatre as university widening participation (WP) for social well-being agendas. *Journal of Applied Arts & Health, 1* (2), 179–191.

Pritzker, S., & Richards-Schuster, K. (2016). Promoting young people's participation: Exploring social work's contribution to the literature. *Social Work, 61* (3), 217–226.

Pryce, J., Giovannetti, S., Spencer, R., Elledge, L. C., Gowdy, G., Whitley, M. L., & Cavell, T. A. (2015). Mentoring in the social context: Mentors' experiences with mentees' peers in a site-based program. *Children and Youth Services Review, 56* (September), 185–192.

Pryor, B. N. K., & Outley, C. W. (2014). Just spaces: Urban recreation centers as sites for social justice youth development. *Journal of Leisure Research, 46* (3), 272–290.

Pulido, I. (2009). "Music fit for us minorities": Latinas/os' use of hip hop as pedagogy and interpretive framework to negotiate and challenge racism. *Equity & Excellence in Education, 42* (1), 67–85.

Purcell, R., & Beck, D. (2010). *Popular education practice for youth and community development work.* London: SAGE.

Puttick, R., Baeck, P., & Colligan, P. (2014). *The teams and funds making innovation happen in governments around the world.* Retrieved from http://www.nesta.org.uk/sites/default/files/i-teams_june_2014.pdf

Pyscher, T., & Lozenski, B. D. (2014). Throwaway youth: The sociocultural location of resistance to schooling. *Equity & Excellence in Education, 47*(4), 531–545.

Quijada Cerecer, D. A., Cahill, C., & Bradley, M. (2013). Toward a critical youth policy praxis: Critical youth studies and participatory action research. *Theory into Practice, 52* (3), 216–223.

Quiroga Murcia, C., Kreutz, G., Clift, S., & Bongard, S. (2010). Shall we dance? An exploration of the perceived benefits of dancing on well-being. *Arts & Health, 2* (2), 149–163.

Raby, R. (2014). Children's participation as neo-liberal governance? *Discourse: Studies in the Cultural Politics of Education, 35* (1), 77–89.

Radano, R. (2016). Black music labor and the animated properties of slave sound. *boundary 2: An International of Literature and Culture, 43* (1), 173–208.

Rahm, J., Lachaîne, A., & Mathura, A. (2014). Youth voice and positive identity building practices: The case of ScienceGirls. *Canadian Journal of Education[Revue canadienne de l'éducation], 37* (1), 209–232.

Rakena, T. O. (2016). Sustaining indigenous performing arts: The potential decolonizing role of arts-based service learning. In B. Bartleet, D. Bennett, A. Power & N. Sunderland

(Eds.), *Engaging first peoples in arts-based service learning: Towards respectful and mutually beneficial educational practices* (pp. 119–131). New York: Springer.

Ramphele, M. (2002). Steering by the stars: Youth in cities. In M. Tienda & W. J. Wilson (Eds.), *Youth in cities: A national perspective* (pp. 21–30). New York: Cambridge University Press.

Randall, L., & Robinson, D. B. (2016). An introduction to social justice in physical education: Critical reflections and pedagogies for change. In D. B. Robinson & L. Randall (Eds.), *Social justice in physical education: Critical reflections and pedagogies for change* (pp. 1–14). New York: Oxford University Press.

Rasquinha, A. M., & Cardinal, B. J. (2015). What if overweight and obese youth were to see themselves as athletes? Sports as a value-added benefit to pediatric tertiary weight-management clinics. *Journal of Physical Education, Recreation and Dance, 86* (1), 6–9.

Rauner, D. M. (2013). *They still pick me up when I fall: The role of caring in youth development and community life.* New York: Columbia University Press.

Rauscher, L., & Cooky, C. (2016). Ready for anything the world gives her? A critical look at sports-based positive youth development for girls. *Sex Roles, 74* (7), 288–298.

Read, J. C., Fitton, D., & Hortton, M. (2014, June). Giving ideas an equal chance: Inclusion and representation in participatory design with children. In *Proceedings of the 2014 conference on Interaction design and children* (pp. 105–114). Aarhus, Denmark: ACM.

Rein, M. (1969). Social planning: The search for legitimacy. *Journal of the American Institute of Planners, 35* (4), 233–244.

Revilla, A. (2012). What happens in Vegas does not stay in vegas: Youth leadership in the immigrant rights movement in Las Vegas, 2006. *Aztlan: A Journal of Chicano Studies, 37* (1), 87–115.

Reynolds, T. (2015). 'Black neighborhoods' and 'race,' placed identities in youth transition to adulthoods. In J. Wyn & H. Cahill (Eds.), *Handbook of children and youth studies* (pp. 651–663). Singapore: Springer.

Rhoades, R. (2016). *Nurturing assets through collaborative arts-based inquiry with youth.* Retrieved from http://qspace.library.queensu.ca/jspui/handle/1974/14037

Richards-Schuster, K., & Pritzker, S. (2015). Strengthening youth participation in civic engagement: Applying the convention on the rights of the child to social work practice. *Children and Youth Services Review, 57* (Oct), 90–97.

Richardson, C., & Reynolds, V. (2012). *"Here we are, amazingly alive": Holding ourselves together with an ethic of social justice in community work.* Retrieved from http://journals.uvic.ca/index.php/ijcyfs/article/view/10471/3103

Richardson, M. (2015). *Youth theatre: Drama for life.* New York: Routledge.

Riggs, N. R., Bohnert, A. M., Guzman, M. D., & Davidson, D. (2010). Examining the potential of community-based after-school programs for Latino youth. *American Journal of Community Psychology, 45* (3-4), 417–429.

Rimmer, M. (2012). The participation and decision making of 'at risk' youth in community music projects: An exploration of three case studies. *Journal of Youth Studies, 15* (3), 329–350.

Rivera-Servera, R. H. (2012). *Movements of hope. Performing queer Latinidad: Dance, sexuality, politics.* Ann Arbor, MI: University of Michigan Press.

Roach, J., Wureta, E., & Ross, L. (2013). Dilemmas of practice in the ecology of emancipatory youth-adult partnerships. *International Journal of Child, Youth and Family Studies, 4* (3.1), 475–488.

Robb, S. L., Burns, D. S., & Carpenter, J. S. (2011). Reporting guidelines for music- based interventions. *Music and medicine, 3* (4), 271–279.

Roberts, L., & Cohen, S. (2014). Unauthorising popular music heritage: Outline of a critical framework. *International Journal of Heritage Studies, 20* (3), 241–261.

Rogers, J., Mediratta, K., & Shah, S. (2012). Building power, learning democracy youth organizing as a site of civic development. *Review of Research in Education, 36* (1), 43–66.

Rhodes, A. M., & Schechter, R. (2014). Fostering resilience among youth in inner city community arts centers: The case of the Artists Collective. *Education and Urban Society, 46* (7), 826–848.

Rieger, K., & Schultz, A. S. (2014). Exploring Arts-Based Knowledge Translation: Sharing Research Findings Through Performing the Patterns, Rehearsing the Results, Staging the Synthesis. *Worldviews on Evidence-Based Nursing, 11*(2), 133–139.

Riele, K. T. (2006). Youth 'at risk': Further marginalizing the marginalized? *Journal of Education Policy, 21* (2), 129–145.

Rios, M., & Vazquez, L. (Eds.). (2012). *Diálogos: placemaking in Latino communities.* New York: Routledge.

Rivas-Drake, D., Syed, M., Umaña-Taylor, A., Markstrom, C., French, S., Schwartz, S. J., & Lee, R. (2014). Feeling good, happy, and proud: A meta-analysis of positive ethnic-racial affect and adjustment. *Child Development, 85* (1), 77–102.

Rizk, B. J. (2015). Milagro Teatro in Portland, Oregon: An interview with founders and artistic director Dañel Malán, José González, and Olga Sánchez. *Latin American Theatre Review, 48* (2), 119–134.

Rizzini, I., & Bush, M. (2013). Affirming the young democracy youth engagement in Rio de Ianeiro. In M. de los Angeles Torres, I. Rizzini & N. Del Rio (Eds.), *Citizens in the present: Youth civic engagement in the Americas* (pp. 60–89). Urbana, IL: University of Illinois Press.

Rogers, A. (2015). Geographies of the performing arts: Landscapes, places and cities. *Geography Compass, 6* (2), 60–75.

Rogers, J., Mediratta, K., & Shah, S. (2012). Building power, learning democracy youth organizing as a site of civic development. *Review of Research in Education, 36* (1), 43–66.

Rogers, K., & Sanders III, J. H. (2012). Moving across the margins: A review of stigma and perseverance in the lives of boys who dance. *Journal of LGBT Youth, 9* (2), 178–181.

Rohd, M. (1998). *Theatre for community, conflict & dialogue: The Hope is Vital training manual.* Portsmouth, NH: Heinemann.

Rondón, J., Campbell, J., Galway, K., & Leavey, G. (2014). Exploring the needs of socially excluded young men. *Children & Society, 28* (2), 104–115.

Ross, L., Capra, S., Carpenter, L., Hubbell, J., & Walker, K. (2015). *Dilemmas in youth work and youth development practice.* New York: Routledge.

Rossiter, K., Gray, J., Kontos, P., Keightley, M., Colantonio, A., & Gilbert, J. (2008). From page to stage dramaturgy and the art of interdisciplinary translation. *Journal of Health Psychology, 13* (2), 277–286.

Roth, J. L., Malone, L. M., & Brooks-Gunn, J. (2010). Does the amount of participation in afterschool programs relate to developmental outcomes? A review of the literature. *American Journal of Community Psychology, 45* (3-4), 310–324.

Rothman, A. J., & Haydon, K. C. (2006). Strategies to motivate behavior change: How can we mobilize adults to promote Positive Youth Development? In E. G. Clary & J. E.

Rhodes (Eds.), *Mobilizing adults for positive youth development: Strategies for closing the gap between beliefs and behaviors* (pp. 101–114). New York: Springer.

Rovito, A. (2012). *A case study of outside looking in (OLI): A youth development through recreation program for aboriginal peoples* (Doctoral dissertation). University of Ottawa, Canada).

Rovito, A., & Giles, A. R. (2016). Outside looking in: Resisting colonial discourses of Aboriginality. *Leisure Sciences, 38* (1), 1–16.

Rubin, D. I. (2012). Critical pedagogy and dialectical thought in the secondary English classroom. *Theory in Action, 5* (2), 70–81.

Ruch, W., Weber, M., & Park, N. (2015). Character strengths in children and adolescents. *European Journal of Psychological Assessment, 30* (1), 57–64.

Ruck, M., Harris, A., Fine, M., & Freudenberg, N. (2008). Youth experiences of surveillance. In M. Flynn & D. C. Brotherton (Eds.), *Globalizing the streets: Cross-cultural perspectives on youth, social control, and empowerment* (pp. 15–30). New York: Columbia University Press.

Runswick-Cole, K., & Goodley, D. (2013). Resilience: A disability studies and community psychology approach. *Social and Personality Psychology Compass, 7* (2), 67–78.

Rusk, N., Larson, R. W., Raffaelli, M., Walker, K., Washington, L., Gutierrez, V., . . . Perry, S. C. (2013). Positive youth development in organized programs: How teens learn to manage emotions. In *Research, applications, and interventions for children and adolescents* (pp. 247–261). Rotterdam: Springer Netherlands.

Rutten, E. A., Biesta, G. J., Deković, M., Stams, G. J. J., Schuengel, C., & Verweel, P. (2010). Using forum theatre in organised youth soccer to positively influence antisocial and prosocial behaviour: A pilot study. *Journal of Moral Education, 39* (1), 65–78.

Ryan, C., & Andrews, N. (2009). An investigation into the choral singer's experience of music performance anxiety. *Journal of Research in Music Education, 57* (2), 108–126.

Sabato, T. M., & Caine, D. (2016). Epidemiology of injury in community club and youth sport organizations. In D. Caine & L. Purcell (Eds.), *Injury in pediatric and adolescent sports*, 33–49. Basel, Switzerland: Springer International Publishing.

Sabo, D., & Veliz, P. (2008). *Go out and play: Youth sports in America*. New York: Women's Sports Foundation.

Saldaña, J. (2011). *Ethnotheatre: Research from page to stage* (Vol. 3). Walnut Creek, CA: Left Coast Press.

Salmon, D., & Rickaby, C. (2014). City of one: A qualitative study examining the participation of young people in care in a theatre and music initiative. *Children & Society, 28* (1), 30–41.

Salusky, I., Larson, R. W., Griffith, A., Wu, J., Raffaelli, M., Sugimura, N., & Guzman, M. (2014). How adolescents develop responsibility: What can be learned from youth programs. *Journal of Research on Adolescence, 24* (3), 417–430.

Sanchez, E. N., Aujla, I. J., & Nordin-Bates, S. (2013). Cultural background variables in dance talent development: Findings from the UK centres for advanced training. *Research in Dance Education, 14* (3), 260–278.

Sánchez, P. (2007). Urban immigrant students: How transnationalism shapes their world learning. *The Urban Review, 39* (5), 489–517.

Sanders, M. (2004). Urban odyssey: Theatre of the oppressed and talented minority youth. *Journal for the Education of the Gifted, 28* (2), 218–241.

Sanderson, R. C., & Richards, M. H. (2010). The after-school needs and resources of a low-income urban community: Surveying youth and parents for community change. *American Journal of Community Psychology, 45* (3-4), 430–440.

Sandhu, P. (2015). Resisting linguistic marginalization in professional spaces: Constructing multi-layered oppositional stances. *Applied Linguistics Review, 6* (3), 369–391.

Santos, F. (2013). Along with dolls and stuffed animals, making time for immigration activism. *The New York Times*, p. A11.

Savage, J. (2007). *Teenage: The prehistory of youth culture 1875–1945*. London: Penguin.

Scales, P. C. (2006).The world of adults today: Implications for positive youth development. In E. G. Clary & J. E. Rhodes (Eds.), *Mobilizing adults for positive youth development: Strategies for closing the gap between beliefs and behaviors* (pp. 41–51). New York: Springer.

Scales, P. C., Syvertsen, A. K., Benson, P. L., Roehlkepartain, E. C., & Sesma, A., Jr. (2014). Relation of spiritual development to youth health and well-being: Evidence from a global study. In A. Ben-Arieh & F. Casas (Eds.), *Handbook of child well-being* (pp. 1101–1135). Rotterdam: Springer Netherlands.

Schaedler, M. T. (2010). Boal's Theater of the Oppressed and how to derail real-life tragedies with imagination. *New Directions for Youth Development, 2010* (125), 141–151.

Schaillée, H., Theeboom, M., & Van Cauwenberg, J. (2015). What makes a difference for disadvantaged girls? Investigating the interplay between group composition and positive youth development in sport. *Social Inclusion, 3* (3), 51–66.

Schiepers, V. (2012). *Challenging youth: Establishing supportive relationships with youth in south Los Angeles* (Doctoral dissertation). University of Humanistic Studies, Utrecht University, Netherlands).

Schilling, T., Martinek, T., & Carson, S. (2007). Youth leaders' perceptions of commitment to a responsibility-based physical activity program. *Research Quarterly for Exercise and Sport, 78* (2), 48–60.

Schneider, W. (2008). *Living with stories: Telling, re-telling, and remembering*. Logan: Utah State University Press. Retrieved from http://digitalcommons.usu.edu/usupress_pubs/56

Schonert-Reichl, K. (Ed.). (2014). *Mindfulness in adolescence: New directions for youth development, number 142*. New York: John Wiley & Sons.

Schroeder-Arce, R. (2016). Zoot suit: Latino/a youth inclusion and exclusion on Texas stages. *Youth Theatre Journal, 30* (1), 35–49.

Schusler, T. M. (2013). Environmental action and positive youth development. In G. A. Boyd & P. R. Eddy (Eds.), *Across the spectrum* (pp. 94–115). Grand Rapids, MI: Baker Publisher.

Schutzman, M., & Cohen-Cruz, J. (1994). Introduction. In J. Cohen-Cruz & M. Schulzman (Eds.), *A Boal companion: Dialogues on theatre and cultural politics* (pp. 1–16). New York: Routledge.

Schweigman, K., Soto, C., Wright, S., & Unger, J. (2011). The relevance of cultural activities in ethnic identity among California Native American youth. *Journal of Psychoactive Drugs, 43* (4), 343–348.

Seaton, E. K., Neblett, E. W., Upton, R. D., Hammond, W. P., & Sellers, R. M. (2011). The moderating capacity of racial identity between perceived discrimination and psychological well-being over time among African American youth. *Child Development, 82* (6), 1850–1867.

Sefton-Green, J. (2006). *New spaces for learning: Developing the ecology of out-of-school education*. McGill, South Australia: Hawke Research Institute for Sustainable Societies.

Sefton-Green, J. (2013). *Learning at not-school: A review of study, theory, and advocacy for education in non-formal settings.* Cambridge, MA: MIT Press.

Segal, E. A. (2011). Social empathy: A model built on empathy, contextual understanding, and social responsibility that promotes social justice. *Journal of Social Service Research, 37* (3), 266–277.

Sekhon, N. (2016). *Blue on Black: An empirical assessment of police shootings.* Available at SSRN. Retrieved from http://papers.ssrn.com/sol3/Papers.cfm?abstract_id=2700724

Semán, P., & Vila, P. (Eds.). (2012). *Youth identities and Argentine popular music: Beyond tango.* New York: Palgrave Macmillan.

Seo, D. C., & Sa, J. (2010). A school-based intervention for diabetes risk reduction. *New England Journal of Medicine, 363* (July), 443–453.

Serido, J., Borden, L. M., & Perkins, D. F. (2011). Moving beyond youth voice. *Youth & Society, 43* (1), 44–63.

Sevdalis, V., & Raab, M. (2014). Empathy in sports, exercise, and the performing arts. *Psychology of Sport and Exercise, 15* (2), 173–179.

Shailor, J. (Ed.). (2011a). *Performing new lives: Prison theatre.* London: Jessica Kingsley Publishers.Shaughnessy, N. (2012). *Applying performance: Live art, socially engaged theatre and affective practice.* New York: Palgrave Macmillan.

Shailor, J. (2011b). Introduction. In J. Shallor (Ed.), *Performing new lives: Prison theatre* (pp. 17–32). London: Jessica Kingsley Publishers.

Shange, S. (2012). "This is not a protest": Managing dissent in racialized San Francisco. *Black California dreamin': The crises of California's African-American communities.* Santa Barbara, CA: University of California, Center for Black Studies Research.

Shank, M., & Schirch, L. (2008). Strategic arts-based peacebuilding. *Peace & Change, 33* (2), 217–242.

Shaw, S. (2014). *Working with Australian church youth to respond to climate change: Improvisational drama as an educational tool.* Retrieved from http://www.jri.org.uk/wp/wp-content/uploads/Shaw-JRI-Briefing-26.pdf

Shaw-Raudoy, K., & McGregor, C. (2013). Co-learning in youth-adult emancipatory partnerships: The way forward? *International Journal of Child, Youth and Family Studies, 4* (3.1), 391–408.

Shay, A. (2006*). Choreographing identities: Folk dance, ethnicity and festival in the United States and Canada.* Jefferson, NC: McFarland.

Shek, D. T., & Sun, R. C. (2014). Promotion of positive youth development and family quality of life in Chinese adolescents. In D. Shek, R. C. Sun, & C. Ma (Eds.), *Chinese adolescents in Hong Kong* (pp. 221–237). Singapore:.

Shelton, J. (2015, January). Understanding programmatic barriers for homeless transgender youth through the lens of cisnormativity. In *Society for Social Work and Research 19th annual conference: The social and behavioral importance of increased longevity.* New Orleans, LA: SSWR.

Shepard, B. (2012*). Play, creativity, and social movements: If I can't dance, it's not my revolution.* New York: Routledge.

Sheppard, G. L. (2013). Closing. In M. S. Hanley, G. W. Nobit, G. L. Sheppard, & T. Barone (Eds.), *Culturally relevant arts education for social justice: A way out* (pp. 224–227). New York: Routledge.

Shernoff, D. J., & Vandell, D. L. (2007). Engagement in after-school program activities: Quality of experience from the perspective of participants. *Journal of Youth and Adolescence, 36* (7), 891–903.

Sherrod, L. (2007). Civic engagement as an expression of positive youth development. In R. K. Silbereison & R. M. Lerner (Eds.), *Approaches to positive youth development* (pp. 59–74). Thousand Oaks, CA: SAGE.

Shiller, J. T. (2013). Preparing for democracy: How community-based organizations build civic engagement among urban youth. *Urban Education, 48* (1), 69–91.

Shinn, M., & Yoshikawa, H. (Eds.). (2008). *Toward positive youth development: Transforming schools and community programs.* New York: Oxford University Press.

Shohat, E., & Stam, R. (2014). *Unthinking Eurocentrism: Multiculturalism and the media.* New York: Routledge.

Siapno, J. (2012). Dance and martial arts in Timor Leste: The performance of resilience in a post-conflict environment. *Journal of Intercultural Studies, 33* (4), 427–443.

Sibthorp, J., Bialeschki, M. D., Stuart, C., & Phelan, J. (2012). Youth work across two diverse domains of practice. In D. Fusco (Ed.), *Advancing youth work: Current trends, critical questions* (pp. 181–189). New York: Routledge.

Sidford, H. (2011). *Arts and culture philanthropy: Fusing arts, culture and social change.* . Washington, DC: National Committee for Responsive Philanthropy.

Silbereisen, R. K., & Lerner, R. M. (Eds). (2007). *Approaches to positive youth development* (1st ed.). Thousand Oaks, CA: SAGE.

Silberg, D. N. (2012). *The utilization of movement and dance to support children in the aftermath of community disaster* (Doctoral dissertation). Drexel University, Philadelphia, PA.

Silver, A. (2012). Aging into exclusion and social transparency: Undocumented immigrant youth and the transition to adulthood. *Latino Studies, 10* (4), 499–522.

Simmonds, J. G., & Southcott, J. E. (2012). Stage fright and joy: Performers in relation to the troupe, audience, and beyond. *International Journal of Applied Psychoanalytic Studies, 9* (4), 318–329.

Singh, A. A. (2013). Transgender youth of color and resilience: Negotiating oppression and finding support. *Sex Roles, 68* (11-12), 690–702.

Singh, A. A., Meng, S. E., & Hansen, A. W. (2014). "I am my own gender": Resilience strategies of trans youth. *Journal of Counseling & Development, 92* (2), 208–218.

Singhal, A. (2004). Entertainment-education through participatory theater: Freirean strategies for empowering the oppressed. In A. Singhal, M. J. Cody, E. M. Rogers, & M. Sabido (Eds.), *Entertainment-education and social change: History, research, and practice* (pp. 377–398). Mahwah, NJ: Lawrence Erlbaum Associates.

Singing. (n. d.). In *Urbandictionary.com.* Retrieved from http://www.urbandictionary.com/define.php?term=singing

Skinner, E. A. (2012). *Aboriginal youth, hip hop, and the right to the city: A participatory action research project* (Doctoral dissertation). University of Manitoba, Canada).

Sládková, J., Mangado, S. M. G., & Quinteros, J. R. (2012). Lowell immigrant communities in the climate of deportations. *Analyses of Social Issues and Public Policy, 12* (1), 78–95.

Slater, J. (2013). Research with dis/abled youth: Taking a critical disability 'critically young' positionality. In T. Curran & K. Runswick-Cole (Eds.), *Disabled children's childhood studies: Critical approaches in a global context* (pp. 180–195). New York: Palgrave Macmillan.

Slater, L. (2014). *'Calling our spirits home': Indigenous cultural festivals and the making of a good life.* Retrieved from http://ro.uow.edu.au/lhapapers/1798/

Sloman, A. (2012). Using participatory theatre in international community development. *Community Development Journal, 47* (1), 42–57.

Smith, A., West, P., & Bozeman, K. (2015). *4-H: Putting the pieces together for positive youth development.* Retrieved from http://digitalcommons.georgiasouthern.edu/nyar_savannah/2015/2015/180/

Smith, E. P., Osgood, D. W., Caldwell, L., Hynes, K., & Perkins, D. F. (2013). Measuring collective efficacy among children in community-based afterschool programs: Exploring pathways toward prevention and positive youth development. *American Journal of Community Psychology, 52* (1-2), 27–40.

Smith, H. (2015). *Neighborhood stories: Creative placemaking for multicultural communities.* Retrieved from the University of Minnesota Digital Conservancy, http://hdl.handle.net/11299/174670

Smith, L. (2012). Sparkling divas! Therapeutic music video groups with at-risk youth. *Music Therapy Perspectives, 30* (1), 17–24.

Smyth, J., Down, B., & McInerney, P. (2014). *The socially just school: Making space for youth to speak back* (Vol. 29). New York: Springer.

Smyth, J., & Robinson, J. (2015). 'Give me air not shelter': Critical tales of a policy case of student re-engagement from beyond school. *Journal of Education Policy, 30* (2), 220–236.

Snyder, M. (2006). Promoting positive youth development: Challenges posed and opportunities provided. In E. G. Clary & J. E. Rhodes (Eds.), *Mobilizing adults for positive youth development: Strategies for closing the gap between beliefs and behaviors* (pp. 257–260). New York: Springer.

Snyder, D. (2008). *The rules that rule their worlds: Urban youth deconstruct their antagonists through Theatre of the Oppressed.* ProQuest. Dissertation, New York University, New York.

Snyder-Young, D. (2012). Youth theatre as cultural artifact: Social antagonism in urban high school environments. *Youth Theatre Journal, 26* (2), 173–183.

Snyder-Young, D. (2013). *Theatre of good intentions: Challenges and hopes for theatre and social change.* New York: Springer.

Soley, G., & Spelke, E. S. (2016). Shared cultural knowledge: Effects of music on young children's social preferences. *Cognition, 148* (March), 106–116.

Solinger, R., Fox, M., & Irani, K. (Eds.). (2010). *Telling stories to change the world: Global voices on the power of narrative to build community and make social justice claims.* New York: Routledge.

Sonn, C. C., Quayle, A. F., Belanji, B., & Baker, A. M. (2015). Responding to racialization through arts practice: The case of Participatory Theater. *Journal of Community Psychology, 43* (2), 244–259.

Sonn, C. C., Quayle, A. F., Mackenzie, C., & Law, S. F. (2014). Negotiating belonging in Australia through storytelling and encounter. *Identities, 21* (5), 551–569.

Sou, S. L. C., DeAngelo, D., Jones, M., & Veth, M. (2012). *How to engage young people: Lessons from Lowell, MA.* Harvard University, Berkman Center Research Publication, (2013–2019).

Southcott, J., & Joseph, D. (2013). Community, commitment and the ten 'command-ments': Singing in the Coro Furlan, Melbourne, Australia. *International Journal of Community Music, 6* (1), 5–21.

Spencer, G., & Doull, M. (2015). Examining concepts of power and agency in research with young people. *Journal of Youth Studies, 18* (7), 900–913.

Spencer, M. B., & Spencer, T. R. (2014). Invited commentary: Exploring the promises, intri-cacies, and challenges to positive youth development. *Journal of Youth and Adolescence, 43* (6), 1027–1035.

Spencer, M. B., & Swanson, D. P. (2013). Opportunities and challenges to the develop-ment of healthy children and youth living in diverse communities. *Development and Psychopathology, 25* (4pt2), 1551–1566.

Spero, A. M. (2012). Human rights education and the performing arts. *Peace Review, 24* (1), 28–35.

Spracklen, K., Richter, A., & Spracklen, B. (2013). The eventization of leisure and the strange death of alternative Leeds. *City: Analysis of Urban Trends, Culture, Theory, Policy, Action, 17* (2), 164–178.

Sprague Martinez, L. S., Reich, A. J., Flores, C. A., Ndulue, U. J., Brugge, D., Gute, D. M., & Peréa, F. C. (2017). Critical Discourse, Applied Inquiry and Public Health Action with Urban Middle School Students: Lessons Learned Engaging Youth in Critical Service-Learning. *Journal of Community Practice, 25* (1), 68–89.

Stanton, C. R. (2012). Context and community. In *The new politics of the textbook* (pp. 173–194). Rotterdam, Netherlands: SensePublishers.

Stanton, N. (2015). *Innovation in youth work: Thinking in practice.* London: YMCA George Williams College.

Stanton-Salazar, R. D. (2011). A social capital framework for the study of institutional agents and their role in the empowerment of low-status students and youth. *Youth & Society, 43* (3), 1066–1109.

Staples, L. (2012). Community organizing for social justice: Grassroots groups for power. *Social Work with Groups, 35* (3), 287–296.

Stark, K. K. (2009). Connecting to dance: Merging theory with practice. *Journal of Dance Education, 9* (2), 61–68.

Stauber, L. S. (2012). *Chicanismo in the new generation: "Youth, identity, power" in the 21st century borderlands* (Doctoral dissertation). University of Arizona, Tempe.

Stephenson M. O., & Tate, A. S. (Eds.). (2015a). *Arts and community change: Exploring cul-tural development policies, practices and dilemmas.* New York: Routledge.

Stephenson, M. O., & Tate, A. S. (2015b). Introduction: The place of the arts in commun-ity identity and social change. In M. O. Stephenson, Jr. & A. S. Tate (Eds.), *Arts and community change: Exploring cultural development policies, practices and dilemmas* (pp. 1–10). New York: Routledge.

Stewart, T., & Alrutz, M. (2012). Meaningful relationships: Cruxes of university- com-munity partnerships for sustainable and happy engagement. *Journal of Community Engagement and Scholarship, 5* (1), 44–55.

Stodolska, M., Sharaievska, I., Tainsky, S., & Ryan, A. (2014). Minority youth participation in an organized sport program: Needs, motivations, and facilitators. *Journal of Leisure Research, 46* (5), 612–634.

Strachan, L., & Davies, K. (2015). Click! Using photo elicitation to explore youth experiences and positive youth development in sport. *Qualitative Research in Sport, Exercise and Health, 7* (2), 170–191.

Strand, K. (2009). Both sides of the coin: Experienced musicians tell of lives lived and shared. In J. L. Kerchner & C. R. Abril (Eds.), *Musical experience in our lives: Things we learn and meanings we make* (pp. 297–311). Lanham, MD: Rowman & Littlefield.

Strobel, K., Kirshner, B., O'Donoghue, J., & Wallin McLaughlin, M. (2008). Qualities that attract urban youth to after-school settings and promote continued participation. *The Teachers College Record, 110* (8), 1677–1705.

Strommen, M. P., Jones, K., & Rahn, D. (Eds.). (2011). *Youth ministry that transforms.* Grand Rapids, MI: Zondervan.

Strong, W. B., Malina, R. M., Blimkie, C. J., Daniels, S. R., Dishman, R. K., Gutin, B., . . . Rowland, T. (2005). Evidence based physical activity for school-age youth. *The Journal of Pediatrics, 146* (6), 732–737.

Struch, R. (2011). *Re-imagining community from the ruins: Explorations of the intersections of the theatre of the oppressed joker, community organizer, and participatory action researcher* (Master's thesis). University of Southern California, Los Angeles.

Stuart, J. (2010). Youth as knowledge producers: Towards changing gendered patterns in rural schools with participatory arts-based approaches to HIV and AIDS. *Agenda, 24* (84), 53–65.

Subrahmanyam, K., & Smahel, D. (2010). *Digital youth: The role of media in development.* New York: Springer Science & Business Media.

Sue, J. L., & Craig, W. M. (2014). *Connecting research and practice in youth mentoring. Do relationships matter? An examination of a school-based intergenerational mentoring program* (Master's thesis). Queens University, Kingston, Canada.

Sullivan, F. M. (2015). 5 Diverse urban youth need a wide range of program opportunities in leadership. One size does not fit all. In M. P. Evans & K. K. Abowitz (Eds.), *Engaging youth in leadership for social and political change* (pp. 59–72). San Francisco, CA: Jossey-Bass Publishers.

Sullivan, J., & Lloyd, R. S. (2006). The Forum Theatre of Augusto Boal: A dramatic model for dialogue and community-based environmental science. *Local Environment, 11* (6), 627–646.

Sullivan, J., Petronella, S., Brooks, E., Murillo, M., Primeau, L., & Ward, J. (2008). Theatre of the oppressed and environmental justice communities: A transformational therapy for the body politic. *Journal of Health Psychology, 13* (2), 166–179.

Sullivan, P. (2016, February 6). A philanthropist drills down to discover why programs work. *The New York Times,* p. D4.

Sun, J., Buys, N. J., & Merrick, J. (2012). Community singing: What does that have to do with health? *International Journal of Adolescent Medicine Health, 24* (4). (Online).

Sun, R. C., & Hui, E. K. (2012). Cognitive competence as a positive youth development construct: A conceptual review. *The Scientific World Journal,* 2012. Retrieved from http://www.hindawi.com/journals/tswj/2012/210953/abs/

Sung, K. K. (2015). "Hella ghetto!" (Dis)locating race and class consciousness in youth discourses of ghetto spaces, subjects and schools. *Race Ethnicity and Education, 18* (3), 363–395.

Swedeen, B. L., Carter, E. W., & Molfenter, N. (2010). Getting everyone involved: Identifying transition opportunities for youth with severe disabilities. *Teaching Exceptional Children, 43* (2), 38–49.

Sy, A., Greaney, M., Nigg, C., & Hirose-Wong, S. M. (2015). Developing a measure to evaluate a positive youth development program for native Hawaiians: The Hui Mālama o ke Kai rubrics of Hawaiian values. *Asia-Pacific Journal of Public Health, 27* (2), NP1517-NP1528.

Syed, M., Azmitia, M., & Cooper, C. R. (2011). Identity and academic success among underrepresented ethnic minorities: An interdisciplinary review and integration. *Journal of Social Issues, 67* (3), 442–468.

Symonds, D., & Taylor, M. (2014). *Gestures of music theater: The performativity of song and dance.* New York: Oxford University Press.

Taft, J. K., & Gordon, H. R. (2013). Youth activists, youth councils, and constrained democracy. *Education, Citizenship and Social Justice, 8* (1), 87–100.

Tansel, C. B. (2015). Deafening silence? Marxism, international historical sociology and the spectre of Eurocentrism. *European Journal of International Relations, 21* (1), 76–100.

Tarasoff, L. A., Epstein, R., Green, D. C., Anderson, S., & Ross, L. E. (2014). Using interactive theatre to help fertility providers better understand sexual and gender minority patients. *Medical Humanities, 40* (2), 135–141.

Taylor, J. (2012). Queerious youth: An empirical study of a queer youth cultural festival and its participants. *Journal of Sociology, 50* (3), 283–298.

Taylor, J., Dworin, J., Buell, B., Sepinuck, T., Palidofsky, M., Tofteland, C., . . . Trounstine, J. (2011). *Performing new lives: Prison theatre.* London: Jessica Kingsley Publishers.

Taylor, J. A. (2008). From the stage to the classroom: The performing arts and social studies. *The History Teacher, 41* (2), 235–248.

Taylor, L. E. (2014). *Acting strengths: The development of resilience and character strengths in actors* (Masters thesis). Penn State University, State College, PA.

Taylor, P. Applied theatre/drama: An e-debate in 2004: Viewpoints. *RIDE: Research in Drama and Education, 11* (1), 90–95. 2006.

Taylor, T. (2012). From social education to positive youth development. In P. Loncie, M. Cuconado, V. Muniglia, & A. Wather (Eds.), *The history of youth work in Europe: Relevance for today's youth work policy* (pp. 117–127). Bristol, UK: Policy Press.

Teater, B., & Baldwin, M. (2012). *Social work in the community: Making a difference.* Bristol, UK: Policy Press.

Teitle, J. R. (2012). *Theorizing hang out: Unstructured youth programs and the politics of representation* (Doctoral dissertation). University of Iowa, Iowa City, IA.

Tello, J., Cervantes, R. C., Cordova, D., & Santos, S. M. (2010). Joven noble: Evaluation of a culturally focused youth development program. *Journal of Community Psychology, 38* (6), 799–811.

Te Riele, K. (2010). Philosophy of hope: Concepts and applications for working with marginalized youth. *Journal of Youth Studies, 13* (1), 35–46.

Thannoo, B. (2012). Rap music in Mauritius: Forging 'connective marginalities' and resistance. *Wasafiri, 27* (4), 35–41.

Tham-Agyekum, E. K., & Loggoh, B. (2011). A review of the use of indigenous communication systems in development work: The case of drama, theatre and puppet shows. *Elixir Social Science, 33,* 2252–2255.

Thaut, M. H., & Hoemberg, V. (Eds.). (2014). *Handbook of neurologic music therapy.* New York: Oxford University Press.

Theorell, T., Lennartsson, A. K., Madison, G., Mosing, M. A., & Ullén, F. (2015). Predictors of continued playing or singing–from childhood and adolescence to adult years. *Acta Paediatrica, 104* (3), 274–284.

Tholley, I. S., Meng, Q. G., & Chung, P. W. (2012, February). Robot dancing: What makes a dance? *Advanced Materials Research, 403,* 4901–4909.

Thomas, N. (2012). *Children's participation: Challenges for research and practice.* Retrieved from http://epubs.scu.edu.au/ccyp_pubs/50/

Thomas, N. D., & León, R. J. (2012). Breaking barriers: Using poetry as a tool to enhance diversity understanding with youth and adults. *Journal of Poetry Therapy, 25* (2), 83–93.

Thomas, T. L. (2013). *"Hey, those are teenagers and they are doing stuff": Youth participation in community development* (Doctoral dissertation). University of Pittsburgh, PA).

Thompson, C. C. (2012). The lessons of non-formal learning for urban youth. *The Educational Forum, 76* (1), 58–68.

Thompson, J. (Ed.). (1998). *Prison theatre: Perspectives and practices.* London: Jessica Kingsley Publishers.

Tienda, M., & Wilson, W. J. (2002). Comparative perspectives of urban youth: Challenges for normative development. In M. Tienda & W. J. Wilson (Eds.), *Youth in cities: A national perspective* (pp. 3–18). New York: Cambridge University Press.

Tillis, S. (2003). East, west, and world theatre. *Asian Theatre Journal, 20* (1), 71–87.

Tilton, J. (2010). *Dangerous or endangered? Race and the politics of youth in urban America.* New York: NYU Press.

Timpe, Z. C., & Lunkenheimer, E. (2015). The long-term economic benefits of natural mentoring relationships for youth. *American Journal of Community Psychology, 56* (1-2), 12–24.

Tinsley, B., Wilson, S., & Spencer, M. B. (2013). Hip-hop culture, youth creativity, and the generational crossroads from a human development perspective. In C. Milbrath & C. Lightfoot (Eds.), *Art and human development* (pp. 83–99). New York: Psychology Press.

To, S. M., Tam, H. L., Ngai, S. S. Y., & Sung, W. L. (2014). Sense of meaningfulness, sources of meaning, and self-evaluation of economically disadvantaged youth in Hong Kong: Implications for youth development programs. *Children and Youth Services Review, 47* (Part 3), 352–361.

Tocci, L. (2007). *The Proscenium Cage: Critical case studies in US prison theatre programs.* Ambria, NY: Cambria Press.

Toivanen, T., Halkilahti, L., & Ruismäki, H. (2013). Creative pedagogy–Supporting children's creativity through drama. *The European Journal of Social & Behavioural Sciences, 7*(4), 1168–1179.

Tolan, P. (2014). Future directions for positive development intervention research. *Journal of Clinical Child & Adolescent Psychology, 43* (4), 686–694.

Tolliver, W. F., Hadden, B. R., Snowden, F., & Brown-Manning, R. (2016). Police killings of unarmed Black people: Centering race and racism in human behavior and the social environment content. *Journal of Human Behavior in the Social Environment, 26* (3-4), 279–286.

Torre, M., & Fine, M. (2006). Researching and resisting: Democratic policy research by and for youth. In S. Ginwright, P. Noguera & J. Cammarota (Eds.), *Beyond resistance* (pp. 269–285). New York: Routledge.

Torres-Fleming, A., Valdes, P., & Pillai, S. (2010). *2010 field scan*. Brooklyn, NY: Funders' Collaborative on Youth Organizing.

Travis R., Jr. (2013). Rap music and the empowerment of today's youth: Evidence in everyday music listening, music therapy, and commercial rap music. *Child and Adolescent Social Work Journal, 30* (2), 139–167.

Travis, R., & Leech, T. G. (2014). Empowerment-based positive youth development: A new understanding of healthy development for African American youth. *Journal of Research on Adolescence, 24* (1), 93–116.

Trayes, J., Harré, N., & Overall, N. C. (2012). A youth performing arts experience: Psychological experiences, recollections, and the desire to do it again. *Journal of Adolescent Research, 27* (2), 155–182.

Tremblay, M. (2016). Cultural resistance. *The Wiley Blackwell encyclopedia of race, ethnicity, and nationalism*. New York: John Wiley.

Trevarthen, C., & Malloch, S. N. (2000). The dance of wellbeing: Defining the musical therapeutic effect. *Nordisk Tidsskrift for Musikkterapi, 9* (2), 3–17.

Trinidad, A. M. O. (2012). Critical indigenous pedagogy of place: A framework to indigenize a youth food justice movement. *Journal of Indigenous Social Development, 1* (1). Retrieved from http://scholarspace.manoa.hawaii.edu/handle/10125/21977

Trounstine, J. (2001). *Shakespeare behind bars: The power of drama in a women's prison*. New York: Macmillan.

Tsai, K. C. (2012). Dance with critical thinking and creative thinking in the classroom. *Journal of Sociological Research, 3* (2), Pages-312. http://www.macrothink.org/journal/index.php/jsr/article/view/2323

Tsang, S. K., Hui, E. K., & Law, B. (2012). Positive identity as a positive youth development construct: A conceptual review. *The Scientific World Journal*, 2012. Retrieved from http://www.hindawi.com/journals/tswj/2012/529691/abs/

Tshabalala, B. G., & Patel, C. J. (2010). The role of praise and worship activities in spiritual well-being: Perceptions of a pentecostal youth ministry group. *International Journal of Children's Spirituality, 15* (1), 73–82.

Tuck. E., & Yang, K. W. (Eds.). (2014). *Youth resistance research and theories of change*. New York: Routledge.

Turner, J. (2007). Making amends: An interventionist theatre programme with young offenders. *Research in Drama Education, 12* (2), 179–194.

Turnnidge, J., Côté, J., & Hancock, D. J. (2014). Positive youth development from sport to life: Explicit or implicit transfer? *Quest, 66* (2), 203–217.

Ungar, M. (2011). Community resilience for youth and families: Facilitative physical and social capital in contexts of adversity. *Children and Youth Services Review, 33* (9), 1742–1748.

Ungar, M. (2014). *Working with children and youth with complex needs: 20 skills to build resilience*. New York: Routledge.

Ungar, M., & Liebenberg, L. (2011). Assessing resilience across cultures using mixed methods: Construction of the child and youth resilience measure. *Journal of Mixed Methods Research, 5* (2), 126–149.

United Nation's Convention on the Rights of the Child (1989). New York: United Nations.

Updegraff, K. A., Umaña-Taylor, A. J., McHale, S. M., Wheeler, L. A., & Perez-Brena, N. J. (2012). Mexican-origin youth's cultural orientations and adjustment: Changes from early to late adolescence. *Child development, 83* (5), 1655–1671.

Urban, A. (2012). *Literacy in ACTion: Using theatre to read the word and the world through critical pedagogy, image theatre and comic creation with youth* (Doctoral dissertation). University of Alberta, Canada.

Urban, J. B., Lewin-Bizan, S., & Lerner, R. M. (2009). The role of neighborhood ecological assets and activity involvement in youth developmental outcomes: Differential impacts of asset poor and asset rich neighborhoods. *Journal of Applied Developmental Psychology, 30* (5), 601–614.

Urban, M. (2016). *New Orleans rhythm and blues after Katrina: Music, magic and myth.* New York: Palgrave Macmillan.

Vadeboncoeur, J. A. (2006). Engaging young people: Learning in informal contexts. *Review of Research in Education, 30* (3), 239–278.

Vaiouli, P., Grimmet, K., & Ruich, L. J. (2015). "Bill is now singing": Joint engagement and the emergence of social communication of three young children with autism. *Autism, 15* (10), 73–83.

Vance, J. L. (2014). *Findings from the field: A pedagogical and cultural study of the North American Drum and Bugle Corps experience* (Doctoral dissertation). Teachers College, Columbia University, New York City).

Vandell, D. L., Larson, R. W., Mahoney, J. L., & Watts, T. W. (2015). Children's organized activities. In R. M. Lerner, L. S. Lieben, & U. Mueller (Eds.), *Handbook of child psychology and developmental science* (Vol. 4, pp. 305–344). New York: John Wiley & Sons.

Vandell, D. L., Pierce, K. M., & Dadisman, K. (2005). Out-of-school settings as a developmental context for children and youth. *Advances in Child Development and Behavior, 33* (1), 43–77.

Van Der Hoeven, A. (2014). Remembering the popular music of the 1990s: Dance music and the cultural meanings of decade-based nostalgia. *International Journal of Heritage Studies,* 20 (3), 316–330.

Van de Water, M. (2012). *Theatre, youth, and culture: A critical and historical exploration.* New York: Palgrave Macmillan.

Van Doorslaer, L. (2012). *The powerful concept of 'eurocentrism'.* Retrieved from https://lirias.kuleuven.be/handle/123456789/386983

Vasudevan, D. S. (2015). *The quest for mastery: Positive youth development through out-of-school programs.* Cambridge, MA: Harvard Education Press.

Vasudevan, L., Stageman, D., Rodriguez, K., Fernandez, E., & Dattatreyan, E. G. (2010). Authoring new narratives with youth at the intersection of the arts and justice. *Penn GSE Perspectives on Urban Education, 7* (1), 54–65.

Vaughan, U. (2012). *Rebel dance, renegade stance: Timba music and Black identity in Cuba.* Ann Arbor, MI: University of Michigan Press.

Vaughn, B. (2005). Afro-Mexico: Blacks, indigenas, politics and the greater diaspora. S. Oboler & A. Dzidzienyo (Eds.), *Neither enemies nor friends: Latinos, Blacks, Afro-Latinos* (pp. 117–136). New York: Pagrave Macmillan.

Veltre, V. J., & Hadley, S. (2012). It's bigger than hip-hop. In S. Sadley & G. Yancy (Eds.), *Therapeutic uses of rap and hip-hop* (pp. 79–98). New York: Routledge.

Vera, A. (2014). Music, Eurocentrism and identity: The myth of the discovery of America in Chilean music history. *Advances in Historical Studies, 3* (05), 298–311.

Viesca, V. H. (2012). Native guns and stray bullets: Cultural activism and Filipino American rap music in post-riot Los Angeles. *Amerasia Journal, 38* (1), 113–142.

Vila, P. (Ed.). (2014). *Music and youth culture in Latin America: Identity construction processes from New York to Buenos Aires.* New York: Oxford University Press.

Vincent, A. P., & Christensen, D. A. (2015). Conversations with parents: A collaborative sport psychology program for parents in youth sport. *Journal of Sport Psychology in Action, 6* (2), 73–85.

Vine, C. (2013). "TIE and the Theatre of the Oppressed" revisited. In A. Jackson & C. Vine (Eds.), *Learning through theatre: The changing face of theatre in education third edition* (pp. 60–80). New York: Routledge.

Vinson, B. (2005). Afro-Mexican history: Trends and directions in scholarship. *History Compass, 3* (1), 1–14.

Wagaman, M. A. (2011). Social empathy as a framework for adolescent empowerment. *Journal of Social Service Research, 37* (3), 278–293.

Wagener, T. L., Fedele, D. A., Mignogna, M. R., Hester, C. N., & Gillaspy, S. R. (2012). Psychological effects of dance-based group exergaming in obese adolescents. *Pediatric obesity, 7* (5), e68-e74.

Waite, S. (2015). Put me in, coach: The political promise of competitive coaching. *Literacy in Composition Studies, 3* (1), 108–121.

Wald, J., & Losen, D. J. (2003). Defining and redirecting a school-to-prison pipeline. *New Directions for Youth Development, 2003* (99), 9–15.

Wales, P. (2012). Telling tales in and out of school: Youth performativities with digital storytelling. *Research in Drama Education: The Journal of Applied Theatre and Performance, 17* (4), 535–552.

Walker, I. J., & Nordin-Bates, S. M. (2010). Performance anxiety experiences of professional ballet dancers: The importance of control. *Journal of Dance Medicine & Science, 14* (4), 133–145.

Walker, I. J., Nordin-Bates, S. M., & Redding, E. (2010). Talent identification and development in dance: A review of the literature. *Research in Dance Education, 11* (3), 167–191.

Walker, K. C. (2011). The multiple roles that youth development program leaders adopt with youth. *Youth & Society, 43* (2), 635–655.

Wallace, M., Weybright, E., Rohner, B., & Crawford, J. (2015). *Over-involved parenting and competition in youth development programs.* Retrieved from https://research.wsulibs.wsu.edu/xmlui/handle/2376/5354

Walsh, D. (2008). Helping youth in underserved communities envision possible futures: An extension of the teaching personal and social responsibility model. *Research Quarterly for Exercise and Sport, 79* (2), 209–221.

Walsh, F. (2012). Facilitating family resilience: Relational resources for positive youth development in conditions of adversity. In M. Unger (Ed.), *The social ecology of resilience* (pp. 173–185). New York: Springer.

Wang, E. L. (2010). The beat of Boyle Street: Empowering aboriginal youth through music making. *New Directions for Youth Development, 2010* (125), 61–70.

Ward, S. A. (2013). African dance aesthetics in a K–12 dance setting: From history to social justice. *Journal of Physical Education, Recreation & Dance, 84* (7), 31–34.

Warrington, J., Hart, J., Daniels, D., & Block, P. (2016). *West African drum therapy and educational empowerment.* Retrieved from http://digitalcommons.georgiasouthern.edu/nyar_savannah/2016/2016/139/

Wartemann, G. (2009). Theatre as interplay: Processes of collective creativity in theatre for young audiences. *Youth Theatre Journal, 23* (1), 6–14.

Waterton, E., & Smith, L. (2010). The recognition and misrepresentation of community heritage. *International Journal of Heritage Studies, 16* (1-2), 4–15.

Watts, R. J., & Flanagan, C. (2007). Pushing the envelope on youth civic engagement: A developmental and liberation psychology perspective. *Journal of Community Psychology, 35* (6), 779–792.

Wei, S. (2013). A multitude of people singing together. *International Journal of Community Music, 6* (2), 183–188.

Weil, M., Reisch, M. S., & Ohmer, M. L. (Eds.). (2012). *The handbook of community practice.* Thousand Oaks, CA: SAGE.

Weiler, L. M., Haddock, S. A., Zimmerman, T. S., Henry, K. L., Krafchick, J. L., & Youngblade, L. M. (2015). Time-limited, structured youth mentoring and adolescent problem behaviors. *Applied Developmental Science, 19* (4), 196–205.

Weinstein, S. (2010). A unified poet alliance: The personal and social outcomes of youth spoken word poetry programming. *International Journal of Education & the Arts, 11* (2), 1–24.

Weis, L., & Dimitriadis, G. (2008). Dueling banjos: Shifting economic and cultural contexts in the lives of youth. *The Teachers College Record, 110* (10), 2290–2316.

Weiss, H. B., Little, P., & Bouffard, S. M. (2005). More than just being there: Balancing the participation equation. *New Directions for Youth Development, 2005* (105), 15–31.

Weiss, J. (2011). Valuing youth resistance before and after public protest. *International Journal of Qualitative Studies in Education, 24* (5), 595–599.

Wembe, C. G. (2013). *The significance of participation in educational theatre for young audiences: The case study of Themba Interactive Theatre Company* (Doctoral dissertation). University of the Witwatersrand, Johannesburg, South Africa).

Wengrower, H. (2015). Widening our lens: The implications of resilience for the professional identity and practice of dance movement therapists. *Body, Movement and Dance in Psychotherapy, 10* (3), 153–168.

Wernick, L. J., Kulick, A., & Woodford, M. R. (2014). How theater within a transformative organizing framework cultivates individual and collective empowerment among LGBTQQ youth. *Journal of Community Psychology, 42* (7), 838–853.

Wernick, L. J., Woodford, M. R., & Kulick, A. (2014). LGBTQQ youth using participatory action research and theater to effect change: Moving adult decision-makers to create youth-centered change. *Journal of Community Practice, 22* (1-2), 47–66.

Westheimer, J., & Kahne, J. (2000). Education for action: Preparing youth for participatory democracy. *The School Field, 11* (1), 21–40.

Wexler, L. (2011). Intergenerational dialogue exchange and action: Introducing a community-based participatory approach to connect youth, adults and elders in an Alaskan Native community. *International Journal of Qualitative Methods, 10* (3), 248–264.

Wexler, L., Jernigan, K., Mazzotti, J., Baldwin, E., Griffin, M., Joule, L., . . . CIPA Team. (2014). Lived challenges and getting through them: Alaska Native youth narratives as a way to understand resilience. *Health Promotion Practice, 15* (1), 10–17.

Whatley, S. (2007). Dance and disability: The dancer, the viewer and the presumption of difference. *Research in Dance Education, 8* (1), 5–25.

Whitaker, N. (2016). Student-created musical as a community of practice: A case study. *Music Education Research, 18* (1), 57–73.

White, D. J., Shoffner, A., Johnson, K., Knowles, N., & Mills, M. (2012). Advancing positive youth development: Perspectives of youth as researchers and evaluators. *Journal of Extension, 50* (4). Retrieved from http://www.joe.org/joe/2012august/pdf/JOE_v50_4a4.pdf

White, R. D., Wyn, J., & Albanese, P. (2008). *Youth and society: Exploring the social dynamics of youth experience.* South Melbourne, NZ: Oxford University Press.

Whitefield, P., & Alvarez, S. (2012). Rethinking organising and leadership. In S. Ledwith & L. L. Hansen (Eds.), *Gendering and diversifying trade union leadership* (pp. 162–180). New York: Routledge.

Whitehead, J., Telfer, H., & Lambert, J. (2013). *Values in youth sport and physical education.* New York: Routledge.

Whittaker, L. (2014). Refining the nation's "new gold": Music, youth development and neoliberalism in South Africa. *Culture, Theory and Critique, 55* (2), 233–256.

Wijnendaele, B. V. (2014). The politics of emotion in participatory processes of empowerment and change. *Antipode, 46* (1), 266–282.

Wilde, O., & Dowling, L. (2001). *The soul of man under socialism and selected critical prose.* London: Penguin.

Williams, J. L., Aiyer, S. M., Durkee, M. I., & Tolan, P. H. (2014). The protective role of ethnic identity for urban adolescent males facing multiple stressors. *Journal of Youth and Adolescence, 43* (10), 1728–1741.

Williams, J. L., Anderson, R. E., Francois, A. G., Hussain, S., & Tolan, P. H. (2014). Ethnic identity and positive youth development in adolescent males: A culturally integrated approach. *Applied Developmental Science, 18* (2), 110–122.

Wilson, B., & Hayhurst, L. (2009). Digital activism: Neoliberalism, the Internet, and sport for youth development. *Sociology of sport journal, 26* (1), 155–181.

Wilson, D. M., Gottfredson, D. C., Cross, A. B., Rorie, M., & Connell, N. (2010). Youth development in after-school leisure activities. *The Journal of Early Adolescence, 30* (5), 668–690.

Winn, M. T. (2011). *Girl time: Literacy, justice, and the school-to-prison pipeline. Teaching for social justice.* New York: Teachers College Press.

Winter, T. (2014). Beyond Eurocentrism? Heritage conservation and the politics of difference. *International Journal of Heritage Studies, 20* (2), 123–137.

Winton, A. (2007). Using 'participatory' methods with young people in contexts of violence: Reflections from Guatemala. *Bulletin of Latin American Research, 26* (4), 497–515.

Wishart, D. J., & D'Elia, L. A. (2013). Engaging disenfranchised urban youth in humanities learning. *Journal of Contemporary Issues in Education, 7* (2), 4–15.

Witt, P. A., & Caldwell, L. L. (2010). *The rationale for recreation services for youth: An evidenced based approach.* Ashburn, VA: National Recreation and Park Association.

Wolf, S., Aber, J. L., & Morris, P. A. (2015). Patterns of time use among low-income urban minority adolescents and associations with academic outcomes and problem behaviors. *Journal of Youth and Adolescence, 44* (6), 1208–1225.

Wood, D., Larson, R. W., & Brown, J. R. (2009). How adolescents come to see themselves as more responsible through participation in youth programs. *Child Development, 80* (1), 295–309.

Woodland, M. H. (2008). Whatcha doin'after school? A review of the literature on the influence of after-school programs on young Black males. *Urban Education, 43* (5), 537–560.

Woodland, M. H. (2016). After-school programs: A resource for young Black males and other urban youth. *Urban Education, 51* (7), 770–796.

Woodland, M. H., Martin, J. F., Hill, R. L., & Worrell, F. C. (2009). The most blessed room in the city: The influence of a youth development program on three young black males. *The Journal of Negro Education, 78* (3), 233–245.

Woodley, H. H. (2013). Embody the dance, embrace the body. In M. S. Hanley, G. W. Nobit, G. L. Sheppard, & T. Barone (Eds.), *Culturally relevant arts education for social justice: A way out* (pp. 216–223). New York: Routledge.

Woodson, S. E. (2015). *Theatre for Youth Third Space: Performance, democracy, and community cultural development*. Chicago: Intellect Books.

Wooster, R. (2009). Creative inclusion in community theatre: A journey with Odyssey Theatre. *RiDE: The Journal of Applied Theatre and Performance, 14* (1), 79–90.

World Health Organization. (2013). *Definition of youth*. Retrieved from http://www.un.org/esa/socdev/documents/youth/fact-sheets/youth-definition.pdf

Wrentschur, M., & Moser, M. (2014). "Stop: Now we are speaking!" A creative and dissident approach of empowering disadvantaged young people. *International Social Work, 57* (4), 398–410.

Wright, P., Davies, C., Haseman, B., Down, B., White, M., & Rankin, S. (2013). Arts practice and disconnected youth in Australia: Impact and domains of change. *Arts & Health, 5* (3), 190–203.

Wylie, T. (2015). Youth work. *Youth & Policy,* (114), 43–54.

Xing, K., Chico, E., Lambouths III, D. L., Brittian, A. S., & Schwartz, S. J. (2015). Identity development in adolescence: Implications for youth policy and practice. In W. P. Powers & G. J. Geldhof (Eds.), *Promoting positive youth development* (pp. 187–208). New York: Springer.

Yohalem, N., & Tseng, V. (2015). Commentary: Moving from practice to research, and back. *Applied Developmental Science, 19* (2), 117–120.

Yohalem, N., & Wilson-Ahlstrom, A. (2010). Inside the black box: Assessing and improving quality in youth programs. *American Journal of Community Psychology, 45* (3-4), 350–357.

Yoon, J. S. (2012). *Courageous conversations in child and youth care: Nothing lost in the telling*. Keynote speech for Child and Youth Care in Action III Conference: Leading conversations in research, practice and policy, April 28 to 30, 2011, University of Victoria.

Yoshihama, M., & Tolman, R. M. (2015). Using interactive theater to create socioculturally relevant community-based intimate partner violence prevention. *American Journal of Community Psychology, 55* (1-2), 136–147.

Young-Law, C. (2012). *Interrupting privilege: White student affairs educators as racial justice allies* (Doctoral dissertation). Mills College, Oakland, CA.

Yu, S. M., Newport-Berra, M., & Liu, J. (2015). Out-of-school time activity participation among US-Immigrant youth. *Journal of School Health, 85* (5), 281–288.

Zaff, J. F., Jones, E. P., Donlan, A. E., & Anderson, S. (Eds.). (2015*). Comprehensive community initiatives for positive youth development.* Washington, DC: Psychology Press.

Zakaras, L., & Lowell, J. F. (2008). *Arts learning, arts engagement and state arts policies.* Santa Monica, CA: Rand Corporation.

Zarrett, N., Fay, K., Li, Y., Carrano, J., Phelps, E., & Lerner, R. M. (2009). More than child's play: Variable-and pattern-centered approaches for examining effects of sports participation on youth development. *Developmental Psychology, 45* (2), 368–382.

Zarrett, N., & Lerner, R. M. (2008). Ways to promote the positive development of children and youth. *Child Trends, 11* (1), 1–5.

Zeldin, S., & Camino, L. (1998). Nothing as theoretical as good practice: Improving partnerships with researchers. *New Designs for Youth Development, 14* (2), 34–36.

Zeldin, S., Camino, L., & Calvert, M. (2012). Toward an understanding of youth in community governance: Policy priorities and research directions. *Análise Psicológica, 25* (1), 77–95.

Zeldin, S., Gauley, J., Krauss, S. E., Kornbluh, M., & Collura, J. (2015). Youth–adult partnership and youth civic development: Cross-national analyses for scholars and field professionals. *Youth & Society,* 0044118X15595153.

Zeldin, S., & Leidheiser, D. (2014). *Youth-adult partnership: A priority for volunteer training and support.* Retrieved from http://fyi.uwex.edu/youthadultpartnership/files/2015/01/Youth-Adult-Parthership_A-Priority-for-Volunteer-Training-and-Support.pdf

Zeldin, S., Petrokubi, J., & MacNeil, C. (2008). Youth-adult partnerships in decision making: Disseminating and implementing an innovative idea into established organizations and communities. *American Journal of Community Psychology, 41* (3-4), 262–277.

Zhang, H., Lu, Y., Gao, P., & Chen, Z. (2014). Social shopping communities as an emerging business model of youth entrepreneurship: Exploring the effects of website characteristics. *International Journal of Technology Management, 66* (4), 319–345.

Zhang, K. C., & Wu, D. I. (2012). Nurturing the spiritual well-being of children with special needs. *Support for Learning, 27* (3), 119–122.

Zitomer, M. R., & Reid, G. (2011). To be or not to be–able to dance: Integrated dance and children's perceptions of dance ability and disability. *Research in Dance Education, 12* (2), 137–156.

INDEX

aboriginal youth
  empowerment of
    hip-hop music in, 122–124
academics
  in collaboration with youth community
    practice, 47
ACE. *see* Arts Council England (ACE)
achievement
  among African-American youth
    perceived racial discrimination
      effects on, 44
action
  theory to
    in social justice youth practice, 219–223 *see*
      also theory to action, in social justice
      youth practice
  youth and, 90
activism
  youth, 63
activity(ies)
  out-of-school *see* out-of-school activities
  values in all, 69
Addams, J., 156
adolescent(s)
  development of
    music in, 122
adulthood
  "emerging"
    socioeconomic status connotation
      associated with, 45
adult-imposed identities
  on youth, 44
adultism
  Eurocentrism and, 17
affirming and structured environment
  early exposure in
    benefits of, 4
African-American blues, 134
African-American community
  music in, 128–129
African-American youth
  well-being and achievement among
    perceived racial discrimination effects on, 44
African drumming
  in ZUMIX, 172
Afrocentric values and culture
  PYD effects of, 42

Afrocentrism, 16
Afroncentric praxis, 16
age generation *vs.* social class
  in youth definition process, 55
age generation *vs.* transition to adulthood
  in youth definition process, 55
agency
  collective, 92
  in critical youth studies, 46
  exercising of
    in youth practice with social justice
      focus, 63
  structure *vs.*
    in youth definition process, 55
agents of control
  as values-based ethical dilemmas, 82
Albanese, P., 45
Allahar, A.L., 56, 63
Alley, A., 144
Alrutz, M., 20, 22, 23
alternative behaviors
  drawn from "tool boxes"
    rationales for, 61
alumni
  of Unusual Suspects Theater Company
    support for, 212–213
Amin, S., 15
Anderson, M.E., 225
A New Youth?: Young People, Generations and
  Family Life, 56
anxiety
  performance, 14
Appert, C.M., 134
applied theatre, 152
Araújo, M., 17
Armin, 17
art(s)
  "high" *vs.* "low," 16
  in integrating heritage language, 65
  performing *see* performing arts
  in shaping human existence, 8
  in shaping human services, 8
Artists Collective, 107
Arts Council England (ACE), 156
arts organizations
  tensions between non-arts organizations and
    in evaluation process, 113

CPSIA information can be obtained
at www.ICGtesting.com
Printed in the USA
BVHW011148240122
627023BV00002B/43